Sleep and Anesthesia

Editor

FRANCES CHUNG

SLEEP MEDICINE CLINICS

www.sleep.theclinics.com

Consulting Editor
TEOFILO LEE-CHIONG Jr

March 2013 • Volume 8 • Number 1

ELSEVIER

1600 John F. Kennedy Boulevard • Suite 1800 • Philadelphia, Pennsylvania, 19103-2899

http://www.theclinics.com

SLEEP MEDICINE CLINICS Volume 8, Number 1
March 2013, ISSN 1556-407X, ISBN-13: 978-1-4557-7330-5

Editor: Katie Saunders
Developmental Editor: Donald E. Mumford

Sleep Medicine Clinics (ISSN 1556-407X) is published quarterly by Elsevier Inc., 360 Park Avenue South, New York, NY 10010-1710. Months of issue are March, June, September and December. Business and Editorial Offices: 1600 John F. Kennedy Blvd., Ste. 1800, Philadelphia, PA 19103-2899. Customer Service Office: 3251 Riverport Lane, Maryland Heights, MO 63043. Periodicals postage paid at New York, NY and additional mailing offices. Subscription prices are $184.00 per year (US individuals), $91.00 (US residents), $383.00 (US institutions), $226.00 (Canadian and foreign individuals), $127.00 (Canadian and foreign residents), and $422.00 (Canadian and foreign institutions). Foreign air speed delivery is included in all *Clinics* subscription prices. All prices are subject to change without notice. **POSTMASTER:** Send change of address to *Sleep Medicine Clinics*, Elsevier Health Sciences Division, Subscription Customer Service, 3251 Riverport Lane, Maryland Heights, MO 63043. Customer Service: **Tel: 1-800-654-2452 (U.S. and Canada); 314-447-8871 (outside U.S. and Canada). Fax: 314-447-8029. E-mail: journals customerservice-usa@elsevier.com (for print support); journalsonlinesupport-usa@elsevier.com (for online support).**

Reprints. For copies of 100 or more of articles in this publication, please contact the Commercial Reprints Department, Elsevier Inc., 360 Park Avenue South, New York, NY 10010-1710. Tel.: 212-633-3812; Fax: 212-462-1935; E-mail: reprints@elsevier.com.

Printed and bound by CPI Group (UK) Ltd, Croydon, CR0 4YY
Transferred to Digital Printing, 2013

PROGRAM OBJECTIVE:
The goal of Sleep Clinics of North America is to keep practicing physicians up to date with current clinical practice by providing timely articles reviewing the state of the art in patient care.

TARGET AUDIENCE
All practicing physicians and other healthcare professionals.

LEARNING OBJECTIVES
Upon completion of this activity, participants should be able to:
1. Explain the differences between home sleep testing versus laboratory testing for preoperative evaluation of obstructive sleep apnea.
2. Describe the use of the STOP-Bang Questionnaire as a screening tool for obstructive sleep apena.
3. Review pathophysiological considerations of perioperative respiratory management of obese patients with obstructive sleep apnea.
4. Recognize the perioperative implications of sleep apnea, chronic sleep restriction and inflammation on anesthesia care.

ACCREDITATION
The Elsevier Office of Continuing Medical Education (EOCME) is accredited by the Accreditation Council for Continuing Medical Education (ACCME) to provide continuing medical education for physicians.

The EOCME designates this journal-based CME activity for a maximum of 16 *AMA PRA Category 1 Credit*(s)™. Physicians should claim only the credit commensurate with the extent of their participation in the activity.

All other health care professionals completing continuing education credit for this activity will be issued a certificate of participation.

DISCLOSURE OF CONFLICTS OF INTEREST
The EOCME assesses conflict of interest with its instructors, faculty, planners, and other individuals who are in a position to control the content of CME activities. All relevant conflicts of interest that are identified are thoroughly vetted by EOCME for fair balance, scientific objectivity, and patient care recommendations. EOCME is committed to providing its learners with CME activities that promote improvements or quality in healthcare and not a specific proprietary business or a commercial interest.

The planning committee, staff, authors and editors listed below have identified no financial relationships or relationships to products or devices they or their spouse/life partner have with commercial interest related to the content of this CME activity:

Norman Bolden, MD; Karen Brown, MD; Stephanie Carter; Edmond H.L. Chau, MD; Frances Chung, MD; Nicole Congleton; Walter Conwell, MD; Nicholas Michael Dalesio, MD; Peter Eastwood; Peter Gay, MD; Tee Lik Han; Shiroh Isono, MD; Mithri Junna, MD; Roop Kaw, MD; Philip Kurien, MD; Sandy Lavery; Atul Malhotra, MD; Mervyn Maze, MB, ChB; Jill McNair; Timothy Morgenthaler, MD; Mahalakshmi Narayanan; Susheel Patil, MD, PhD; Satya K. Ramachandran, MBBS; Alan Schwartz, MD; Edwin Seet, MBBS, M.Med; Bernardo Selim, MD; Tracey Stierer, MD; Kingman Strohl, MD; Eswar Sundar, MBBS; Susana Vacas, MD; and Yiliang Yang, MD, PhD.

The planning committee, staff, authors and editors listed below have identified financial relationships or relationships to products or devices they or their spouse/life partner have with commercial interest related to the content of this CME activity:

David Hillman, MBBS is a consultant/advisor for APNEX Medical, Inc. and has a research grant from ResMed, Inc. Babak Mokhlesi, MD, MSc is a consultant/advisor for Philips/Respironics. Lee-Chiong Teofilo, MD has stock ownership, a research grant and an employment affiliation with Philips Respironics, and is a consultant/advisor for Carecore National.

UNAPPROVED/OFF-LABEL USE DISCLOSURE
The EOCME requires CME faculty to disclose to the participants:
1. When products or procedures being discussed are off-label, unlabelled, experimental, and/or investigational (not US Food and Drug Administration (FDA) approved; and
2. Any limitations on the information presented, such as data that are preliminary or that represent ongoing research, interim analyses, and/or unsupported opinions. Faculty may discuss information about pharmaceutical agents that is outside of DA-approved labelling. This information is intended solely for CME and is not intended to promote off-label use of these medications. If you have any questions, contact the medical affairs department of the manufacturer for the most recent prescribing information.

TO ENROLL
To enroll in the Sleep Medicines Clinic Continuing Medical Education program, call customer service at 1-800-654-2452 or sign up online at http://www.theclinics.com/home/cme. The CME program is available to subscribers for an additional annual fee of USD 126.

METHOD OF PARTICIPATION
In order to claim credit, participants must complete the following:
1. Complete enrolment as indicated above.
2. Read the activity.
3. Complete the CME Test and Evaluation. Participants must achieve a score of 70% on the test. All CME Tests and Evaluations must be completed online.

CME INQUIRIES/SPECIAL NEEDS
For all CME inquiries or special needs, please contact elsevierCME@elsevier.com.

SLEEP MEDICINE CLINICS

FORTHCOMING ISSUES

June 2013
Fatigue
Max Hirshkowitz, MD, *Editor*

September 2013
Insomnia
Jack Edinger, MD, *Editor*

December 2013
Obstructive Sleep Apnea
Shirley Jones, MD and
James Barker, MD, *Editors*

March 2014
Central Sleep Apnea
Peter Gay, MD, *Editor*

RECENT ISSUES

December 2012
Sleep and Neurorehabilitation
Richard J. Castriotta and
Mark C. Wilde, *Editors*

September 2012
Biology of Sleep
Teofilo Lee Chiong Jr, MD, *Editor*

June 2012
Hypersomnia
Alon Y. Avidan, MD, MPH, *Editor*

Contributors

CONSULTING EDITOR

TEOFILO LEE-CHIONG Jr, MD
Professor of Medicine, Department of
Medicine, Division of Pulmonary, Critical Care
and Sleep Medicine, National Jewish Health
and University of Colorado, Denver, Colorado

EDITOR

FRANCES CHUNG, MBBS, FRCPC
Professor, Department of Anesthesia, Toronto
Western Hospital, University Health Network,
University of Toronto, Toronto, Ontario,
Canada

AUTHORS

NORMAN BOLDEN, MD
Assistant Professor of Anesthesiology,
Vice-Chairman, Department of Anesthesiology,
MetroHealth Medical Center, Case Western
Reserve University, Cleveland, Ohio

KAREN A. BROWN, MD
Professor and Queen Elizabeth Hospital
Foundation of Montreal Chair in Pediatric
Anesthesia, Department of Pediatric
Anesthesia, Montreal Children's Hospital,
McGill University Health Center, Montreal,
Quebec, Canada

EDMOND H.L. CHAU, MD
Resident, Department of Anesthesiology,
Toronto Western Hospital, University Health
Network, University of Toronto, Toronto,
Ontario, Canada

FRANCES CHUNG, MBBS, FRCPC
Professor, Department of Anesthesia, Toronto
Western Hospital, University Health Network,
University of Toronto, Toronto, Ontario,
Canada

WALTER CONWELL, MD
Fellow, Division of Pulmonary Sciences and
Critical Care Medicine, University of Colorado,
Denver, Colorado

NICHOLAS M. DALESIO, MD
Assistant Professor, Division of Pediatric
Anesthesiology, Department of Anesthesiology
and Critical Care Medicine, Johns Hopkins
School of Medicine, Baltimore, Maryland

PETER R. EASTWOOD, PhD
Professor, Department of Pulmonary
Physiology and Sleep Medicine, West
Australian Sleep Disorders Research Institute,
Sir Charles Gairdner Hospital; Centre for Sleep
Science, School of Anatomy and Human
Biology, University of Western Australia, Perth,
Australia

PETER C. GAY, MD
Professor of Medicine, Pulmonary, Critical
Care and Sleep Medicine, Mayo Clinic,
Rochester, Minnesota

TEE LIK HAN, MBBS
Medical Officer, Department of Anesthesia, Khoo Teck Puat Hospital, Alexandra Health Private Limited, Singapore

DAVID R. HILLMAN, MD
Professor, Department of Pulmonary Physiology and Sleep Medicine, West Australian Sleep Disorders Research Institute, Sir Charles Gairdner Hospital, Perth, Australia

SHIROH ISONO, MD
Professor, Department of Anesthesiology, Graduate School of Medicine, Chiba University, Chiba, Japan

MITHRI R. JUNNA, MD
Instructor in Neurology, Department of Neurology, Mayo Clinic Center for Sleep Medicine, Mayo Clinic, Rochester, Minnesota

ROOP KAW, MD
Associate Professor, Departments of Hospital Medicine and Outcomes Research, Anesthesiology, Cleveland Clinic, Cleveland, Ohio

PHILIP KURIEN, MD
Department of Anesthesia and Perioperative Care, University of California San Francisco, San Francisco, California

TEOFILO LEE-CHIONG Jr, MD
Professor of Medicine, Department of Medicine, Division of Pulmonary, Critical Care and Sleep Medicine, National Jewish Health and University of Colorado, Denver, Colorado

ATUL MALHOTRA, MD
Associate Professor in Medicine, Brigham and Women's Hospital, Harvard Medical School, Boston, Massachusetts

MERVYN MAZE, MB ChB, FRCA, FRCP, FMedSci
Department of Anesthesia and Perioperative Care, University of California San Francisco, San Francisco, California

BABAK MOKHLESI, MD, MSc
Associate Professor, Section of Pulmonary and Critical Care Medicine, Department of Medicine, Sleep Disorders Center, University of Chicago Pritzker School of Medicine, Chicago, Illinois

TIMOTHY I. MORGENTHALER, MD
Patient Safety Officer and Associate Professor in Medicine, Division of Pulmonary and Critical Care Medicine, Mayo Clinic Center for Sleep Medicine, Mayo Clinic, Rochester, Minnesota

SUSHEEL P. PATIL, MD, PhD
Assistant Professor of Medicine, Division of Pulmonary and Critical Care Medicine, Johns Hopkins Sleep Disorders Center, Johns Hopkins School of Medicine, Baltimore, Maryland

SATYA KRISHNA RAMACHANDRAN, MD, FRCA
Assistant Professor, Director, Quality Assurance and Post Anesthesia Care, Department of Anesthesiology, University of Michigan Medical School, Ann Arbor, Michigan

ALAN R. SCHWARTZ, MD
Professor of Medicine, Sleep Medicine Section, Division of Pulmonary and Critical Care Medicine, Department of Medicine, Johns Hopkins School of Medicine, Baltimore, Maryland

EDWIN SEET, MBBS, MMed (Anesthesia)
Consultant Anesthesiologist, Department of Anesthesia, Khoo Teck Puat Hospital, Alexandra Health Private Limited, Singapore

BERNARDO J. SELIM, MD
Assistant Professor in Medicine, Division of Pulmonary and Critical Care Medicine, Mayo Clinic Center for Sleep Medicine, Mayo Clinic, Rochester, Minnesota

TRACEY L. STIERER, MD
Assistant Professor of Anesthesiology, Department of Anesthesiology and Critical Care Medicine; Assistant Professor of Otolaryngology-Head and Neck Surgery, Johns Hopkins School of Medicine, Baltimore, Maryland

KINGMAN P. STROHL, MD
Professor of Medicine, Physiology & Biophysics, and Oncology, Director, Center for Sleep Disorders Research, Louis Stokes Cleveland DVA Medical Center, Case Western Reserve University, Cleveland, Ohio

ESWAR SUNDAR, MD
Department of Anesthesia, Critical Care and
Pain Medicine, Beth Israel Deaconess Medical
Center, Harvard Medical School, Boston,
Massachusetts

SUSANA VACAS, MD
Department of Anesthesia and Perioperative
Care, University of California San Francisco,

San Francisco, California; Programme for
Advance Medical Education, Lisbon,
Portugal

YILIANG YANG, MD, PhD
Department of Anesthesia, Toronto Western
Hospital, University Health Network, University
of Toronto, Toronto, Ontario, Canada

Contents

Preface: Sleep and Anesthesia   xiii

Frances Chung

Sleep and Anesthesia: Common Mechanisms of Action   1

Susana Vacas, Philip Kurien, and Mervyn Maze

> Appropriate sleep hygiene is crucial for repair in states of disease and injury and in restoring function especially in the central nervous and immune systems. Anesthetics have different action targets and ultimately different consequences. The effects of anesthetics on circadian rhythm possibly also lead to immune deregulation. α_2-adrenergic agonists converge on sleep pathways within the brainstem and are associated with changes in neuronal activity similar to those seen in deeper stages of NREM sleep. Thoughtful attention must be made in selecting an anesthetic agent that best mimics natural sleep. Future studies will further elucidate the benefits of dexmedetomidine as a good anesthetic/sedative candidate.

Sleep Apnea, Chronic Sleep Restriction, and Inflammation: Perioperative Implications   11

Walter Conwell and Teofilo Lee-Chiong Jr

> Obstructive sleep apnea (OSA) and chronic sleep restriction can lead to adverse consequences on various organ systems, including cardiovascular, neuroendocrine, and immune. There are bidirectional relationships among OSA, chronic sleep restriction, and the metabolic syndrome. Several mechanisms are responsible for these relationships, including intermittent hypoxia, systemic inflammation, activation of the sympathetic nervous system, and changes in neuroendocrine function. Intermittent hypoxia and systemic inflammation also play central roles in endothelial dysfunction and accelerated atherosclerosis associated with both OSA and chronic sleep restriction.

Upper Airway, Obstructive Sleep Apnea, and Anesthesia   23

David R. Hillman and Peter R. Eastwood

> The tendencies to upper airway obstruction during sleep and anesthesia are related. Loss of consciousness in either state increases upper airway collapsibility and anesthesia-related suppression of rousability confers great vulnerability to its effects. This vulnerability increases perioperative risk of obstruction in patients with predisposed airways, such as those with obstructive sleep apnea. This risk diminishes with emergence from anesthesia and return of arousal responses but is likely to recur with postoperative sedation/narcotics. It can be adversely influenced by individual drug sensitivities, posture, postsurgical upper airway edema/hematoma, or hypoventilation/hypercapnia. Close postoperative observation is required until consistent rousability returns.

Upper Airway Physiology in Sleep and Anesthesia   29

Nicholas M. Dalesio, Tracey L. Stierer, and Alan R. Schwartz

> The optimal perioperative management of the patient with, or at risk for, obstructive sleep apnea (OSA) requires a multidisciplinary approach. Further studies are needed to facilitate a better understanding of the factors that place a patient with OSA at risk for adverse outcome and of the methods and duration of monitoring that confer optimal patient safety.

Medical Sedation and Sleep Apnea   43

Mithri R. Junna, Bernardo J. Selim, and Timothy I. Morgenthaler

The effects of hypnosedatives and opioids on breathing control may share common pathophysiologic pathways with obstructive sleep apnea (OSA), resulting in additive adverse consequences. Current understanding of the complex interaction of these medications across multiple systems is not only limited to muscle tone and anatomic considerations but also to dynamic ventilatory control and how they modulate the sleep state. This review article provides a systematic review of the most recent clinical and pharmacologic literature published regarding the effects of opioids and hypnosedatives on the clinical manifestation of OSA.

Pathophysiologic Considerations of Perioperative Respiratory Managements of Obese Patients with Obstructive Sleep Apnea   59

Shiroh Isono

Anesthesia and surgical interventions significantly alter structures and neural control of the respiratory system, resulting in adverse postoperative respiratory complications, particularly in obese patients with obstructive sleep apnea. Current understanding of the pathophysiology of obstructive sleep apnea supports perioperative lung volume maintenance strategies, optimal postoperative positioning such as sniffing head position and sitting posture, and oxygen administration in addition to application of continuous positive airway pressure. These strategies are speculative and need collaborative investigations between anesthesiologists and sleep physicians.

A Screening Tool of Obstructive Sleep Apnea: STOP-Bang Questionnaire   65

Yiliang Yang and Frances Chung

The STOP-Bang questionnaire is a concise and easy-to use screening tool to identify patients with obstructive sleep apnea (OSA). The questionnaire has been validated in medical and surgical patients and in different ethnic groups. A STOP-Bang score of 0 to 2 indicates a low risk of OSA; a STOP-Bang score of 3 to 4 indicates an intermediate risk of OSA; and a STOP-Bang score of 5 to 8 indicates a high risk of OSA; a STOP-Bang score of 3 or greater plus a high serum HCO_3^- level also increases the specificity for moderate/severe OSA.

Preoperative Evaluation of Obstructive Sleep Apnea: Home Sleep Testing Versus Laboratory Testing   73

Susheel P. Patil

Obstructive sleep apnea (OSA), a highly prevalent condition affecting 24% of men and 9% of women, is associated with many comorbidities. Patients with OSA are at increased risk for postoperative respiratory and cardiovascular complications, resulting in the need for increased levels of monitoring and longer hospitalizations. Most patients at risk for OSA, however, remain undiagnosed or untreated, placing the surgical patient with OSA at risk for postoperative complications. Diagnostic testing for OSA can be performed using in-laboratory polysomnography (PSG) or limited-channel portable monitoring (PM). This article addresses the use of PM and in-laboratory PSG in the assessment of OSA.

Obstructive Sleep Apnea and Perioperative Complications: From Mechanisms to Risk Modification   93

Satya Krishna Ramachandran

Obstructive sleep apnea (OSA) is prevalent in a significant proportion of surgical patients, although most of these patients are undiagnosed. Interest into OSA as an independent risk factor for adverse perioperative outcomes is fairly recent. Although the specific mechanisms of adverse outcomes are yet unclear, specialty bodies have recognized the challenges and provided expert guidance on the perioperative risk assessment and management of these complex patients. This article reviews the key putative mechanisms for adverse outcomes and provides an overview of the effectiveness of risk-modification strategies.

Perioperative Clinical Pathways to Manage Sleep-Disordered Breathing 105

Edwin Seet, Tee Lik Han, and Frances Chung

The obstructive sleep apnea (OSA) syndrome is prevalent yet underdiagnosed. A significant number of patients with OSA are undiagnosed when they present for surgery. Clinical features of OSA include repeated nocturnal arousals and increased sympathetic output, daytime hypersomnolence, memory loss, and executive and psychomotor dysfunction. OSA can lead to several systemic complications and is also linked to increased perioperative morbidity. This article reviews the evidence behind the perioperative management of OSA patients and proposes an approach to the screening, evaluation, and management of known and suspected OSA patients, with the intention of mitigating the perioperative risks to such patients.

Positive Airway Pressure Therapy for Perioperative Patients 121

Peter C. Gay

Positive airway pressure (PAP) therapy can be administered as a fixed pressure level, a variable autotitrating pressure, or a bilevel setting. Evidence for use of PAP therapy in postoperative patients comes from patients with postextubation respiratory failure or from preemptive efforts to prevent reintubation. Patients with obstructive sleep apnea (OSA) or other forms of sleep-disordered breathing are recognized as having additional risks for postoperative complications. Protocols are being proposed to manage postoperative patients with known or suspected OSA with PAP therapy. The role of preoperative diagnosis of OSA and preoperative PAP therapy treatment is also being explored.

Perioperative Complications in Patients with Obstructive Sleep Apnea 129

Roop Kaw

Factors to consider when evaluating how patients with suspected obstructive sleep apnea (OSA) should be monitored postoperatively include the preclinical suspicion of the severity of OSA, type of surgery, the anticipated need for pain medications, and the availability of emergency airway and respiratory equipment. In general, all patients with OSA undergoing upper airway surgery should be strongly considered for inpatient surgery. Minor surgeries requiring local or regional anesthesia only can be safely performed on an outpatient basis in patients with OSA. Minor outpatient procedures that require IV sedation or IV analgesia can also be safely performed in patients with OSA.

Obesity Hypoventilation Syndrome and Anesthesia 135

Edmond H.L. Chau, Babak Mokhlesi, and Frances Chung

Patients with obesity hypoventilation syndrome (OHS) have a higher burden of co-morbidities and increased risk for perioperative morbidity and mortality. Therefore, a thorough plan of evaluation and management is essential for patients with OHS who undergo surgery. Currently, information on the perioperative management of OHS is extremely limited in the literature. As the prevalence of OHS is likely to increase as a result of the current global obesity epidemic, it is crucial for physicians to recognize and manage patients with this syndrome. This review examines the current data on OHS and discusses its optimal perioperative management.

Evaluation of the Child with Sleep-Disordered Breathing Scheduled for Adenotonsillectomy   149

Karen A. Brown

Assessment with a combination of sleep-disordered breathing questionnaires and the McGill Oximetry Score identifies the child with severe obstructive sleep apnea syndrome, and provides a prediction of the risk for perioperative adverse respiratory events. This approach allows (1) exclusion of the at-risk child from ambulatory surgical programs, (2) triage of patient priority, and (3) implementation of risk-reduction strategies.

Curricular Elements for Circadian Rhythm and Sleep Disorders in Anesthesiology Training Programs   157

Norman Bolden and Kingman P. Strohl

Sleep apnea is an underrecognized chronic disorder that is immediately relevant to perioperative risk and specific plans to postoperatively recognize and manage respiratory disorders of sleep. Although an anesthesia residency is one pathway for advanced training for those interested sleep medicine, there are basic knowledge and skills that are highly relevant to today's general practice of anesthesiology. After a discussion of the ways that sleep influences anesthetic practice, this article proposes an outline for content, examples of current resources and assessment tools, and strategies one might use to implement instruction in the context of an accredited residency program.

Unanswered Questions in Sleep and Anesthesia   165

Eswar Sundar and Atul Malhotra

This article attempts to synthesize current research around the following topics of sleep, obstructive sleep apnea (OSA), and anesthesia. Does OSA or even risk of OSA increase the perioperative morbidity? Does use of continuous positive airway pressure (CPAP) reduce these complications? Is a questionnaire-based screening tool alone sufficient to prevent resource use associated with increased monitoring and CPAP usage in the postoperative setting? Are sleep and anesthesia the same condition? Can we prevent extubation failures in the intensive care unit? What is the best modality of sedation for intubated patients?

Index   177

Preface
Sleep and Anesthesia

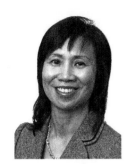

Frances Chung, MBBS, FRCPC
Editor

Sleep medicine and anesthesiology both are concerned with the significant changes in autonomic control associated with the loss of waking consciousness. There are similarities and differences between sleep and anesthesia. Sleep and anesthesia may have a common mechanism of action. The tendencies to upper airway obstruction during sleep and anesthesia are interrelated.

Many patients with obstructive sleep apnea remain underdiagnosed and may be first recognized in the perioperative setting. Sedatives and opioids may suppress arousals, resulting in postoperative deaths or significant morbidities. Given the significant morbidity associated with obstructive sleep apnea syndrome, it is incumbent that the anesthesiologist and sleep medicine collaborate to ensure that arrangements are made for appropriate diagnosis and treatment when such possibilities exist.

This issue serves several purposes. It promotes the cross-fertilization of ideas between sleep medicine and anesthesiology. The screening of patients at risk of obstructive sleep apnea and preoperative evaluation of obstructive sleep apnea and home sleep testing vs laboratory testing are examined. The methods of minimizing perioperative risk of upper airway obstruction or ventilatory insufficiency in predisposed patients are explored. The use of noninvasive positive airway pressure therapies to prevent and treat perioperative upper airway obstruction or hypoventilation is examined. There are a number of unanswered questions in sleep and anesthesia. Further research is required.

Frances Chung, MBBS, FRCPC
Department of Anesthesiology
University of Toronto
Ambulatory Surgical Unit
and Combined Surgical Unit
Toronto Western Hospital
University Health Network
Toronto, Ontario, Canada

E-mail address:
Frances.chung@uhn.ca

Sleep Med Clin 8 (2013) xiii
http://dx.doi.org/10.1016/j.jsmc.2013.01.001
1556-407X/13/$ – see front matter © 2013 Published by Elsevier Inc.

Sleep and Anesthesia
Common Mechanisms of Action

Susana Vacas, MD[a,b], Philip Kurien, MD[a],
Mervyn Maze, MB ChB, FRCA, FRCP, FMedSci[a,*]

KEYWORDS

- Anesthesia • Sleep • Circadian rhythm • Dexmedetomidine

KEY POINTS

- Anesthetic drugs induce unconsciousness by altering neurotransmission at multiple sites.
- α_2-Agonists, such as dexmedetomidine, are associated with changes in neuronal activity similar to those seen in deeper stages of non–rapid eye movement sleep.
- The effects of anesthetics on circadian rhythm possibly lead to immune deregulation.
- Thoughtful attention must be paid to selecting an anesthetic agent that best mimics natural sleep.

INTRODUCTION

"You are going to go to sleep now" is an oft-repeated colloquialism in every anesthesiologist's daily practice. The phrase might be useful in allaying the fears of nervous patients, but does general anesthesia actually mimic sleep? Do they travel on the same neural pathways? To what degree does the comparison accurately reflect the underlying mechanisms involved?

Sleep, especially non–rapid eye movement (NREM) sleep, and anesthesia may use common neuronal and genetic substrates. Anesthetics act through sleep neural circuits but not necessarily in the same way.

AROUSAL PATHWAYS

To promote and sustain cortical arousal, neuronal pathways have developed two parallel ascending neuronal pathways. The first branch activates the thalamic relay neurons that are crucial for transmission of information to the cortex. Cholinergic signaling originating from the laterodorsal tegmental (LDT) and pedunculopontine tegmental (PPT) nuclei and the basal forebrain promote the cortically activated states of wakefulness and rapid eye movement (REM) sleep. The second branch bypasses the thalamus, activating neurons in the lateral hypothalamic area and basal forebrain (BF), and throughout the cortex. This pathway originates from monoaminergic neurons in the upper brainstem and caudal hypothalamus. The locus coeruleus (LC) provides norepinephrine-mediated inhibition of the ventrolateral preoptic (VLPO) nucleus in the hypothalamus.[1,2] Therefore, γ-aminobutyric acid (GABA$_A$)-mediated and galanin-mediated inhibition of the ascending arousal circuits by the VLPO nucleus is inhibited and the awake state is promoted.

SLEEP PATHWAYS

Sleep is under the control of two processes, a circadian clock that regulates the appropriate timing of sleep and wakefulness across the 24-hour day and a homeostatic process (sleep homeostasis) that regulates sleep need and intensity according to the time spent awake or asleep.[3] Sleep is a nonhomogeneous state that can be divided into NREM sleep and REM (paradoxic) sleep. The brain areas identified as important in sleep fall into 2

[a] Department of Anesthesia and Perioperative Care, University of California San Francisco, 521 Parnassus Avenue, San Francisco, CA 94143-0648, USA; [b] Programme for Advanced Medical Education, Calouste Gulbenkian Foundation Av, 45-A Berna, Lisbon 1067-001, Portugal
* Corresponding author.
E-mail address: MazeM@anesthesia.ucsf.edu

Sleep Med Clin 8 (2013) 1–9
http://dx.doi.org/10.1016/j.jsmc.2012.11.009
1556-407X/13/$ – see front matter © 2013 Elsevier Inc. All rights reserved.

general groups: those with an arousing influence and active during wakefulness, namely the LC, dorsal raphe (DR), tuberomammillary (TMN), and BF; and those active primarily during sleep, namely the VLPO. The median preoptic area contains both wake-active and sleep-active neurons.

Discrete neurochemical changes accompany the different types of sleep with cholinergic (in brainstem and forebrain), noradrenergic (LC), and serotonergic (DR) all becoming less active in NREM sleep, whereas cholinergic activity increases in REM sleep.[4] Activity in the VLPO is increased in NREM sleep and the GABAergic/galanin input from VLPO inhibits the histaminergic TMN nucleus. Orexinergic pathways from the perifornical nucleus are inactive during NREM sleep (**Fig. 1**).

The relatively quiescent LC facilitates a series of changes that includes activation of the galanin/GABA-containing neurons of the VLPO nucleus that terminate on and inhibit aminergic neurons within the tuberomammillary nucleus.[5]

Anesthetic-induced unconsciousness results from specific interactions of anesthetics, with the neural circuits regulating sleep and wakefulness.

WHERE DO ANESTHETICS COLLIDE IN SLEEP PATHWAYS?

The currently available imaging techniques can only indirectly measure neuronal activity, for example through changes in blood flow, glucose metabolism, or oxygen concentration. One can then understand the difficulty in fully comprehending the mechanisms by which anesthesia induces sleep/unconsciousness. A common finding between NREM sleep and anesthesia in imaging studies is the deactivation of the thalamus leading to cortical inhibition. Anesthetic drugs induce unconsciousness by altering neurotransmission at multiple sites in the cerebral cortex, brainstem, and thalamus. The different actions of the different available anesthetics have made the understanding of the exact mechanism even more difficult. Effects of modern anesthetics on subsequent sleep behavior are known for some, but not all, anesthetics. No one electroencephalogram (EEG) pattern characterizes the anesthetized state. Different anesthetics and doses have distinct profiles with respect to the EEG activity.

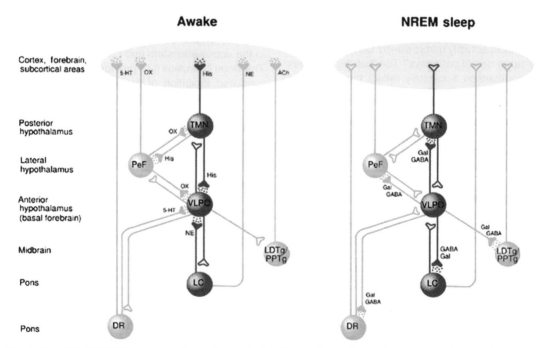

Fig. 1. Simplified NREM sleep-promoting pathway. An inhibition of noradrenergic neurons in the LC, which accompanies endogenous NREM sleep, releases a tonic noradrenergic inhibition of the VLPO. The activated VLPO is believed to release GABA into the TMN which inhibits its release of arousal-promoting histamine into the cortex, and thus induces loss of consciousness. A number of pathways are involved in NREM sleep; the sleep-active VLPO projects to all the ascending monoaminergic, cholinergic and orexinergic arousal nuclei (TMN, LC, DR, PPTg, LDTg, PeF), which project to the cortex where they release arousal-promoting neurotransmitters to promote wakefulness. (*From* Nelson LE, Guo TZ, Lu J, et al. The sedative component of anesthesia is mediated by GABA(A) receptors in an endogenous sleep pathway. Nat Neurosci 2002;5(10):979–84; with permission.)

Although some agents act on excitatory synapses, others act through potentiation of inhibitory synaptic receptors. The GABA_A receptors are neurotransmitter-gated chloride channels that exist on cells that may also contain nicotinic acetylcholine receptors, glycine receptors, and serotonin type 3 receptors. Anesthetics such as propofol, etomidate, and barbiturates exert their effect through enhancement of GABA-mediated channel activation and prolong postsynaptic inhibitory currents, suppressing neuronal excitability. In brain regions containing neurons that promote wakefulness, GABAergic inhibition has been shown to cause an increase in sleep. These brain regions include the DR nucleus, TMN, medial preoptic area, and ventrolateral periaqueductal gray.[6,7] In a series of studies involving GABAergic agents, it was reported that unlike in NREM sleep, these hypnotic agents did not alter noradrenergic activity in the LC (see **Fig. 1**).[1] Instead these agents converged on the NREM sleep pathway at the level of the hypothalamus.[8] However, short-term administration of the GABAergic agent propofol permitted normal recovery after a period of sleep deprivation.[9,10]

At clinical concentrations, drugs such as N_2O, xenon, and ketamine have little or no effect on GABA_A receptors. Instead, these anesthetics potently inhibit N-methyl-D-aspartate (NMDA) receptors, which are excitatory cation channels activated by glutamate. These agents reduce excitatory signals in critical neuronal circuits, causing unconsciousness. Glutamate levels in the PPT are greater during wakefulness as opposed to NREM and REM sleep.[11,12] The dissociative state that is produced by ketamine anesthesia can be in part attributed to the different regions to which ketamine promotes glutamate release (nucleus accumbens,[13] prefrontal cortex,[14] and anterior cingulate[15]). It has been shown that isoflurane and sevoflurane reduce glutamate release[16–18] and inhibit its uptake,[19] but few in vivo studies elaborated on understanding the exact mechanism by which isoflurane modulates glutamatergic transmission.

REM sleep rebound after exposure to volatile anesthetics suggests that these volatile anesthetics do not fully substitute for natural sleep.[20] In humans, isoflurane anesthesia alone (without surgery) results in no change in subsequent REM or NREM sleep, but a shift in NREM sleep from slow-wave sleep to lighter (I and II) stages.[21] On the other hand, it has been shown that wake-active orexinergic neurons are inhibited by isoflurane and sevoflurane, and that waking up from anesthesia uses neural circuits distinct from those necessary to become anesthetized but similar to the neural circuitry that promotes arousal.[22] Furthermore, isoflurane depresses

serotonin levels on hypoglossal motoneurons in dogs[23] and on mice hippocampus.[24]

The molecular targets for dexmedetomidine are central α_2-adrenergic receptors. It has been shown that α_2-agonists transduce its hypnotic response after binding to the α_{2A}-receptor subtype[25] in the LC.[26] Through signaling processes that involve both pertussis toxin–sensitive G proteins[27] and effector mechanisms that include inhibition of adenylyl cyclase[27] and ligand-gated calcium channels as well as activation of inwardly rectifying potassium channels,[28] the noradrenergic neurons become hyperpolarized and are less likely to achieve an action potential. α_2-Agonists such as dexmedetomidine are associated with similar changes in neuronal activity, as is seen in deeper stages of NREM sleep[2,29] apart from the absence of inhibitory effect on the orexinergic neurons in the perifornical nucleus.[8] A functional magnetic resonance study showed that a thalamic nucleus, which receives afferent input from orexinergic neurons, is activated during an arousal stimulus in α_2-agonist–sedated subjects.[30] Children sedated with dexmedetomidine showed an EEG pattern that was identical to that seen in stage 2 NREM sleep.[31]

Although acetylcholine (ACh) plays a primary role in generating the brain-activated states of wakefulness and REM sleep, cholinergic receptors are not a main target of common anesthetics. Nonetheless, ACh interacts with other transmitter systems that are targets of sleep pharmacology, for example the GABAergic agents. The clinical finding that physostigmine (acetylcholinesterase inhibitor) reverses propofol sedation, causing arousal, suggests that propofol produces unconsciousness, in part, by disrupting cholinergic neurotransmission.[32] In vitro studies showed that propofol, isoflurane, sevoflurane, and ketamine inhibit muscarinic and nicotinic ACh receptors,[33–37] providing support that these agents cause sedation, in part, by inhibiting cholinergic neurotransmission in brain regions that regulate arousal.

CIRCADIAN RHYTHM

The 2-process model of sleep homeostasis as described by Borbely and Wirz-Justice[38] integrates sleep debt ("process-s") and circadian rhythm ("process-c"). This model implicates circadian rhythm and sleep as intertwined, codependent processes. Experimentally, distinguishing process-c from process-s presents a challenge in deconstructing causative factors in sleep disorders. Nevertheless, there is a growing body of evidence that suggests circadian rhythm can be altered independent of sleep deprivation and that anesthetics can specifically change circadian rhythm.

Circadian rhythmicity is thought to be controlled by the suprachiasmatic nucleus and is established by processing external cues (zeitgebers), such as light, into systemic mediators, such as temperature, adrenergic signaling, and circulating hormones (eg, cortisol and melatonin). This process serves to maintain a diurnal pattern, presumably to coordinate intracellular or intersystem function by re-synchronizing intrinsic cellular molecular clocks. In brief, the molecular core of the circadian clock involves the heterodimerization of CLOCK and BMAL1, which act as the canonical arm of the clock, and the heterodimerization of PER1/2 and CRY1/2, which are critical components of the negative feedback arm[18]; stabilizing proteins RORα, REV-ERB, DEC, DBP, and E4BP4 act as additional repressors or activators of the canonical arm,[39] and these proteins oscillate through the day and translocate from the cytoplasm to the nucleus in a highly coordinated fashion to provide a reliable rhythm of approximately 24 hours. Disruption of circadian processes is being studied as a relevant contributing factor to multiple human conditions altering, among others, immunity.

CIRCADIAN RHYTHM AND ANESTHESIA

An initial indication that circadian rhythm is important in anesthetic delivery is the time-of-day variance in susceptibility to general anesthetics.[40,41] Indeed, the greatest therapeutic effect of general anesthetics in animal models occurs during the animals' rest phase for propofol[42] and ketamine.[43] A volatile anesthetic effect may also vary according to a diurnal pattern; halothane administration in rats varied with a lower minimum alveolar concentration requirement during the rest phase in comparison with the active phase.[44] Recently, using bees as a model system, 6-hour isoflurane administration during the rest phase failed to alter the circadian activity patterns of the hive, whereas isoflurane administered in the active phase significantly altered the circadian activity of the hive.[45] Taken together, the time-of-day administration of anesthesia is likely important in both the dose-dependent effect and the maintenance of circadian rhythm.

As parameters for outlining circadian rhythm, cortisol and melatonin levels can be used to make assumptions about the effect of general anesthesia on daily cycling in human subjects. Most human studies following these variables involve general anesthesia with the confounding aspect of surgery, and do not incorporate the natural underlying cycling of these hormones adequately. Given these and other significant caveats, a propofol-based anesthetic appears to decrease the amount of plasma cortisol during surgery in comparison with sevoflurane.[46] Postoperatively, following a thiopental/sevoflurane-based or thiopental/isoflurane-based anesthetic, cortisol levels are elevated in men who underwent long-duration surgery for larynx or pharynx cancer.[47] Conversely, in women undergoing laparoscopic procedures for pelvis surgery, anesthesia with thiopental/sevoflurane reduced amounts of cortisol 2 to 4 hours after surgery compared with thiopental/isoflurane anesthesia.[48] Given that these studies were designed to investigate the anesthetic effects on stress responses and not on circadian rhythm directly, there remains only a suggestion that altered cortisol levels may interfere with circadian rhythm after anesthesia and surgery.

Investigation into the effect of anesthesia on the cycling of melatonin points more directly to a circadian rhythm effect. A comparison of general anesthesia (thiopental/isoflurane) with spinal anesthesia for orthopedic procedures showed a significant reduction in melatonin levels in the first postsurgical night compared with baseline levels; interestingly, there was no significant difference in the reduction of melatonin between the experimental groups, indicating that the effect was independent of the anesthesia, and pointing to the possibility of a significant surgical influence of postoperative opiate use on melatonin secretion.[49] In patients undergoing general anesthesia (thiopental/isoflurane/fentanyl) for laparoscopy, a modest reduction in 13-hour average melatonin secretion was noted in the evening after surgery compared with the presurgical night, with a large increase in melatonin secretion the second night after surgery.[50] Corroborating these data, in patients undergoing major abdominal surgery with general anesthesia and concomitant use of a thoracic epidural, there was a similar modest reduction in basal melatonin secretion on the first postoperative day, followed by a significant increase on the second postoperative day.[51] Following urine metabolites of melatonin (aMT6s), general anesthesia (thiopental/propofol) decreased the maximal concentration and delayed the peak of aMT6s.[52] Short mask-inhalation anesthetics (21 minutes average duration) for dilation and curettage showed no difference in melatonin secretion compared with nonsurgical controls.[53] Experimental models allow for more precise examination of melatonin secretion and general anesthesia apart from surgical effect. Rats anesthetized with propofol for 25 to 30 minutes around the peak of serum melatonin secretion showed a significant reduction in melatonin secretion for the 3 hours following anesthesia, a subsequent increase 20 hours after the anesthetic, and a phase advance of cyclical melatonin secretion of 40 minutes consistent with the approximate duration of anesthesia.[40] Whether in humans or rats, it seems consistent that melatonin levels are reduced in the immediate postoperative/anesthetic period with a rebound phenomenon observed thereafter, although it remains unclear in human subjects which component of the observed effect can be attributable to either surgery or anesthesia.

The effect of anesthetics on intrinsic molecular circadian clocks is beginning to be explored in experimental models. In rats, 6 hours of sevoflurane anesthesia changed the expression pattern of approximately 1.5% of 10,000 genes surveyed. Of interest, the expression of Per2 was the only circadian protein in the brain that was significantly reduced after the anesthetic.[54] The effect of reduced expression of Per2 and an auxiliary clock gene Dbp persists for 24 hours.[55] Infusions of both propofol and dexmedetomidine likewise reduced the expression of Per2 in rat brain 6 hours after anesthetic delivery, but the effect persisted for only 24 hours in the case of dexmedetomidine.[56] Further investigation demonstrated that a 4-hour sevoflurane anesthetic blunted Per2 mRNA production in the suprachiasmatic nucleus in response to a light stimulus, and created a delayed activity rhythm in anesthetized mice.[57] Repression of Per2 expression by sevoflurane anesthesia was most significant when administered between the hours of 8 AM and 12 PM in comparison with other time points, but activity patterns of anesthetized animals were delayed for all time points of anesthetic administration.[58] Bees anesthetized with a 6-hour course of isoflurane during the day had a reduction in the amplitude of Cry expression and phase delay of both Cry and Per2 expression in whole bee brains in comparison with bees anesthetized during the evening, leading to alterations in circadian governed homing patterns and foraging times.[45] With respect to the molecular clock, general anesthesia appears to significantly affect critical clock proteins in a time-of-day–dependent fashion, and corresponds to changes in activity patterns consistent with circadian disruption.

CIRCADIAN CONTROL OF IMMUNE FUNCTION

A separate line of investigation has focused on the influence of circadian rhythm on immune function. Clinically, timing is relevant in terms of susceptibility to infection,[59] asthma attacks,[60] or flares of rheumatic arthritis,[61] all of which suggest circadian principles underlying these immune-mediated processes.

Circulating pools of many immune cells' cycle throughout the day indicate the influence of circadian timing. Natural killer (NK) cells peak in both activity and numbers in the human circulation in the early morning, and likely marginate away from circulation during other times of the day.[62] In mouse models, after lipopolysaccharide (LPS) administration, macrophages circulate cyclically to the spleen.[63] Of importance, the circadian molecular clock exists and functions in NK cells,[64,65] macrophages, dendritic cells, and B cells.[63,66] Indeed, approximately 8% of the macrophage genome is classified as falling under the control of circadian transcription factors,[63] and critical immune transcription factors such as signal transducer and activator of transcription family (STATs) and nuclear factor κB (NF-κB) are regulated by clock proteins.[67] Study of the functional consequence of disturbing circadian molecular clock proteins in immune subsets is generating interesting data. Injection of LPS at specific time points caused significantly elevated cytokine production in both macrophage-restricted Bmal1 knockout (KO), and systemic Rev-Erbα KO mice, compared with the chronometric 12-hour opposite time point (antiphasic control).[68] Cry1/2 double KO mice have elevated NF-κB activity causing increased baseline inflammatory cytokine expression in vitro, and generated greater inflammation when challenged with LPS in vitro and in vivo.[69] Examining lymphocyte function has similarly elucidated at least some aspect of circadian gating. Per2 KO mouse lymphocytes had a robust increase in proliferative capacity after being immunized in vivo when compared with their antiphasic control.[70] Isolated T cells cultured from mouse lymph nodes proliferated after stimulation in a circadian manner, an effect that was abolished in Clock mutant mice.[71] Whether by observation or direct experimentation these data showed that certain immune cells traffic according to apparent circadian parameters, possess oscillating intrinsic molecular clocks, have critical transcription factors controlled by clock proteins, and have altered function when clock proteins are perturbed.

SLEEP DISRUPTION AND COGNITIVE DYSFUNCTION IN SEDATED PATIENTS IN THE INTENSIVE CARE UNIT

Sleep disruption in critically ill patients is a common occurrence in the intensive care unit (ICU), with the potential to adversely affect patients' outcome and also to provide a direct financial detriment with respect to the length of hospital stay and depletion of health care resources. Early polysomnographic studies had revealed extreme sleep disruption in ICU patients with decreases in total sleep time, altered sleep architecture (predominance of stage 1 and 2 sleep, decreased or absent stages 3 and 4 NREM and REM sleep), and sleep fragmentation[72,73]; also, up to 50% of the total sleep time occurred during daytime. Among the possible causes that contribute to sleep disruption in the ICU are those related to the patient's acute illness and comorbidities, environmental factors (including noise and inappropriate light), and iatrogenic factors including frequent care-related interruptions and medications prescribed for analgesia and sedation.[74,75] Among those that are potentially amenable to modification, excessive noise does not contribute as much as was anticipated,[76] and attention has focused on sedative practices.[77] Sedative-hypnotic agents are widely used to facilitate sleep in the ICU; however, depending on the sedative agent, it may not produce appropriate sleep hygiene and instead will aggravate the problem by producing fewer of the restorative properties of natural sleep.

Several studies have now demonstrated the association between the use of benzodiazepines (BZDs) and increased incidence[78] and duration[79] of delirium in medical ICU patients, although the relationship of the development and duration of delirium with sleep disruption was not ascertained. Acute withdrawal from long-term sedation with BZDs and opiate narcotics results in profound sleep disruption.[80] The pivotal work of the MENDs trial[78,81,82] indicated the benefits of a specific anesthetic agent, dexmedetomidine, in the outcome of the ICU population.

SUMMARY

Appropriate sleep hygiene is crucial for repair in states of disease and injury, and in restoring function especially in the central nervous and immune systems. Lack of sleep hygiene results in cognitive dysfunction, contributes to the delirium that is prevalent in patients within the ICU, adversely affects immunity, and independently increases both morbidity and mortality. Anesthetics used in hospital care have different action targets and, ultimately, different consequences. Those which act by modulating the $GABA_A$ receptor converge at the level of the hypothalamus, whereas α_2-adrenergic agonists converge on sleep pathways within the brainstem. Thus, thoughtful attention must be paid to selecting an anesthetic agent that best mimics natural sleep. Future studies will further elucidate the benefits of dexmedetomidine as a good anesthetic/sedative candidate to mimic natural sleep.

While the fields of investigation into the anesthetic effect on circadian rhythm and the circadian influence on immune function remain disparate, there exists the plausible concatenation that anesthetics, by altering circadian rhythm (possibly independent of sleep deprivation), affect immune function. Given that anesthetics are often used adjunctively to facilitate therapeutic interventions, it would be worthwhile to elucidate whether more precise applications of anesthesia could improve immunologic outcomes for patients who require them.

Anesthesia is not the same as sleep. The actions of anesthetics on sleep pathways and the restorative properties of natural sleep for the central nervous system are undeniable and essential, yet they also advance a concomitant advantage to the immune system, with fewer infections and a greater likelihood of survival from sepsis.

REFERENCES

1. Nelson LE, Guo TZ, Lu J, et al. The sedative component of anesthesia is mediated by GABA(A) receptors in an endogenous sleep pathway. Nat Neurosci 2002; 5(10):979–84.
2. Saper CB, Scammell TE, Lu J. Hypothalamic regulation of sleep and circadian rhythms. Nature 2005; 437(7063):1257–63.
3. Borbely AA, Achermann P. Sleep homeostasis and models of sleep regulation. J Biol Rhythms 1999; 14(6):557–68.
4. Walker MP, Stickgold R. Sleep-dependent learning and memory consolidation. Neuron 2004;44(1): 121–33.
5. Nelson LE, Lu J, Guo T, et al. The alpha2-adrenoceptor agonist dexmedetomidine converges on an endogenous sleep-promoting pathway to exert its sedative effects. Anesthesiology 2003; 98(2):428–36.
6. Szymusiak R, McGinty D. Hypothalamic regulation of sleep and arousal. In: Pfaff DW, Kieffer BL, editors. Molecular and biophysical mechanisms of arousal, alertness, and attention, vol. 1129. Malden (MA): Wiley-Blackwell; 2008. p. 275–86.
7. Vanini G, Torterolo P, McGregor R, et al. GABAergic processes in the mesencephalic tegmentum modulate the occurrence of active (rapid eye movement) sleep in guinea pigs. Neuroscience 2007;145(3): 1157–67.
8. Zecharia AY, Nelson LE, Gent TC, et al. The involvement of hypothalamic sleep pathways in general anesthesia: testing the hypothesis using the GABAA receptor beta3N265M knock-in mouse. J Neurosci 2009;29(7):2177–87.
9. Tung A, Bergmann BM, Herrera S, et al. Recovery from sleep deprivation occurs during propofol anesthesia. Anesthesiology 2004;100(6):1419–26.

10. Tung A, Lynch JP, Mendelson WB. Prolonged sedation with propofol in the rat does not result in sleep deprivation. Anesth Analg 2001;92(5):1232–6.

11. Datta S, Spoley EE, Patterson EH. Microinjection of glutamate into the pedunculopontine tegmentum induces REM sleep and wakefulness in the rat. Am J Physiol Regul Integr Comp Physiol 2001;280(3): R752–9.

12. Kodama T, Honda Y. Acetylcholine and glutamate release during sleep-wakefulness in the pedunculopontine tegmental nucleus and norepinephrine changes regulated by nitric oxide. Psychiatry Clin Neurosci 1999;53(2):109–11.

13. Razoux F, Garcia R, Lena I. Ketamine, at a dose that disrupts motor behavior and latent inhibition, enhances prefrontal cortex synaptic efficacy and glutamate release in the nucleus accumbens. Neuropsychopharmacology 2007;32(3):719–27.

14. Lorrain DS, Baccei CS, Bristow LJ, et al. Effects of ketamine and N-methyl-D-aspartate on glutamate and dopamine release in the rat prefrontal cortex: modulation by a group II selective metabotropic glutamate receptor agonist LY379268. Neuroscience 2003;117(3):697–706.

15. Rowland LM, Bustillo JR, Mullins PG, et al. Effects of ketamine on anterior cingulate glutamate metabolism in healthy humans: a 4-T proton MRS study. Am J Psychiatry 2005;162(2):394–6.

16. Lingamaneni R, Birch ML, Hemmings HC. Widespread inhibition of sodium channel-dependent glutamate release from isolated nerve terminals by isoflurane and propofol. Anesthesiology 2001;95(6):1460–6.

17. Larsen M, Valo ET, Berg-Johnsen J, et al. Isoflurane reduces synaptic glutamate release without changing cytosolic free calcium in isolated nerve terminals. Eur J Anaesthesiol 1998;15(2):224–9.

18. Moe MC, Berg-Johnsen J, Larsen GA, et al. Sevoflurane reduces synaptic glutamate release in human synaptosomes. J Neurosurg Anesthesiol 2002;14(3): 180–6.

19. Liachenko S, Tang P, Somogyi GT, et al. Concentration-dependent isoflurane effects on depolarization-evoked glutamate and GABA outflows from mouse brain slices. Br J Pharmacol 1999;127(1):131–8.

20. Pick J, Chen YH, Moore JT, et al. Rapid eye movement sleep debt accrues in mice exposed to volatile anesthetics. Anesthesiology 2011;115(4):702–12.

21. Moote CA, Knill RL. Isoflurane anesthesia causes a transient alteration in nocturnal sleep. Anesthesiology 1988;69(3):327–31.

22. Kelz MB, Sun Y, Chen J, et al. An essential role for orexins in emergence from general anesthesia. Proc Natl Acad Sci U S A 2008;105(4):1309–14.

23. Brandes IF, Zuperku EJ, Stucke AG, et al. Isoflurane depresses the response of inspiratory hypoglossal motoneurons to serotonin in vivo. Anesthesiology 2007;106(4):736–45.

24. Whittington RA, Virag L. Isoflurane decreases extracellular serotonin in the mouse hippocampus. Anesth Analg 2006;103(1):92–8.

25. Lakhlani PP, MacMillan LB, Guo TZ, et al. Substitution of a mutant alpha2a-adrenergic receptor via "hit and run" gene targeting reveals the role of this subtype in sedative, analgesic, and anesthetic-sparing responses in vivo. Proc Natl Acad Sci U S A 1997; 94(18):9950–5.

26. Correa-Sales C, Rabin BC, Maze M. A hypnotic response to dexmedetomidine, an alpha 2 agonist, is mediated in the locus coeruleus in rats. Anesthesiology 1992;76(6):948–52.

27. Correa-Sales C, Reid K, Maze M. Pertussis toxin-mediated ribosylation of G proteins blocks the hypnotic response to an alpha 2-agonist in the locus coeruleus of the rat. Pharmacol Biochem Behav 1992;43(3):723–7.

28. Nacif-Coelho C, Correa-Sales C, Chang LL, et al. Perturbation of ion channel conductance alters the hypnotic response to the alpha 2-adrenergic agonist dexmedetomidine in the locus coeruleus of the rat. Anesthesiology 1994;81(6):1527–34.

29. Huupponen E, Kulkas A, Tenhunen M, et al. Diffuse sleep spindles show similar frequency in central and frontopolar positions. J Neurosci Methods 2008;172(1):54–9.

30. Coull JT, Jones ME, Egan TD, et al. Attentional effects of noradrenaline vary with arousal level: selective activation of thalamic pulvinar in humans. Neuroimage 2004;22(1):315–22.

31. Mason KP, O'Mahony E, Zurakowski D, et al. Effects of dexmedetomidine sedation on the EEG in children. Paediatr Anaesth 2009;19(12):1175–83.

32. Meuret P, Backman SB, Bonhomme V, et al. Physostigmine reverses propofol-induced unconsciousness and attenuation of the auditory steady state response and bispectral index in human volunteers. Anesthesiology 2000;93(3):708–17.

33. Nagase Y, Kaibara M, Uezono Y, et al. Propofol inhibits muscarinic acetylcholine receptor-mediated signal transduction in Xenopus oocytes expressing the rat M1 receptor. Jpn J Pharmacol 1999;79(3): 319–25.

34. Flood P, RamirezLatorre J, Role L. alpha 4 beta 2 neuronal nicotinic acetylcholine receptors in the central nervous system are inhibited by isoflurane and propofol, but alpha 7-type nicotinic acetylcholine receptors are unaffected. Anesthesiology 1997;86(4):859–65.

35. Furuya R, Oka K, Watanabe I, et al. The effects of ketamine and propofol on neuronal nicotinic acetylcholine receptors and P-2X purinoceptors in PC12 cells. Anesth Analg 1999;88(1):174–80.

36. Coates KM, Flood P. Ketamine and its preservative, benzethonium chloride, both inhibit human recombinant alpha 7 and alpha 4 beta 2 neuronal nicotinic

acetylcholine receptors in Xenopus oocytes. Br J Pharmacol 2001;134(4):871–9.

37. Scheller M, Bufler J, Schneck H, et al. Isoflurane and sevoflurane interact with the nicotinic acetylcholine receptor channels in micromolar concentrations. Anesthesiology 1997;86(1):118–27.

38. Borbely AA, Wirz-Justice A. Sleep, sleep deprivation and depression. A hypothesis derived from a model of sleep regulation. Hum Neurobiol 1982;1(3):205–10.

39. Ueda HR, Hayashi S, Chen WB, et al. System-level identification of transcriptional circuits underlying mammalian circadian clocks. Nat Genet 2005; 37(2):187–92.

40. Dispersyn G, Pain L, Challet E, et al. General anesthetics effects on circadian temporal structure: an update. Chronobiol Int 2008;25(6):835–50.

41. Chassard D, Duflo F, Bouvet L, et al. Chronobiology of postoperative pain: it's time to wake up! Can J Anaesth 2007;54(9):685–8.

42. Challet E, Gourmelen S, Pevet P, et al. Reciprocal relationships between general (propofol) anesthesia and circadian time in rats. Neuropsychopharmacology 2007;32(3):728–35.

43. Rebuelto M, Ambros L, Waxman S, et al. Chronobiological study of the pharmacological response of rats to combination ketamine-midazolam. Chronobiol Int 2004;21(4–5):591–600.

44. Munson ES, Martucci RW, Smith RE. Circadian variations in anesthetic requirement and toxicity in rats. Anesthesiology 1970;32(6):507–14.

45. Cheeseman JF, Winnebeck EC, Millar CD, et al. General anesthesia alters time perception by phase shifting the circadian clock. Proc Natl Acad Sci U S A 2012;109(18):7061–6.

46. Ledowski T, Bein B, Hanss R, et al. Neuroendocrine stress response and heart rate variability: a comparison of total intravenous versus balanced anesthesia. Anesth Analg 2005;101(6):1700–5.

47. Nishiyama T, Yamashita K, Yokoyama T. Stress hormone changes in general anesthesia of long duration: isoflurane-nitrous oxide anesthesia oxide vs sevoflurane-nitrous. J Clin Anesth 2005;17(8):586–91.

48. Marana E, Annetta MG, Meo F, et al. Sevoflurane improves the neuroendocrine stress response during laparoscopic pelvic surgery. Can J Anaesth 2003;50(4):348–54.

49. Karkela J, Vakkuri O, Kaukinen S, et al. The influence of anaesthesia and surgery on the circadian rhythm of melatonin. Acta Anaesthesiol Scand 2002;46(1):30–6.

50. Ram E, Vishne TH, Weinstein T, et al. General anesthesia for surgery influences melatonin and cortisol levels. World J Surg 2005;29(7):826–9.

51. Gogenur I, Ocak U, Altunpinar O, et al. Disturbances in melatonin, cortisol and core body temperature rhythms after major surgery. World J Surg 2007; 31(2):290–8.

52. Gogenur I, Middleton B, Kristiansen VB, et al. Disturbances in melatonin and core body temperature circadian rhythms after minimal invasive surgery. Acta Anaesthesiol Scand 2007;51(8):1099–106.

53. Fassoulaki A, Kostopanagiotou G, Meletiou P, et al. No change in serum melatonin, or plasma beta-endorphin levels after sevoflurane anesthesia. J Clin Anesth 2007;19(2):120–4.

54. Sakamoto A, Imai J, Nishikawa A, et al. Influence of inhalation anesthesia assessed by comprehensive gene expression profiling. Gene 2005;356:39–48.

55. Kobayashi K, Takemori K, Sakamoto A. Circadian gene expression is suppressed during sevoflurane anesthesia and the suppression persists after awakening. Brain Res 2007;1185:1–7.

56. Yoshida H, Kubota T, Krueger JM. A cyclooxygenase-2 inhibitor attenuates spontaneous and TNF-alpha-induced non-rapid eye movement sleep in rabbits. Am J Physiol Regul Integr Comp Physiol 2003; 285(1):R99–109.

57. Ohe Y, Iijima N, Kadota K, et al. The general anesthetic sevoflurane affects the expression of clock gene mPer2 accompanying the change of NAD(+) level in the suprachiasmatic nucleus of mice. Neurosci Lett 2011;490(3):231–6.

58. Kadota K, Iijima N, Ohe-Hayashi Y, et al. Time-dependent repression of mPer2 expression in the suprachiasmatic nucleus by inhalation anesthesia with sevoflurane. Neurosci Lett 2012; 528(2):153–8.

59. Pollmacher T, Mullington J, Korth C, et al. Diurnal variations in the human rest response to endotoxin. J Infect Dis 1996;174(5):1040–5.

60. Ferraz E, Borges MC, Terra Filho J. Comparison of 4 AM and 4 PM bronchial responsiveness to hypertonic saline in asthma. Lung 2006;184(6):341–6.

61. Cutolo M, Straub RH. Circadian rhythms in arthritis: hormonal effects on the immune/inflammatory reaction. Autoimmun Rev 2008;7(3):223–8.

62. Lange T, Dimitrov S, Born J. Effects of sleep and circadian rhythm on the human immune system. Ann N Y Acad Sci 2010;1193:48–59.

63. Keller M, Mazuch J, Abraham U, et al. A circadian clock in macrophages controls inflammatory immune responses. Proc Natl Acad Sci U S A 2009;106(50):21407–12.

64. Arjona A, Sarkar DK. Circadian oscillations of clock genes, cytolytic factors, and cytokines in rat NK cells. J Immunol 2005;174(12):7618–24.

65. Arjona A, Sarkar DK. Evidence supporting a circadian control of natural killer cell function. Brain Behav Immun 2006;20(5):469–76.

66. Silver AC, Arjona A, Hughes ME, et al. Circadian expression of clock genes in mouse macrophages, dendritic cells, and B cells. Brain Behav Immun 2012;26(3):407–13.

67. Bozek K, Relogio A, Kielbasa SM, et al. Regulation of clock-controlled genes in mammals. PloS One 2009;4(3):e4882.

68. Gibbs JE, Blaikley J, Beesley S, et al. The nuclear receptor REV-ERB alpha mediates circadian regulation of innate immunity through selective regulation of inflammatory cytokines. Proc Natl Acad Sci U S A 2012;109(2):582–7.

69. Narasimamurthy R, Hatori M, Nayak SK, et al. Circadian clock protein cryptochrome regulates the expression of proinflammatory cytokines. Proc Natl Acad Sci U S A 2012;109(31):12662–7.

70. Silver AC, Arjona A, Walker WE, et al. The circadian clock controls toll-like receptor 9-mediated innate and adaptive immunity. Immunity 2012; 36(2):251–61.

71. Fortier EE, Rooney J, Dardente H, et al. Circadian variation of the response of T cells to antigen. J Immunol 2011;187(12):6291–300.

72. Aurell J, Elmqvist D. Sleep in the surgical intensive care unit: continuous polygraphic recording of sleep in nine patients receiving postoperative care. Br Med J (Clin Res Ed) 1985;290(6474):1029–32.

73. Hilton BA. Quantity and quality of patients' sleep and sleep-disturbing factors in a respiratory intensive care unit. J Adv Nurs 1976;1(6):453–68.

74. Gabor JY, Cooper AB, Hanly PJ. Sleep disruption in the intensive care unit. Curr Opin Crit Care 2001;7(1):21–7.

75. Krachman SL, D'Alonzo GE, Criner GJ. Sleep in the intensive care unit. Chest 1995;107(6):1713–20.

76. Freedman NS, Gazendam J, Levan L, et al. Abnormal sleep/wake cycles and the effect of environmental noise on sleep disruption in the intensive care unit. Am J Respir Crit Care Med 2001;163(2):451–7.

77. Bourne RS, Mills GH. Sleep disruption in critically ill patients—pharmacological considerations. Anaesthesia 2004;59(4):374–84.

78. Pandharipande P, Ely EW. Sedative and analgesic medications: risk factors for delirium and sleep disturbances in the critically ill. Crit Care Clin 2006; 22(2):313–27, vii.

79. Pisani MA, Murphy TE, Araujo KL, et al. Benzodiazepine and opioid use and the duration of intensive care unit delirium in an older population. Crit Care Med 2009;37(1):177–83.

80. Cammarano WB, Pittet JF, Weitz S, et al. Acute withdrawal syndrome related to the administration of analgesic and sedative medications in adult intensive care unit patients. Crit Care Med 1998;26(4):676–84.

81. Pandharipande PP, Pun BT, Herr DL, et al. Effect of sedation with dexmedetomidine vs lorazepam on acute brain dysfunction in mechanically ventilated patients—the MENDS randomized controlled trial. JAMA 2007;298(22):2644–53.

82. Pandharipande PP, Sanders RD, Girard TD, et al. Effect of dexmedetomidine versus lorazepam on outcome in patients with sepsis: an a priori-designed analysis of the MENDS randomized controlled trial. Crit Care 2010;14(2):R38.

Sleep Apnea, Chronic Sleep Restriction, and Inflammation
Perioperative Implications

Walter Conwell, MD[a], Teofilo Lee-Chiong Jr, MD[a,b],*

KEYWORDS

- Obstructive sleep apnea • Chronic sleep restriction • Inflammation

KEY POINTS

- Obstructive sleep apnea, chronic sleep restriction, and obesity increase the risk for cardiovascular disease and mortality via several mechanisms, including intermittent hypoxia (oxidative stress), systemic inflammation, neuroendocrine changes (ie, metabolic syndrome), and hypercoagulability.
- These disorders should be aggressively identified and treated to prevent downstream complications.

INTRODUCTION

Obstructive sleep apnea (OSA), chronic sleep restriction, and obesity are epidemic in the United States. Two percent to 4% of the US population has OSA, defined as having an apnea-hypopnea index (AHI) of greater than 5 events per hour.[1] One-fifth of the general population suffers from chronic sleep restriction, and habitually sleeps for only 4 to 7 hours nightly.[2] An alarming 70% of the US population is overweight, and 33% falls under the obese range with a body mass index (BMI) of more than 30 kg/m^2.[3,4] These disease processes can exist in isolation of one another; however, when all 3 entities are present, they interact in a cyclical, and often bidirectional, manner (**Fig. 1**). Patients with obesity may go on to develop OSA, and the latter can result in chronic sleep restriction, daytime hypersomnolence, and further weight gain. The story is likely more complicated, as a growing body of evidence implicates chronic inflammation as an important sequela and possible contributor of each disease process.[4–13] In the present review, we discuss the evidence for the role of inflammation in these pathophysiologic states and discuss how these physiologic derangements may interact and lead to increased morbidity and mortality.

OSA, CHRONIC SLEEP RESTRICTION, AND THE METABOLIC SYNDROME

The metabolic syndrome consists of the clinical tetrad of visceral adiposity, hypertension, insulin resistance, and dyslipidemia[14]; however, there are many other associated features, including hyperuricemia, coagulopathy, and secondary disorders, such as polycystic ovarian syndrome and nonalcoholic steatohepatitis. Notably, all of these components have individually been associated with markers of chronic inflammation. In this regard, the metabolic syndrome, as a whole, may be considered a chronic inflammatory disorder.[14] Whether inflammation is a cause or an effect of the metabolic syndrome remains unclear; however, it has become more apparent that there is considerable interplay with the clinical entities of OSA and metabolic syndrome. In fact, there appears to be a bidirectional relationship. One study estimated that metabolic syndrome was present in 59% of children with OSA (ie, AHI >5) compared with only 16% of those without OSA. Conversely, about 25% of children with metabolic syndrome had OSA.[12] Another study reported a prevalence of OSA (AHI ≥15) of 60% in 152 adult patients with newly diagnosed metabolic syndrome irrespective

[a] Division of Pulmonary Sciences and Critical Care Medicine, University of Colorado, Denver, CO, USA;
[b] Department of Medicine, Division of Pulmonary, Critical Care and Sleep Medicine, National Jewish Health, 1400 Jackson Street, Denver, CO 80206, USA
* Corresponding author.
E-mail address: Lee-chiongt@njhealth.org

Sleep Med Clin 8 (2013) 11–21
http://dx.doi.org/10.1016/j.jsmc.2012.11.003
1556-407X/13/$ – see front matter © 2013 Elsevier Inc. All rights reserved.

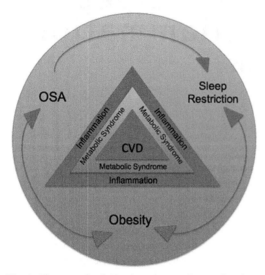

Fig. 1. The complex interplay among obstructive sleep apnea, chronic sleep restriction, and obesity. All 3 have been shown to promote systemic inflammation, which in turn, promotes the metabolic syndrome and contributes increased cardiovascular risk and mortality.

of sleep complaints. Those with OSA had significantly higher blood pressure and levels of glucose, triglycerides, cholesterol, low-density lipoproteins (LDL), cholesterol/high-density lipoprotein (HDL) ratio, triglycerides/HDL ratio, uric acid, and C-reactive protein (CRP) compared with patients without OSA. OSA and indices of disease severity (AHI and minimum oxygen saturation [SaO2]) were independently associated with glucose, triglycerides, cholesterol/HDL ratio, uric acid, and CRP levels.[13] Obesity is an obvious connection between OSA and the metabolic syndrome, given that the former is the most important risk factor for the development of OSA. Approximately 70% of persons with OSA are either overweight or obese, and the prevalence of OSA has been noted to increase with greater obesity.[15,16] There are several mechanisms by which excess weight can give rise to OSA, including decrease in size of the upper airway (UA) as a result of local fat deposition and reduction in lung volumes, as well as decreased UA muscle tone secondary to fatty infiltration of the musculature.

OSA can, in turn, contribute to sustained or progressive obesity via its effects on leptin and ghrelin levels, development of insulin resistance and diabetes, sleep deprivation, and sleepiness and physical inactivity.[15] Leptin is an adipokine produced by adipocytes and acts to regulate appetite and metabolism. It is anorexigenic and increases energy expenditure. Leptin also stimulates respiration and its activity affects pulmonary disorders, including chronic obstructive pulmonary disease and asthma.[17] Leptin has direct effects on the vasculature and leptin resistance is present in a number of disorders, such as metabolic syndrome, endothelial dysfunction, and cardiovascular disease (CVD).[18,19] Despite multiple studies, the relationship between leptin and OSA remains uncertain. In some reports, leptin levels are elevated in persons with OSA compared with BMI-matched controls, and are reduced by positive airway pressure (PAP) therapy in both obese and nonobese patients.[20–22] Confusing the matter are other studies that describe a correlation of elevated leptin levels with visceral fat and certain cytokines (tumor necrosis factor alpha [TNF-α] and interleukin 6 [IL-6]) but not with AHI.[23] Ghrelin is a peptide produced mainly in the stomach; its main action is stimulation of appetite. Ghrelin levels are higher in OSA compared with healthy controls, and decrease with PAP treatment.[24] Glucose metabolism is also altered in OSA, most likely because of intermittent hypoxia (IH), insulin insensitivity, and sleep deprivation.[25]

Chronic sleep restriction, independent of OSA, has also been linked to the development of metabolic syndrome. An observational study showed that a well-validated measure of sleep quality, the Pittsburgh Sleep Quality Index, was significantly related to waist circumference, BMI, percentage of body fat, serum levels of insulin and glucose, and estimated insulin resistance.[26] Of note, numerous other studies have also shown a close correlation between short sleep times (<6 hours) and increased BMI.[27] Conversely, obesity independent of OSA may also affect sleep quality and lead to chronic sleep restriction. One study showed that obese patients without OSA have increased sleep fragmentation, poor sleep quality, and daytime hypersomnolence compared with nonobese patients.[28] Additionally, a significant number of patients with obesity and OSA remain hypersomnolent despite compliance with appropriate PAP therapy.[29]

MECHANISMS LINKING METABOLIC SYNDROME WITH OSA AND SLEEP RESTRICTION

Several mechanisms have been proposed to explain the increased prevalence of metabolic syndrome in persons with OSA. These include IH, systemic inflammation, activation of the sympathetic nervous system, changes in neuroendocrine function, and sleep loss because of sleep fragmentation.

IH refers to the repetitive short cycles of oxygen desaturation followed by rapid reoxygenation, comparable to the phenomenon seen with ischemic-reperfusion injury in atherosclerosis.[30] IH plays a significant role in initiation of inflammation. Oxidative stress from IH results in depletion of adenosine triphosphate (ATP) and activation of xanthine oxidase. Reactive oxygen species (ROS) are produced during the next period of reoxygenation. These, in turn, result in adaptive responses via activation of hypoxia inducible factor-1 (HIF-1), as well as inflammatory responses with generation of nuclear factor kappa beta (NF-κβ) and activator protein 1 (AP-1). Activation of HIF-1 leads to increased expression of products, such as erythropoietin, vascular endothelial growth factor (VEGF), and inducible nitric oxide synthase (iNOS), to improve tissue adaptation to hypoxia. On the other hand, activation of NF-κβ augments production of proinflammatory cytokines, including TNF-α, IL-6, and IL-8; stimulates activation of endothelial cells, leukocytes, and platelets; and gives rise to endothelial dysfunction.[31] It is believed that there is preferential activation of the inflammatory NF-κβ–dependent pathway over the adaptive HIF-1–dependent pathway in OSA. Increased oxidative stress in OSA, therefore, results from decreased antioxidant capacity in the face of greater ROS production, increased lipid peroxidation, and elevated levels of xanthine oxidoreductase. IH can also give rise to activation of the renin-angiotensin system.[32] In summary, the development of key components of the metabolic syndrome in OSA is believed to be directly related to IH. The latter alters glucose metabolism via its effects on systemic inflammation, sympathetic activation, pancreatic beta cell injury, and greater activation of counter-regulatory hormones. On the other hand, IH also upregulates lipid biosynthesis in the liver, enhances lipolysis in peripheral adipose tissues, and inhibits lipoprotein clearance, all of which lead to dyslipidemia.[33]

OSA may additionally exacerbate the chronic inflammation seen in obese individuals. It has been shown that TNF-α is overexpressed in the adipose tissue of diet-induced obese mice, as well as in macrophage infiltrated into these tissues.[11] One possible mechanism for the adipose tissue inflammation in the setting of obesity is believed to be hypoxia in hypertrophied adipocytes that are farther away from the tissue blood supply.[7] This may lead to an increased TNF-α generation, apoptosis, and chemotaxic cytokine release and subsequent inflammatory cell infiltration. It is likely that cyclical hypoxia in the setting of OSA would only worsen this process.

Sleep restriction, independent of OSA, also has bidirectional interplay with both obesity and inflammation. Markers of inflammation have a normal variation with the sleep-wake cycle, with innate immune cells and inflammatory cytokines being lowest during the morning and highest in the evening. Sleep restriction and sleep deprivation have pronounced effects on the immune system and are associated with increases in monocyte and natural killer (NK) cells, as well as TNF-α, IL-6, and CRP levels.[34–36] Conversely, sleep deprivation has been associated with decreased adaptive immune response in the form of less antibody production post vaccination.[37,38] Inflammation may also affect sleep. Animal studies have demonstrated increased total sleep time with injection of IL-1. Humans injected with lipopolysaccharides (LPS) develop increased sleepiness and enhanced slow-wave sleep with low levels of the agent, and increased sleep fragmentation with higher levels.[39–41] Patients with OSA, treated with etanercept (a TNF-α antagonist) report decreased subjective sleepiness.[42] This evidence argues for an important role of inflammation in normal sleep promotion. This consequence, however, can become pathologic in the setting of sleep restriction or deprivation or during inflammation due to other causes.

OSA, CHRONIC SLEEP RESTRICTION, AND CARDIOVASCULAR DISORDERS

Cardiovascular consequences of OSA include hypertension, cardiac arrhythmias, ischemic heart disease, heart failure, stroke, and increased CVD-related mortality.[43]

OSA increases the likelihood of hypertension independent of known confounding factors. The disorder increases both systolic and diastolic blood pressures and abolishes the normal nocturnal fall in blood pressure, referred to as the "dipping" phenomenon. It is believed that the risk of CVD may be greater among "nondippers" compared with "dippers." The odds of hypertension are increased by 1% for each additional apnea event per hour of sleep, and by 13% by each 10% decrease in nocturnal SaO2 level. In the Wisconsin Sleep Cohort Study, 709 participants were followed for 4 years, and relative to a reference category of AHI = 0, the odds ratios for the presence of hypertension at 4-year follow-up were 1.42 for AHI of 0.1 to 4.9 at baseline, 2.03 for AHI of 5.0 to 14.9, and 2.89 for AHI of 15.0 or more.[44] Not all studies have supported the correlation between OSA and hypertension, however. In the Sleep Heart Health Study, AHI was not a significant predictor of future hypertension among middle-aged and older persons after adjustment for BMI at 5-year follow-up; subjects in this study were, on average, 14 years older and less obese compared with the Wisconsin sleep cohort.[45] Last, some reports have indicated an improvement in blood pressure during PAP therapy in persons with OSA and hypertension. In one meta-analysis of 16 randomized controlled trials published from 1980 to 2006 and that involved 818 subjects, the mean net change in blood pressure with continuous positive airway pressure (CPAP) therapy compared with controls was −2.46 mm Hg (systolic blood pressure), −1.83 mm Hg (diastolic blood pressure), and −2.2 mm Hg (mean arterial pressure).[46]

The risk of ischemic heart disease (IHD) is also increased in middle-aged adults with OSA independent of age, BMI, blood pressure, and smoking. OSA may influence the timing of myocardial infarction (MI) and sudden cardiac death. The incidence of MI and sudden cardiac death peaks between 6:00 AM and noon in the general population with a nadir from midnight to 6:00 AM. In contrast, in patients with OSA, the incidence of MI is most common between midnight and 6:00 AM.[47] Finally, the risk of strokes in persons with OSA, and the risk of OSA following strokes are both increased. OSA is associated with increased carotid artery intima-media thickness (IMT), a marker of atherosclerosis, and IMT values are positively related with both disease severity (AHI) and duration (in months).[48]

Sleep deprivation is associated with increased mortality. In a retrospective study of 1.1 million patients, those who received 7 hours of sleep per night had the lowest all-cause mortality. Those who slept less than 3.5 to 4.5 hours per night (or more than 8.5 hours) had an adjusted mortality of greater than 15%.[2] Another study evaluating women health care professionals found that those who slept less than 5 hours per night had an approximate relative risk of 1.5 for developing coronary heart disease during the 10-year follow-up.[49] Sleep restriction has also been associated with increased risk of hypertension in patients sleeping fewer than 6 hours per night compared with those patients sleeping 7 hours per night.[50,51]

In the perioperative setting, anesthesia has several adverse effects on persons with OSA, some of whom may have undiagnosed disease at the time of surgery. The administration of anesthetic, sedative, and analgesic agents can reduce UA muscle tone that, in turn, can prolong the duration and increase the frequency of apneas-hypopneas as well as decrease arousal responses to UA occlusion, hypoxia, and hypercapnia. The potency of anesthetic agents is affected by prior sleep disturbance, a common occurrence in the preoperative period. Finally, sleep-disordered breathing may become more pronounced during rapid eye movement sleep rebound commonly noted postoperatively and by the supine posture the patients are asked to maintain.[52]

MECHANISMS FOR ENDOTHELIAL DYSFUNCTION IN OSA AND CHRONIC SLEEP RESTRICTION

As in the case with metabolic syndrome, systemic inflammation plays a central role in the development of endothelial dysfunction in OSA and chronic sleep restriction. Other factors are equally important in the genesis of accelerated atherosclerosis, including hypertension; dyslipidemia; insulin resistance; increased activation of monocytes, lymphocytes, and vascular smooth muscle cells; increased expression of adhesion molecules; hypercoagulability; sympathetic overactivity; and intrathoracic pressure swings.[53] For instance, reflex sympathetic activation during arousals in response to obstructive apneas-hypopneas can result in repetitive rises in blood pressure, whereas large thoracic pressure changes can lead to extreme mechanical stress on the heart (ie, transmural pressure) and vessels.[54,55] Elevations in heart rate and systolic blood pressure in the setting of sleep restriction and sleep deprivation can also increase cardiac stress.

Both local (UA) and systemic inflammation have been described in persons with OSA. Several mechanisms might be responsible for the UA inflammation in OSA. Intermittent UA obstruction can give rise to muscular and soft tissue injury. Systemic hypoxia may also play a role in local inflammation.[56] There are many published reports supporting the presence of considerable local inflammation in OSA, including (1) increase in polymorphonuclear leukocytes, bradykinin, and vasoactive intestinal peptide in nasal lavage fluid[57]; (2) greater percentage of neutrophils in induced sputum[58]; (3) increased exhaled markers of airway inflammation, such as 8-isopetane, IL-6, and nitric oxide (NO)[59–62]; (4) presence of subepithelial edema and inflammatory cell infiltration in soft tissues removed during uvulopalatopharyngoplasty[63]; (5) increase in CD4+ and activated CD25+ T cells in the soft palate muscles and UA mucosa[64]; (6) greater UA connective tissue deposition[65]; and (7) increased UA oxidative stress (via protein carbonyl group detection by immunoblotting).[65]

Of greater significance in the role of OSA in endothelial dysfunction and accelerated atherosclerosis is systemic inflammation. OSA can be regarded as a chronic low-grade inflammatory condition in which numerous circulating inflammatory markers are increased, including high-sensitivity CRP (hsCRP), TNF-α, IL-6, IL-8, intercellular adhesion molecule-1 (ICAM-1), vascular cell adhesion molecule-1 (VCAM-1), and selectins. OSA is also associated with activation of several cell lines. These include enhanced expression of adhesion molecules by activated endothelial cells,[66] greater production of ROS and selectins by activated neutrophils,[67,68] increased ROS production and adhesion molecule expression by monocytes,[66] and phenotypic and functional changes in CD4+ T cells (higher % CD4+CD28null and cytotoxicity) and CD8+ T cells (increase in TNF-α and CD40 ligand and greater OSA severity-dependent cytotoxicity against endothelial cells).[69,70]

Cytokines are intercellular mediator proteins that have multiple biologic actions. They act as mediators of fatigue and sleepiness. Not only is sleep increased by certain cytokines, the latter are, in turn, increased by sleep loss. This communication between the innate immune system and sleep-wake centers in the central nervous system (CNS) is medicated by cytokines as well as by endocrine hormones and the autonomic nervous system.[71] In the presence of local injury or infection, cytokines from peripheral immune cells send signals to various areas of the CNS, including the cortex, limbic region, and autonomic and neuroendocrine systems.[72]

Cytokines are also biomarkers of inflammation and predictive of risk of CVD. There are 2 general classes of cytokines, namely proinflammatory (TNF-α, IL-6, and IL-8) and anti-inflammatory (IL-10). Both classes are regulated by oxidative stress and IH, and are generated via activation of NF-κβ and AP-1. Different patterns of deoxyribonucleic acid (DNA) methylation in genes responsible for the immune response may be present. Children with OSA and increased inflammation (high hsCRP) have been noted to be more likely to have greater Forkhead box P3 (FOXP3) and interferon regulatory factor 1 DNA methylation levels. The FOXP3 gene regulates expression of T regulatory lymphocytes, and DNA methylation levels of this gene are related to AHI, hsCRP, BMI z score, and apolipoprotein-B levels.[73]

IL-6 is also a proinflammatory cytokine, levels of which correlate with atherosclerosis and greater likelihood for future ischemic CVD.[74–76] Earlier studies suggested that IL-6 levels are increased in OSA.[77,78] More recent studies, however, indicate no difference in IL-6 after adjustment for BMI. Similarly, some studies noted decrease in IL-6 levels with PAP therapy or tonsillo-adenoidectomy but other studies show no effect.[78–81] IL-6 has also been shown to be increased in the setting of moderate sleep restriction.

IL-8 has been noted to enhance oxidative stress, and elevated levels are associated with increased risk of CVD.[82,83] Levels of IL-8 are increased in OSA compared with controls and are reduced with PAP therapy.[79,84,85]

TNF-α is a proinflammatory cytokine. Levels of TNF-α have been shown to correlate with early atherosclerosis, and increased activity of this cytokine predicts greater risk for future ischemic CVD (ischemic heart disease and heart failure).[86,87] In OSA, circulating levels of TNF-α and serum-soluble TNF receptor are increased independent of obesity.[88] The degree of hypoxia is the strongest predictor of TNF-α levels in persons with OSA, and levels of TNF-α decrease or normalize after correction of hypoxia with PAP treatment.[77,79,89] Conversely, it has been proposed that TNF-α can contribute to pathogenesis of OSA by promoting UA inspiratory muscle dysfunction and by worsening somnolence and fatigue.[90] In multivariate analysis, TNF-α levels were independently associated with excessive daytime sleepiness (Epworth sleepiness scale) and were greater in persons with OSA compared with both sleepy nonapneic subjects who snored and healthy controls.[79] It is important to note, however, that not all studies have described a correlation between OSA and TNF-α; in one report, OSA was not associated with changes in stimulated TNF-α production from peripheral blood mononuclear cells compared with controls matched to major CVD risk factors and cardio-metabolic therapies.[91]

NF-κβ is a proinflammatory, oxidant-sensitive transcription factor. Increased activity of NF-κβ in monocytes and neutrophils are seen in OSA and are correlated with disease severity. One study noted that NF-κβ binding activity in neutrophils was 4.8- and 7.9-fold greater in mild-moderate (AHI 11–40) and severe (AHI >40) OSA, respectively, compared with controls (AHI <5).[92] PAP therapy reduces NF-κβ levels.[93]

CRP is an acute phase reactant and is a nonspecific biomarker of inflammation. CRP may, itself, contribute to systemic inflammation and accelerated atherosclerosis. Level of hsCRP is an important independent predictor of future CVD events.[94] The evidence linking CRP to OSA is inconsistent. Some investigators have reported that CRP levels are higher in moderate-severe OSA compared with mild OSA and healthy controls, and that PAP treatment decreased the former.[95–98] Other studies, however, failed to demonstrate this relationship. In the Wisconsin Sleep Cohort Study, there was no independent association noted between OSA and CRP after adjustment for BMI.[99] The differences in these outcomes might simply reflect the poor specificity of CRP as an inflammatory marker.

CRP elevations are also noted in the setting of sleep restriction. In one study, healthy young men were exposed to 5 nights of moderate sleep restriction (4 hours of sleep per night) followed by 2 nights of recovery sleep. Levels of CRP were increased to 145% above baseline at the end of sleep restriction and continued to rise to 231% above baseline by the end of the recovery period.[100] In another study involving young healthy volunteers, moderate sleep restriction for 10 days and severe sleep deprivation (no sleep for >4 days) were both associated with significant elevations in CRP to levels equivalent to mild cardiovascular risk.[8]

Pentraxin-3, like CRP, is made up of 5 identical subunits. Whereas CRP (also referred to as short pentraxin) is produced primarily by hepatocytes, pentraxin-3 is produced by vascular endothelial cells, macrophages, and smooth muscle cells, and is considered as a more specific marker of inflammation. Levels of pentraxin-3 are higher in moderate-severe OSA compared with mild OSA and healthy controls, and decrease after CPAP therapy.[101] In one study, levels of both plasma pentraxin-3 and arterial stiffness (cardio-ankle vascular index [CAVI]) were greater in moderate-to-severe OSA than in controls, and decreased after 1 month of PAP therapy. Pentraxin-3 levels were independently correlated with CAVI.[101]

Xanthine oxidoreductase, an enzyme involved in the catalytic conversion of hypoxanthine to uric acid, can contribute to endothelial dysfunction by reducing molecular oxygen, yielding superoxide and hydrogen peroxide. Increased levels of uric acid are present in OSA and levels decreased with PAP therapy.[102] Linear regression analysis has shown an association between uric acid(log) and oxygen desaturation index(log). Uric acid levels also decreased after weight loss in obese children with sleep-disordered breathing.[103]

VEGF enhances proliferation of endothelial cells and is involved with vessel growth and development. Like TNF-α, expression of VEGF is primarily stimulated by hypoxia.[104] Levels of VEGF are increased in OSA, are correlated with AHI, and are reduced with treatment.[105–108]

Vascular homeostasis depends on the balance between vasoconstrictive (endothelin-1, renin-angiotensin-aldosterone system, and thromboxane) and vasorelaxant (NO and prostacyclin) factors. NO is a potent endothelial vasoactive and airway inflammatory mediator that has a key role in flow-mediated dilation of peripheral arteries. Nitric oxide and neuronal NO-synthase (NOS) are also involved in the homeostatic sleep drive and may contribute to the increase in slow-wave sleep during inflammatory states. Several processes regulate NO/NOS output, such as the L-arginine/arginase substrate-competing system, L-citrulline/arginosuccinate-recycling system and asymmetric dimethyl-/monomethyl-L-arginine-inhibiting system.[109] The combination of decreased levels of circulating NO and increased plasma levels of asymmetric NG, NG-dimethylarginine supports the notion of OSA as a vasoconstrictive disorder and may contribute, at least partly, to the development of hypertension in this disorder.[110,111] NO levels return to normal levels and asymmetric NG, NG-dimethylarginine levels are reduced after PAP treatment.[112] As mentioned earlier, higher airway and lower alveolar levels of NO in exhaled breath have been described in OSA, and both airway and alveolar levels correlate with AHI and normalize after PAP treatment.[113]

Dysfunctional interaction of endothelial cells, leukocytes, and platelets is important in atherosclerosis. This interaction consists of 3 stages, occurring sequentially, namely rolling, firm adhesion, and leukocyte migration to the interstitium. Each stage is associated with specific adhesion molecules, which facilitate the various cellular interactions.[114] Rolling refers to the slowing of the flow of leukocytes in the circulation and is mediated by selectins (ie, L-selectins expressed in leukocytes, E-selectins in endothelial cells, and P-selectins in platelets and endothelial cells). The next stage, firm adhesion, involves attachment of leukocytes to endothelial cells via integrins on leukocytes and ICAM-1 and VCAM-1 on endothelial cells. Finally, release of cytokines and free radicals facilitates leukocyte migration into the interstitium. Many of these factors are upregulated in response to IH, including endothelial (ICAM-1, VCAM-1, and E-selectin), monocytic (CD15 moiety on selectins and CD11c, a subunit of integrins), and platelet (P-selectin) adhesion molecules. PAP therapy has been demonstrated to reduce levels of ICAM-1, percentage of monocytes expressing CD15 and CD11c, and platelets expressing P-selectin.[66,115–123]

Other modulators of inflammation affected by OSA include peroxisome proliferator-activated receptor-gamma (PPAR-γ) and macrophage migratory inhibitory factor (MIF). A negative regulator of inflammation, PPAR-γ is expressed in alveolar macrophages and helps in the regulation of lipid and glucose metabolism. Functional activity and mRNA levels of PPAR-γ are decreased in obese persons with OSA compared with controls.[124] Macrophage MIF is a cytokine that may contribute to inflammation by desensitizing the organism to the anti-inflammatory effects of glucocorticoids. Compared with healthy controls, levels of MIF over a 24-hour period are higher in

OSA and are significantly associated with AHI and total arousal index even after adjusting for BMI.[125]

Finally, OSA is associated with increases in platelet aggregability and blood viscosity, the latter secondary to hypoxia-induced polycythemia. Increased levels of activated coagulation factors XIIa and VIIa, fibrinogen, plasminogen activator inhibitor 1 (PAI-1), soluble P-selectin, and thrombin/antithrombin III complexes have been described in OSA. PAP treatment results in a reduction of fibrinogen levels and PAI-1 activity.[126,127]

SUMMARY

In summary, OSA, chronic sleep restriction, and obesity increase the risk for CVD and mortality via several mechanisms, including intermittent hypoxia (oxidative stress), systemic inflammation, neuroendocrine changes (ie, metabolic syndrome), and hypercoagulability. These disorders should therefore be aggressively identified and treated to prevent downstream complications.

REFERENCES

1. Punjabi NM. The epidemiology of adult obstructive sleep apnea. Proc Am Thorac Soc 2008; 5(2):136–43.
2. Kripke DF, Garfinkel L, Wingard DL, et al. Mortality associated with sleep duration and insomnia. Arch Gen Psychiatry 2002;59(2):131–6.
3. Flegal KM, Carrol MD, Kit BK, et al. Prevalence of obesity and trends in the distribution of body mass index among US adults, 1999–2010. JAMA 2012;307(5):491–7.
4. Patel SR, Zhu X, Strofer-Isser A, et al. Sleep duration and biomarkers of inflammation. Sleep 2009; 32(2):200–4.
5. Simpson N, Dinges DF. Sleep and inflammation. Nutr Rev 2007;65(12 Pt 2):S244–52.
6. Hotamisligil GS. Inflammation and metabolic disorders. Nature 2006;444(7121):860–7.
7. Trayhurn P, Wang B, Wood IS. Hypoxia in adipose tissue: a basis for the dysregulation of tissue function in obesity? Br J Nutr 2008;100(2):227–35.
8. Meier-Ewert HK, Ridker PM, Rifai N, et al. Effect of sleep loss on C-reactive protein, an inflammatory marker of cardiovascular risk. J Am Coll Cardiol 2004;43(4):678–83.
9. Mullington JM, Haack M, Toth M, et al. Cardiovascular, inflammatory, and metabolic consequences of sleep deprivation. Prog Cardiovasc Dis 2009; 51(4):294–302.
10. Magee CA, Huang XF, Iverson DC, et al. Examining the pathways linking chronic sleep restriction to obesity. J Obes 2010;2010. pii: 821710.
11. Piva SJ, Tatsch E, De Carvalho JA, et al. Assessment of inflammatory and oxidative biomarkers in obesity and their associations with body mass index. September 9, 2012. Inflammation 2012. Available at: http://link.springer.com.proxy.uchicago.edu/article/10.1007/s10753-012-9538-2/fulltext.html. Accessed October 10, 2012 [Epub ahead of print].
12. Redline S, Storfer-Isser A, Rosen CL, et al. Association between metabolic syndrome and sleep-disordered breathing in adolescents. Am J Respir Crit Care Med 2007;176(4):401–8.
13. Drager LF, Lopes HF, Maki-Nunes C, et al. The impact of obstructive sleep apnea on metabolic and inflammatory markers in consecutive patients with metabolic syndrome. PLoS One 2010;5(8):e12065.
14. Sutherland JP, McKinley B, Eckel RH. The metabolic syndrome and inflammation. Metab Syndr Relat Disord 2004;2(2):82–104.
15. Pillar G, Shehadeh N. Abdominal fat and sleep apnea: the chicken or the egg? Diabetes Care 2008;31(Suppl 2):S303–9.
16. Daltro C, Gregorio PB, Alves E, et al. Prevalence and severity of sleep apnea in a group of morbidly obese patients. Obes Surg 2007;17(6):809–14.
17. Malli F, Papaioannou AI, Gourgoulianis KI, et al. The role of leptin in the respiratory system: an overview. Respir Res 2010;11:152.
18. Galletti F, Barbato A, Versiero M, et al. Circulating leptin levels predict the development of metabolic syndrome in middle-aged men: an 8-year follow-up study. J Hypertens 2007;25(8):1671–7.
19. Luo JD, Zhang GS, Chen MS. Leptin and cardiovascular diseases. Drug News Perspect 2005; 18(7):427–31.
20. McArdle N, Hillman D, Beilin L, et al. Metabolic risk factors for vascular disease in obstructive sleep apnea: a matched controlled study. Am J Respir Crit Care Med 2007;175(2):190–5.
21. Barceló A, Barbé F, Llompart E, et al. Neuropeptide Y and leptin in patients with obstructive sleep apnea syndrome: role of obesity. Am J Respir Crit Care Med 2005;171(2):183–7.
22. Sanner BM, Kollhosser P, Buechner N, et al. Influence of treatment on leptin levels in patients with obstructive sleep apnoea. Eur Respir J 2004;23(4):601–4.
23. Vgontzas AN, Papanicolaou DA, Bixler EO, et al. Sleep apnea and daytime sleepiness and fatigue: relation to visceral obesity, insulin resistance, and hypercytokinemia. J Clin Endocrinol Metab 2000; 85(3):1151–8.
24. Harsch IA, Konturek PC, Koebnick C, et al. Leptin and ghrelin levels in patients with obstructive sleep apnoea: effect of CPAP treatment. Eur Respir J 2003;22(2):251–7.
25. Tasali E, Mokhlesi B, Van Cauter E. Obstructive sleep apnea and type 2 diabetes: interacting epidemics. Chest 2008;133(2):496–506.

26. Jennings JR, Muldoon MF, Hall M, et al. Self-reported sleep quality is associated with the metabolic syndrome. Sleep 2007;30(2):219–23.

27. Magee CA, Iverson DC, Huang XF, et al. A link between chronic sleep restriction and obesity: methodological considerations. Public Health 2008;122(12):1373–81.

28. Resta O, Barbaro MP, Bonfitto P, et al. Low sleep quality and daytime sleepiness in obese patients without obstructive sleep apnoea syndrome. J Intern Med 2003;253(5):536–43.

29. Antic NA, Catcheside P, Buchan C, et al. The effect of CPAP in normalizing daytime sleepiness, quality of life, and neurocognitive function in patients with moderate to severe OSA. Sleep 2011;34:111–9.

30. Lavie L. Oxidative stress—a unifying paradigm in obstructive sleep apnea and comorbidities. Prog Cardiovasc Dis 2009;51(4):303–12.

31. Lavie L. Sleep-disordered breathing and cerebrovascular disease: a mechanistic approach. Neurol Clin 2005;23(4):1059–75.

32. Ramar K, Caples SM. Vascular changes, cardiovascular disease and obstructive sleep apnea. Future Cardiol 2011;7(2):241–9.

33. Drager LF, Jun JC, Polotsky VY. Metabolic consequences of intermittent hypoxia: relevance to obstructive sleep apnea. Best Pract Res Clin Endocrinol Metab 2010;24(5):843–51.

34. Redwine L, Dang J, Irwin M. Cellular adhesion molecule expression, nocturnal sleep and partial sleep deprivation. Brain Behav Immun 2004;18: 333–40.

35. Born J, Lange T, Hansen K, et al. Effects of sleep and circadian rhythm on human circulating immune cells. J Immunol 1997;158:4454–64.

36. Redwine L, Hauger RL, Gillin JC, et al. Effects of sleep and sleep deprivation on interleukin-6, growth hormone, cortisol and melatonin levels in humans. J Clin Endocrinol Metab 2000;83:1573–9.

37. Spiegel K, Sheridan JF, Van Cauter E. Effect of sleep deprivation on response to immunization. JAMA 2002;288:1471–2.

38. Lange T, Perras B, Fehm HL, et al. Sleep enhances the human antibody response to hepatitis A vaccination. Psychosom Med 2003;65:831–5.

39. Opp MR. Cytokines and sleep. Sleep Med Rev 2005;9(5):355–64.

40. Opp MR. Sleeping to fuel the immune system: mammalian sleep and resistance to parasites. BMC Evol Biol 2009;9:8.

41. Krueger JM. The role of cytokines in sleep regulation. Curr Pharm Des 2008;14(32):3408–16.

42. Vgontzas AN, Zoumakis E, Lin HM, et al. Marked decrease in sleepiness in patients with sleep apnea by etanercept, a tumor necrosis factor-alpha antagonist. J Clin Endocrinol Metab 2004; 89(9):4409–13.

43. Levy P, Tamisier R, Arnaud C, et al. Sleep deprivation, sleep apnea and cardiovascular diseases. Front Biosci (Elite Ed) 2012;4:2007–21.

44. Peppard PE, Young T, Palta M, et al. Prospective study of the association between sleep-disordered breathing and hypertension. N Engl J Med 2000;342(19):1378–84.

45. O'Connor GT, Caffo B, Newman AB, et al. Prospective study of sleep-disordered breathing and hypertension: the Sleep Heart Health Study. Am J Respir Crit Care Med 2009;179(12): 1159–64.

46. Bazzano LA, Khan Z, Reynolds K, et al. Effect of nocturnal nasal continuous positive airway pressure on blood pressure in obstructive sleep apnea. Hypertension 2007;50(2):417–23.

47. Gami AS, Howard DE, Olson EJ, et al. Day-night pattern of sudden death in obstructive sleep apnea. N Engl J Med 2005;352(12):1206–14.

48. Ciccone MM, Scicchitano P, Mitacchione G, et al. Is there a correlation between OSAS duration/severity and carotid intima-media thickness? Respir Med 2012;106(5):740–6.

49. Ayas NT, White DP, Mason JE, et al. A prospective study of sleep duration and coronary heart disease in women. Arch Intern Med 2003;163(2):205–9.

50. Gottlieb DJ, Redline S, Nieto FJ, et al. Association of usual sleep duration with hypertension: the Sleep Heart Health Study. Sleep 2006;29(8): 1009–14.

51. Magee CA, Kritharides L, Attia J, et al. Short and long sleep duration are associated with prevalent cardiovascular disease in Australian adults. J Sleep Res 2012;21(4):441–7.

52. Kaw R, Michota F, Jaffer A, et al. Unrecognized sleep apnea in the surgical patient: implications for the perioperative setting. Chest 2006;129(1): 198–205.

53. Lurie A. Endothelial dysfunction in adults with obstructive sleep apnea. Adv Cardiol 2011;46: 139–70.

54. Kohler M, Stradling JR. Mechanisms of vascular damage in obstructive sleep apnea. Nat Rev Cardiol 2010;7(12):677–85.

55. Drager LF, Polotsky VY, Lorenzi-Filho G. Obstructive sleep apnea: an emerging risk factor for atherosclerosis. Chest 2011;140(2):534–42.

56. Sabato R, Guido P, Salerno FG, et al. Airway inflammation in patients affected by obstructive sleep apnea. Monaldi Arch Chest Dis 2006; 65(2):102–5.

57. Rubinstein I. Nasal inflammation in patients with obstructive sleep apnea. Laryngoscope 1995; 105(2):175–7.

58. Salerno FG, Carpagnano E, Guido P, et al. Airway inflammation in patients affected by obstructive sleep apnea syndrome. Respir Med 2004;98(1):25–8.

59. Olopade CO, Christon JA, Zakkar M, et al. Exhaled pentane and nitric oxide levels in patients with obstructive sleep apnea. Chest 1997;111(6):1500–4.

60. Carpagnano GE, Kharitonov SA, Resta O, et al. Increased 8-isoprostane and interleukin-6 in breath condensate of obstructive sleep apnea patients. Chest 2002;122(4):1162–7.

61. Carpagnano GE, Spanevello A, Sabato R, et al. Exhaled pH, exhaled nitric oxide, and induced sputum cellularity in obese patients with obstructive sleep apnea syndrome. Transl Res 2008; 151(1):45–50.

62. Petrosyan M, Perraki E, Simoes D, et al. Exhaled breath markers in patients with obstructive sleep apnoea. Sleep Breath 2008;12(3):207–15.

63. Sekosan M, Zakkar M, Wenig BL, et al. Inflammation in the uvula mucosa of patients with obstructive sleep apnea. Laryngoscope 1996;106(8): 1018–20.

64. Boyd JH, Petrof BJ, Hamid Q, et al. Upper airway muscle inflammation and denervation changes in obstructive sleep apnea. Am J Respir Crit Care Med 2004;170(5):541–6.

65. Kimoff RJ, Hamid Q, Divangahi M, et al. Increased upper airway cytokines and oxidative stress in severe obstructive sleep apnoea. Eur Respir J 2011;38(1):89–97.

66. Dyugovskaya L, Lavie P, Lavie L. Increased adhesion molecules expression and production of reactive oxygen species in leukocytes of sleep apnea patients. Am J Respir Crit Care Med 2002;165(7): 934–9.

67. Dyugovskaya L, Polyakov A, Lavie P, et al. Delayed neutrophil apoptosis in patients with sleep apnea. Am J Respir Crit Care Med 2008;177(5): 544–54.

68. Schulz R, Mahmoudi S, Hattar K, et al. Enhanced release of superoxide from polymorphonuclear neutrophils in obstructive sleep apnea. Impact of continuous positive airway pressure therapy. Am J Respir Crit Care Med 2000;162(2 Pt 1):566–70.

69. Dyugovskaya L, Lavie P, Hirsh M, et al. Activated CD8+ T-lymphocytes in obstructive sleep apnea. Eur Respir J 2005;25(5):820–8.

70. Dyugovskaya L, Lavie P, Lavie L. Lymphocyte activation as a possible measure of atherosclerotic risk in patients with sleep apnea. Ann N Y Acad Sci 2005;1051:340–50.

71. Motivala SJ. Sleep and inflammation: psychoneuroimmunology in the context of cardiovascular disease. Ann Behav Med 2011;42(2):141–52.

72. Lorton D, Lubahn CL, Estus C, et al. Bidirectional communication between the brain and the immune system: implications for physiological sleep and disorders with disrupted sleep. Neuroimmunomodulation 2006;13(5–6):357–74.

73. Kim J, Bhattacharjee R, Khalyfa A, et al. DNA methylation in inflammatory genes among children with obstructive sleep apnea. Am J Respir Crit Care Med 2012;185(3):330–8.

74. Eckel RH, Grundy SM, Zimmet PZ. The metabolic syndrome. Lancet 2005;365(9468):1415–28.

75. Alam I, Lewis K, Stephens JW, et al. Obesity, metabolic syndrome and sleep apnoea: all proinflammatory states. Obes Rev 2007;8(2):119–27.

76. Luc G, Bard JM, Juhan-Vague I, et al. C-reactive protein, interleukin-6, and fibrinogen as predictors of coronary heart disease: the PRIME Study. Arterioscler Thromb Vasc Biol 2003;23(7):1255–61.

77. Ciftci TU, Kokturk O, Bukan N, et al. The relationship between serum cytokine levels with obesity and obstructive sleep apnea syndrome. Cytokine 2004;28(2):87–91.

78. Yokoe T, Minoguchi K, Matsuo H, et al. Elevated levels of C-reactive protein and interleukin-6 in patients with obstructive sleep apnea syndrome are decreased by nasal continuous positive airway pressure. Circulation 2003;107(8):1129–34.

79. Ryan S, Taylor CT, McNicholas WT. Predictors of elevated nuclear factor-kappaB-dependent genes in obstructive sleep apnea syndrome. Am J Respir Crit Care Med 2006;174(7):824–30.

80. Burioka N, Miyata M, Fukuoka Y, et al. Day-night variations of serum interleukin-6 in patients with severe obstructive sleep apnea syndrome before and after continuous positive airway pressure (CPAP). Chronobiol Int 2008;25(5):827–34.

81. Gozal D, Serpero LD, Sans Capdevila O, et al. Systemic inflammation in non-obese children with obstructive sleep apnea. Sleep Med 2008;9(3): 254–9.

82. Boekholdt SM, Peters RJ, Hack CE, et al. IL-8 plasma concentrations and the risk of future coronary artery disease in apparently healthy men and women: the EPIC-Norfolk prospective population study. Arterioscler Thromb Vasc Biol 2004; 24(8):1503–8.

83. Romuk E, Skrzep-Poloczek B, Wojciechowska C, et al. Selectin-P and interleukin-8 plasma levels in coronary heart disease patients. Eur J Clin Invest 2002;32(9):657–61.

84. Alzoghaibi MA, Bahammam AS. Lipid peroxides, superoxide dismutase and circulating IL-8 and GCP-2 in patients with severe obstructive sleep apnea: a pilot study. Sleep Breath 2005;9(3): 119–26.

85. Ohga E, Tomita T, Wada H, et al. Effects of obstructive sleep apnea on circulating ICAM-1, IL-8, and MCP-1. J Appl Physiol 2003;94(1):179–84.

86. Cesari M, Penninx BW, Newman AB, et al. Inflammatory markers and onset of cardiovascular events: results from the Health ABC study. Circulation 2003;108(19):2317–22.

87. Ridker PM, Rifai N, Pfeffer M, et al. Elevation of tumor necrosis factor-alpha and increased risk of recurrent coronary events after myocardial infarction. Circulation 2000;101(18):2149–53.

88. Arias MA, García-Río F, Alonso-Fernández A, et al. CPAP decreases plasma levels of soluble tumour necrosis factor-alpha receptor 1 in obstructive sleep apnoea. Eur Respir J 2008;32(4):1009–15.

89. Minoguchi K, Tazaki T, Yokoe T, et al. Elevated production of tumor necrosis factor-alpha by monocytes in patients with obstructive sleep apnea syndrome. Chest 2004;126(5):1473–9.

90. Reid MB, Lännergren J, Westerblad H. Respiratory and limb muscle weakness induced by tumor necrosis factor-alpha: involvement of muscle myofilaments. Am J Respir Crit Care Med 2002; 166(4):479–84.

91. Guasti L, Marino F, Cosentino M, et al. Cytokine production from peripheral blood mononuclear cells and polymorphonuclear leukocytes in patients studied for suspected obstructive sleep apnea. Sleep Breath 2011;15(1):3–11.

92. Htoo AK, Greenberg H, Tongia S, et al. Activation of nuclear factor kappaB in obstructive sleep apnea: a pathway leading to systemic inflammation. Sleep Breath 2006;10(1):43–50.

93. Yamauchi M, Tamaki S, Tomoda K, et al. Evidence for activation of nuclear factor kappaB in obstructive sleep apnea. Sleep Breath 2006; 10(4):189–93.

94. Willerson JT, Ridker PM. Inflammation as a cardiovascular risk factor. Circulation 2004;109(21 Suppl 1): II2–10.

95. Dorkova Z, Petrasova D, Molcanyiova A, et al. Effects of continuous positive airway pressure on cardiovascular risk profile in patients with severe obstructive sleep apnea and metabolic syndrome. Chest 2008;134(4):686–92.

96. Gozal D, Kheirandish-Gozal L. Cardiovascular morbidity in obstructive sleep apnea: oxidative stress, inflammation, and much more. Am J Respir Crit Care Med 2008;177(4):369–75.

97. Drager LF, Bortolotto LA, Figueiredo AC, et al. Effects of continuous positive airway pressure on early signs of atherosclerosis in obstructive sleep apnea. Am J Respir Crit Care Med 2007;176(7): 706–12.

98. Steiropoulos P, Tsara V, Nena E, et al. Effect of continuous positive airway pressure treatment on serum cardiovascular risk factors in patients with obstructive sleep apnea-hypopnea syndrome. Chest 2007;132(3):843–51.

99. Taheri S, Austin D, Lin L, et al. Correlates of serum C-reactive protein (CRP)—no association with sleep duration or sleep disordered breathing. Sleep 2007;30(8):991–6.

100. van Leeuwen WM, Lehto M, Karisola P, et al. Sleep restriction increases the risk of developing cardiovascular diseases by augmenting proinflammatory responses through IL-17 and CRP. PLoS One 2009; 4(2):e4589.

101. Kasai T, Inoue K, Kumagai T, et al. Plasma pentraxin3 and arterial stiffness in men with obstructive sleep apnea. Am J Hypertens 2011;24(4):401–7.

102. Steiropoulos P, Kotsianidis I, Nena E, et al. Long-term effect of continuous positive airway pressure therapy on inflammation markers of patients with obstructive sleep apnea syndrome. Sleep 2009; 32(4):537–43.

103. Van Hoorenbeeck K, Franckx H, Debode P, et al. Weight loss and sleep-disordered breathing in childhood obesity: effects on inflammation and uric acid. Obesity (Silver Spring) 2012;20(1):172–7.

104. Cherniack NS. Inflammatory ideas about sleep apnea. Respiration 2004;71(1):20–1.

105. Schulz R, Hummel C, Heinemann S, et al. Serum levels of vascular endothelial growth factor are elevated in patients with obstructive sleep apnea and severe nighttime hypoxia. Am J Respir Crit Care Med 2002;165(1):67–70.

106. Imagawa S, Yamaguchi Y, Higuchi M, et al. Levels of vascular endothelial growth factor are elevated in patients with obstructive sleep apnea–hypopnea syndrome. Blood 2001;98(4):1255–7.

107. Gozal D, Lipton AJ, Jones KL. Circulating vascular endothelial growth factor levels in patients with obstructive sleep apnea. Sleep 2002;25(1):59–65.

108. Lavie L, Kraiczi H, Hefetz A, et al. Plasma vascular endothelial growth factor in sleep apnea syndrome: effects of nasal continuous positive air pressure treatment. Am J Respir Crit Care Med 2002; 165(12):1624–8.

109. Cespuglio R, Amrouni D, Meiller A, et al. Nitric oxide in the regulation of the sleep-wake states. Sleep Med Rev 2012;16(3):265–79.

110. Ip MS, Lam B, Chan LY, et al. Circulating nitric oxide is suppressed in obstructive sleep apnea and is reversed by nasal continuous positive airway pressure. Am J Respir Crit Care Med 2000;162(6):2166–71.

111. Schulz R, Schmidt D, Blum A, et al. Decreased plasma levels of nitric oxide derivatives in obstructive sleep apnoea: response to CPAP therapy. Thorax 2000;55(12):1046–51.

112. Ohike Y, Kozaki K, Iijima K, et al. Amelioration of vascular endothelial dysfunction in obstructive sleep apnea syndrome by nasal continuous positive airway pressure—possible involvement of nitric oxide and asymmetric NG, NG-dimethylarginine. Circ J 2005;69(2):221–6.

113. Fortuna AM, Miralda R, Calaf N, et al. Airway and alveolar nitric oxide measurements in obstructive

sleep apnea syndrome. Respir Med 2011;105(4): 630–6.

114. Libby P. Inflammation in atherosclerosis. Nature 2002;420(6917):868–74.

115. Carpagnano GE, Spanevello A, Sabato R, et al. Systemic and airway inflammation in sleep apnea and obesity: the role of ICAM-1 and IL-8. Transl Res 2010;155(1):35–43.

116. O'Brien LM, Serpero LD, Tauman R, et al. Plasma adhesion molecules in children with sleep-disordered breathing. Chest 2006;129(4):947–53.

117. Zamarrón-Sanz C, Ricoy-Galbaldon J, Gude-Sampedro F, et al. Plasma levels of vascular endothelial markers in obstructive sleep apnea. Arch Med Res 2006;37(4):552–5.

118. Robinson GV, Pepperell JC, Segal HC, et al. Circulating cardiovascular risk factors in obstructive sleep apnoea: data from randomised controlled trials. Thorax 2004;59(9):777–82.

119. Granger DN, Vowinkel T, Petnehazy T. Modulation of the inflammatory response in cardiovascular disease. Hypertension 2004;43(5):924–31.

120. Hui DS, Ko FW, Fok JP, et al. The effects of nasal continuous positive airway pressure on platelet activation in obstructive sleep apnea syndrome. Chest 2004;125(5):1768–75.

121. Geiser T, Buck F, Meyer BJ, et al. In vivo platelet activation is increased during sleep in patients with obstructive sleep apnea syndrome. Respiration 2002;69(3):229–34.

122. El-Solh AA, Mador MJ, Sikka P, et al. Adhesion molecules in patients with coronary artery disease and moderate-to-severe obstructive sleep apnea. Chest 2002;121(5):1541–7.

123. Chin K, Nakamura T, Shimizu K, et al. Effects of nasal continuous positive airway pressure on soluble cell adhesion molecules in patients with obstructive sleep apnea syndrome. Am J Med 2000;109(7):562–7.

124. Sharma S, Malur A, Marshall I, et al. Alveolar macrophage activation in obese patients with obstructive sleep apnea. Surgery 2012;151(1): 107–12.

125. Edwards KM, Tomfohr LM, Mills PJ, et al. Macrophage migratory inhibitory factor (MIF) may be a key factor in inflammation in obstructive sleep apnea. Sleep 2011;34(2):161–3.

126. von Känel R, Loredo JS, Ancoli-Israel S, et al. Association between sleep apnea severity and blood coagulability: treatment effects of nasal continuous positive airway pressure. Sleep Breath 2006;10(3): 139–46.

127. Chin K, Ohi M, Kita H, et al. Effects of NCPAP therapy on fibrinogen levels in obstructive sleep apnea syndrome. Am J Respir Crit Care Med 1996;153(6 Pt 1):1972–6.

Upper Airway, Obstructive Sleep Apnea, and Anesthesia

David R. Hillman, MD[a,*], Peter R. Eastwood, PhD[a,b]

KEYWORDS

- Sleep • Anesthesia • Upper airway • Obstructive sleep apnea • Physiology

KEY POINTS

- The tendencies to upper airway obstruction during sleep and anesthesia are related.
- Loss of consciousness is associated with a decrease in activation of upper airway (and other) muscles and an increase in pharyngeal collapsibility.
- Individuals with obstructive sleep apnea have abnormally collapsible upper airways and are at increased risk of obstruction in both states.
- Although the capacity to arouse protects the sleeping individual, anesthesia involves suppression of arousals, which greatly magnifies the risk of asphyxia.
- This risk diminishes with the emergence from anesthesia and return of arousal responses but may recur with postoperative sedation or narcotic analgesia, particularly in those sensitive to their sedative or respiratory depressant effects.
- Close observation is required postoperatively until the patient is consistently rousable.
- Although helpful in treating upper airway obstruction, positive airway pressure therapy does not prevent the need for this careful monitoring.

INTRODUCTION

In recent years the neurophysiologic mechanisms governing sleep and wakefulness have become increasingly well understood. These developments have provided new insights into mechanisms of anesthesia as many anesthetic drugs are now known to activate key components of sleep-related neuronal circuits. Examination of the *similarities* between sleep and anesthesia helps explain why individuals vulnerable to upper airway obstruction or hypoventilation in one state are predisposed to these ventilatory problems in the other state. Consideration of the *differences* between these states explains why vulnerability to these problems is so much greater during anesthesia than during sleep.

SLEEP AND ANESTHESIA: SIMILARITIES AND DIFFERENCES

Sleep is a natural state of unconsciousness, the propensity for which is governed by homeostatic drive (which increases with lengthening time without sleep) and circadian variation. Anesthesia is a drug-induced state that is largely independent of homeostatic and circadian influences. Although sleep is readily disrupted by psychological and environmental disturbances, these factors do not affect anesthesia. Sleep is an inhomogeneous state with distinct stages, periodic arousals, and variable postures, whereas, although its depth can vary, anesthesia is relatively homogeneous. Sufficient stimulation causes the sleeping subject to arouse, whereas suppression of arousals is

[a] Department of Pulmonary Physiology and Sleep Medicine, West Australian Sleep Disorders Research Institute, Sir Charles Gairdner Hospital, Hospital Avenue, Nedlands, Perth 6009, Western Australia, Australia;
[b] Centre for Sleep Science, School of Anatomy and Human Biology, University of Western Australia, Stirling Highway, Crawley, Perth 6009, Western Australia, Australia
* Corresponding author.
E-mail address: David.Hillman@health.wa.gov.au

Sleep Med Clin 8 (2013) 23–28
http://dx.doi.org/10.1016/j.jsmc.2012.11.002
1556-407X/13/$ – see front matter Crown Copyright © 2013 Published by Elsevier Inc. All rights reserved.

a basic characteristic (and objective) of anesthesia. After the restorative need is met, sleep reverses spontaneously. With anesthesia, reversal requires anesthetic drug elimination.

Recognizing that sleep and anesthesia have these differences, it is important to note their similarities. There is some evidence to suggest that anesthesia, when undisturbed by surgery and its sequelae, has some sleeplike restorative properties and that sedative drug requirements decrease with both sleep deprivation and circadian dips in alertness.[1,2] Common neurophysiologic mechanisms are involved: neural pathways engaged in sleep are activated by anesthetic drugs and increased knowledge of these has provided new insights into the mechanisms of sedation and anesthesia.[3,4] Sleep and anesthesia have similar effects on upper airway and ventilatory function: they both reduce wakeful cortical influences, reflex gain, and ventilatory drive predisposing to upper airway obstruction and hypoventilation. However, the effects of anesthesia are greater in these respects because the decrease in tonic and phasic muscle activity is profound and abolition of arousal responses removes the protection against prolonged obstruction and asphyxia that they provide for the sleeping subject.

SHARED NEUROBIOLOGY: A COMMON NARCOTIC SWITCH

Although different anesthetic agents may activate a variety of neuronal targets, Propofol provides an archetypical example of activation of key sleep centers by them.

Ascending activation of the cortex by activity generated in subcortical centers is important in the maintenance of wakefulness. Thalamic and extrathalamic pathways are involved.[5] During wakefulness, the locus coeruleus (LC) is active and exerts an inhibitory influence on the hypothalamic ventrolateral preoptic nucleus (VLPO). With sleep onset, the activity of the LC decreases, disinhibiting the VLPO, which now exerts an inhibitory influence on key brainstem and thalamic centers, inhibiting the ascent of activating stimuli to the cortex through them (Fig. 1). It also projects back onto the LC, tending to inhibit its activity. The result is a diminution in ascending activation of the cortex together with reinforcement of inhibition of LC output, with the result being sleep. The mutual inhibition between VLPO and LC acts to produce bistable states of wakefulness (when the LC is ascendant) and sleep (when the VLPO is ascendant) with switchlike changes between the states once a threshold sufficient for change has been reached.[6]

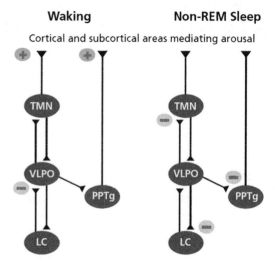

Fig. 1. Cartoon demonstrating key neural centers involved in the regulation of sleep and wakefulness. LC, locus coeruleus; PPTg, pedunculopontine tegmental nuclei; TMN, tuberomammillary nucleus; VLPO, ventrolateral preoptic nucleus. (*From* Harrison NL. General anesthesia research: aroused from a deep sleep? Nat Neurosci 2002;5:928; with permission.)

These VLPO-associated inhibitory pathways are populated by GABAa-ergic neurons. Their action is replicated by Propofol and other sedative agents (such as the benzodiazepines), which stimulate the same target receptors. Hence neural pathways integral to sleep and wakefulness are used by anesthetic agents in production of the anesthetic state.

UPPER AIRWAY COLLAPSIBILITY DURING SLEEP

With a change in state comes a change in upper airway collapsibility, because consciousness is an important protector against upper airway narrowing and collapse. Sleep onset is identifiable from electroencephalographic changes in which there is a transition from the alpha rhythm (frequency range of 8–12 Hz) of relaxed wakefulness to a slower theta rhythm (frequency range 4–7 Hz). Coincident with this switchlike "alpha-theta transition" is a switchlike marked decrease in inspiratory phasic activity in the pharyngeal musculature that helps stabilize the upper airway, with resultant increased upper airway collapsibility.[7] Some tonic muscle activity persists through this transition, affording protection from collapse for less vulnerable airways. This tonic activity diminishes in deeper sleep and is absent in rapid eye movement sleep, the stage of sleep in which airway collapsibility is greatest.

UPPER AIRWAY COLLAPSIBILITY DURING ANESTHESIA

Switchlike precipitate changes in upper airway muscle activation and upper airway collapsibility are also evident at the induction of anesthesia.[8,9] As with sleep, loss of consciousness (often defined in terms of anesthetic induction as loss of response to loud spoken command) is a critical interface. When anesthesia is induced in a slow stepwise fashion, an abrupt decrease in phasic activity of the genioglossus muscle (the major upper airway dilator muscle) is seen at the time that consciousness is lost, with an accompanying increase in collapsibility. The abruptness of the changes and their coincidence highlights the importance of conscious state in the maintenance of upper airway stability and the strong parallels between the effects of sleep and anesthesia, as might be expected given the similar neural pathways involved.

AIRWAYS THAT ARE DIFFICULT UNDER ANESTHESIA ARE DIFFICULT DURING SLEEP

Given this, it might be expected that airways that are obstruction-prone ("difficult" in anesthesiology parlance) during anesthesia are also obstruction-prone during sleep. There is plenty of evidence to support this suggestion. Increased airway collapsibility under anesthesia is associated with a substantially increased risk of obstructive sleep apnea (**Fig. 2**).[10] Conversely those with sleep apnea are at increased risk of airway difficulty during anesthesia. Not surprisingly, not only is obstructive sleep apnea (OSA) associated with increased collapsibility during anesthesia, but also, those who have OSA also present anatomic

challenges during anesthesia because they are more likely to be difficult to intubate tracheally.[11] Equally, those that prove difficult to intubate are at high risk of OSA, often quite severe.[12]

CROSSING THE CONSCIOUSNESS DIVIDE

Hence with both sleep onset and anesthetic induction, as the divide from consciousness to unconsciousness is crossed, there is a relatively abrupt change in upper airway behavior, with decreased muscle activation and increased collapsibility. This abruptness is consistent with the behavior of a narcotic "switch," as described earlier. The purpose of such a bistable flip-flop switch is to produce a stable state of wakefulness on one side of the divide and sleep on the other side of the divide. The similarities in behavior between sleep onset and anesthetic induction reflect the common neural pathways involved in both states with activation of sleep circuits by anesthetic drugs.

However the critical difference between the states is the capacity to arouse.[13] In the case of sleep, physiologic or environmental disturbance causes arousal, which protects against the danger of asphyxia from prolonged episodes of partial or complete upper airway obstruction. In contrast it is a basic objective of anesthesia to suppress arousal responses and this protection is lost as the divide is crossed from consciousness to unconsciousness, coincident with the occurrence of muscle relaxation and increased airway collapsibility. It can then only return with drug elimination, a finite process which, somewhat ironically given the potential for compromise of it, requires ventilation in the case of

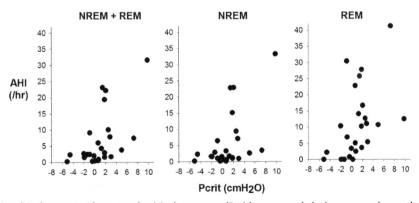

Fig. 2. Relationship between pharyngeal critical pressure (Pcrit) measured during general anesthesia and AHI measured during non–rapid eye movement (NREM) and rapid eye movement (REM) sleep in 25 normal subjects. Increased collapsibility under anesthesia (elevated Pcrit) was associated with increased AHI. The relationship is closer for REM than non-REM sleep because the profound muscle relaxation of REM sleep more closely approximates that of anesthesia. (*From* Eastwood PR, Szollosi I, Platt PR, et al. Comparison of upper airway collapse during general anaesthesia and sleep. Lancet 2002;359:1208; with permission.)

inhalational anesthetic agents. Suppression of arousal is a particular danger for individuals with upper airways that are vulnerable to collapse, such as those with OSA.

In the absence of neurologic injury, there are 3 ways to cross the divide from consciousness to unconsciousness in the perioperative period: (1) by natural sleep, in which case the individual readily arouses to threat of asphyxia; (2) by drug-induced sleep (ie, mild [conscious] sedation + sleep), in which the individual remains rousable, although arousal responses may obtunded; and (3) by drug-induced deep (unconscious) sedation whereby the individual is unrousable and remains so until drug elimination occurs.

Clearly it is in this latter circumstance that danger is most apparent. In patients with a propensity to upper airway collapse, this situation presents a potentially lethal combination of increased collapsibility and obtunded arousal responses, which occur contemporaneously as sedative levels deepen. Managing these issues under the controlled circumstances of anesthetic induction and emergence is the daily business of anesthesiologists. The concern is to ensure this combination does not occur in less rigorously controlled circumstances, such as lie beyond the post-anesthesia care unit or other high acuity areas where intensive observation and the capacity to intervene decisively are readily available.

This problem can be addressed by ensuring intensive monitoring of patients continues following anesthesia until consciousness and ready rousability return and by using sedating drugs, including narcotic analgesics, conservatively beyond this point. Variability between patients in their vulnerability to upper airway obstruction, hypoventilation, or the sedating effect of drugs needs to be taken into account. There are great differences in individual susceptibility to sedatives, which requires careful observation to help define. Age is a factor. Sedative effects can be compounded by unfavorable drug combinations and by pathophysiologic changes, such as hypercapnia resulting from drug-induced respiratory depression and/or obstructed breathing, which has its own narcotic effects. As with OSA, patients with preexistent sleep hypoventilation and/or respiratory failure are at increased risk of these problems. Intensive observation is required together with the use of treatment strategies, such as continuous positive airway pressure or bilevel ventilatory assistance, where ventilatory problems arise. In managing postoperative pain, regional analgesic techniques are very helpful, circumventing these difficulties by reducing or eliminating the need for systemic narcotics.

PERIOPERATIVE PROBLEMS FOR PATIENTS WITH SLEEP APNEA

There is plenty of evidence to demonstrate that patients with OSA present more difficulties during and immediately after the conduct of anesthesia. They are more difficult to intubate, have more episodes of hypoxemia and obstruction during emergence, and require more medical interventions during this time.[11,12] Because of their relatively small airways relative to body size, children present special difficulties.[14] Given the protection that returns with the return of rousability, it is perhaps not surprising that OSA does not seem to be a substantial risk factor for adverse events after outpatient surgery, where no further narcotic analgesia or sedation is administered following emergence. In a retrospective case control study of 234 OSA patients, matched for type and time of procedure, age, gender, and body mass index, Sabers and colleagues[15] were unable to demonstrate any significant difference in perioperative adverse events, unplanned hospital admissions, or death. However OSA does seem to be a risk factor for complications following more involved anesthesia and surgery associated with multiday admissions. Early concern was raised by the work of Gupta and colleagues,[16] who demonstrated, also in a retrospective case control study, an increased occurrence of serious complications requiring medical intervention, unplanned ICU admission, and length of stay in OSA patients following hip or knee arthroplasty. More recently a series of articles have emerged substantiating these concerns: these have been summarized in several useful reviews and will be outlined later in this monograph.[17,18] Upper airway surgery is of additional concern because postoperative edema, hematoma, or the presence of nasal packing may increase the vulnerability to airway obstruction. This increased vulnerability may continue for several days postoperatively.

PERIOPERATIVE OSA MANAGEMENT

Several principles emerge from this examination of the pathophysiologic factors that place OSA patients at increased risk of perioperative complications (**Box 1**).[19]

First, those at increased risk must be identified. Given its high prevalence and relevance to airway management, OSA should be considered in all patients presenting for anesthesia. The STOP-Bang questionnaire is a useful method that allows basic screening to be performed simply and systematically.[20] Where a high likelihood of OSA is present (eg, loud habitual snoring, witnessed

---

Box 1
Principles for perioperative management of patients with OSA

OSA and Anesthesia Management

- Identify those at risk of OSA preoperatively by routinely using screening questions (eg, STOP-Bang).
- Where OSA is strongly suspected but not previously diagnosed, refer patients for preoperative evaluation of sleep where circumstances allow (eg, if surgery is elective) and there is a likely need for postoperative narcotic analgesia or sedation.
- Be particularly cautious in the case of morbidly obesity; ventilatory impairment; respiratory or right heart failure; sensitivity to narcotic effects of sedatives and analgesics; or upper airway surgery.
- When OSA has been previously diagnosed and the patient is compliant with CPAP, ensure it is available for perioperative use.
- Where previously diagnosed but not CPAP compliant, reinstruct in its use.
- Where CPAP has not been previously used but is indicated, ensure patient is familiarized with it preoperatively where possible.
- Avoid sedative premedication.
- Use regional anesthesia and analgesia where feasible.
- When general anesthesia is used, be prepared for difficulty with airway maintenance. Use techniques that allow early return of consciousness.
- Try to minimize postoperative sedation.
- Have CPAP available for early postoperative use.
- Nurse in a high-dependency area with continuous monitoring until the patient is sentient and able to self-administer CPAP. Patients requiring ongoing narcotic analgesia or sedation should remain in a high-dependency area until this need abates.
- Use lateral positioning, a nasopharyngeal airway, and oxygen therapy where CPAP is refused and upper airway obstruction is problematic.
- Where not already diagnosed, consider OSA in patients with difficult to manage airways perioperatively. Refer for investigation where indicated.

---

apneas, excessive daytime sleepiness) further investigation should be pursued where circumstances allow, as with elective surgery. Particular concern exists when the patient has morbid obesity, ventilatory impairment (forced expiratory volume$_1$ or forced vital capacity less than 80% of predicted normal), respiratory or right heart failure, or polycythemia. Sensitivity to the narcotic effects of sedatives, hypnotics, and analgesics poses additional risk, as does surgery in the upper airway.

Where OSA is identified, continuous positive airway pressure (CPAP) therapy should be considered and started preoperatively where possible. It is far easier to use this intrusive therapy postoperatively, when the patient is already familiar with it. If OSA has been previously diagnosed and the patient is compliant with CPAP, it must be available for perioperative use. If the patient has been previously diagnosed but is not CPAP compliant, then steps should be taken to reinstruct in its use.

When general anesthesia is undertaken in patients with OSA, preparations should be made

for difficulty with intraoperative and perioperative airway management. Techniques that allow early return of consciousness are desirable. Preoperative and postoperative use of sedatives and sedative narcotics should be minimized in vulnerable patients. Use of non-narcotic analgesics and regional analgesic techniques are helpful strategies to achieve this.

Careful observation is required postoperatively until the patient is sentient with the capacity to arouse restored and not likely to be subject to further compromise. This observation entails initial care in a high dependency area with a high nurse: patient ratio, nurses in close proximity, and monitoring equipment (pulse oximetry at a minimum) in place.

CPAP should be used postoperatively in patients who are vulnerable to obstructed breathing when asleep or sedated. Nursing in the lateral posture may help, as may the use of other aids, such as a nasopharyngeal airway, where the patient is sedated, tending to obstruct, and unable to tolerate CPAP.

If a patient presents difficulties with airway management intraoperatively but has not previously been diagnosed with OSA, then the possibility that he or she has OSA should be considered. Where indicated, the patient should be referred for further investigation.

SUMMARY

In conclusion, it is evident that the tendencies to upper airway obstruction during sleep and anesthesia are related. The loss of consciousness that accompanies sleep onset and anesthetic induction has a powerful influence on upper airway collapsibility and anesthesia-related suppression of rousability confers great vulnerability to its effects. This vulnerability increases the perioperative risk of obstruction in patients with predisposed airways. The magnitude of risk diminishes with the emergence from anesthesia and the return of arousal responses but is likely to recur with postoperative sedation/narcotics. Individual variation in drug sensitivities, airway collapsibility, posture, postsurgery upper airway edema/hematoma, and hypoventilation/hypercapnia can compound these effects. Close observation is required postoperatively until the patient is consistently rousable. Positive airway pressure therapy, while helpful, does not prevent the need for this.

REFERENCES

1. Tung A, Lynch JP, Mendelson WB. Prolonged sedation with propofol in the rat does not result in sleep deprivation. Anesth Analg 2001;92:1232–6.
2. Tung A, Bergmann BM, Herrera S, et al. Recovery from sleep deprivation occurs during propofol anesthesia. Anesthesiology 2004;100:1419–26.
3. Allada R. An emerging link between general anesthesia and sleep. Proc Natl Acad Sci U S A 2008; 105:2257–8.
4. Brown EN, Lydic R, Schiff ND. General anesthesia, sleep, and coma. N Engl J Med 2010;363:2638–50.
5. Saper CB, Scammell TE, Lu J. Hypothalamic regulation of sleep and circadian rhythms. Nature 2005; 437:1257–63.
6. Harrison NL. General anesthesia research: aroused from a deep sleep? Nat Neurosci 2002; 5:928–9.
7. Wilkinson V, Malhotra A, Nicholas CL, et al. Discharge patterns of human genioglossus motor units during sleep onset. Sleep 2008;31:525–33.
8. Hillman DR, Walsh JH, Maddison KJ, et al. Evolution of changes in upper airway collapsibility during slow induction of anesthesia with propofol. Anesthesiology 2009;111:63–71.
9. Franks NP. General anaesthesia: from molecular targets to neuronal pathways of sleep and arousal. Nat Rev Neurosci 2008;9:370–86.
10. Eastwood PR, Szollosi I, Platt PR, et al. Comparison of upper airway collapse during general anaesthesia and sleep. Lancet 2002;359:1207–9.
11. Kim JA, Lee JJ. Preoperative predictors of difficult intubation in patients with obstructive sleep apnea syndrome. Can J Anaesth 2006;53:393–7.
12. Hiremath AS, Hillman DR, James AL, et al. Relationship between difficult tracheal intubation and obstructive sleep apnoea. Br J Anaesth 1998;80:606–11.
13. Tung A, Mendelson WB. Anesthesia and sleep. Sleep Med Rev 2004;8:213–25.
14. Sanders JC, King MA, Mitchell RB, et al. Perioperative complications of adenotonsillectomy in children with obstructive sleep apnea syndrome. Anesth Analg 2006;103:1115–21.
15. Sabers C, Plevak DJ, Schroeder DR, et al. The diagnosis of obstructive sleep apnea as a risk factor for unanticipated admissions in outpatient surgery. Anesth Analg 2003;96:1328–35.
16. Gupta RM, Parvizi J, Hanssen AD, et al. Postoperative complications in patients with obstructive sleep apnea syndrome undergoing hip or knee replacement: a case-control study. Mayo Clin Proc 2001; 76:897–905.
17. Kaw R, Chung F, Pasupuleti V, et al. Meta-analysis of the association between obstructive sleep apnoea and postoperative outcome. Br J Anaesth 2012; 109:897–906.
18. Kaw R, Pasupuleti V, Walker E, et al. Postoperative complications in patients with obstructive sleep apnea. Chest 2012;141:436–41.
19. Gross JB, Bachenberg KL, Benumof JL, et al. American Society of Anesthesiologists Task Force on Perioperative Management of Patients with Obstructive Sleep Apnea: Practice guidelines for the perioperative management of patients with obstructive sleep apnea. Anesthesiology 2006;104:1081–91.
20. Chung F, Subramanyam R, Liao P, et al. High STOP-Bang score indicates a high probability of obstructive sleep apnoea. Br J Anaesth 2012;108:768–75.

Upper Airway Physiology in Sleep and Anesthesia

Nicholas M. Dalesio, MD[a],*, Tracey L. Stierer, MD[b],
Alan R. Schwartz, MD[c]

KEYWORDS

- Sleep • Anesthesia • Upper airway obstruction • Pharynx • Obstructive sleep apnea

KEY POINTS

- The optimal perioperative management of the patient with, or at risk for, obstructive sleep apnea (OSA) requires a multidisciplinary approach.
- Further studies are needed to facilitate a better understanding of the factors that place a patient with OSA at risk for adverse outcome and of the methods and duration of monitoring that confer optimal patient safety.

INTRODUCTION

Upper airway patency, during periods of sleep and anesthesia, is an area of study gaining interest in many fields of medicine. Disturbances in ventilatory control that occur during various stages of sleep and anesthesia are well recognized. These alterations can involve the upper airway, leading to increases in upper airway collapsibility and airflow obstruction. Comorbid conditions including obesity, craniofacial disorders, and Down syndrome as well as the administration of respiratory depressants markedly increase the individual's susceptibility to upper airway obstruction.[1–7] These conditions are known risk factors for obstructive sleep apnea (OSA), a chronic condition that is characterized by recurrent episodes of pharyngeal obstruction with ensuing oxyhemoglobin desaturations and arousals from sleep. Furthermore, anesthetic and sedative agents can precipitate upper airway obstruction acutely in the perioperative period,[8–11] leading to potentially catastrophic respiratory complications, especially in patients undergoing upper airway surgery.[12–15] Regardless of the clinical setting, similar mechanisms govern the development of upper airway obstruction in the perioperative period and during sleep. In this article, we draw on work elucidating underlying mechanisms of upper airway obstruction during sleep and anesthesia and develop insights required for the prevention, detection, and management of upper airway obstruction and its attendant respiratory complications in the perioperative period.

CONTROL OF UPPER AIRWAY PATENCY
Overview

The upper airway is a complex structure designed to support a variety of respiratory, linguistic, and alimentary functions. Such versatility in function is supported by a complex interplay of soft tissue, bony, neuromuscular structures, which can markedly alter the pliability of the conduit from the nares to the larynx. Airway patency is controlled dynamically along the length of the upper airway as a function of sleep-wake state and respiratory phase, with multiple sites of potential collapse.[16] Major dilator muscles including the alae nasi,

[a] Division of Pediatric Anesthesiology, Department of Anesthesiology and Critical Care Medicine, Johns Hopkins School of Medicine, Baltimore, MD 21287-4904, USA; [b] Department of Anesthesiology and Critical Care Medicine, Johns Hopkins School of Medicine, Johns Hopkins Outpatient Center, 601 N. Caroline Street, Baltimore, MD 21287–0712, USA; [c] Sleep Medicine Section, Division of Pulmonary and Critical Care Medicine, Department of Medicine, Johns Hopkins School of Medicine, Johns Hopkins Sleep Disorders Center, 5501 Hopkins Bayview Circle, Baltimore, MD 21224, USA
* Corresponding author. The Charlotte R. Bloomberg Children's Center, 1800 Orleans Street, Suite 6368, Baltimore, MD 21287-4904.
E-mail address: ndalesi1@jhmi.edu

Sleep Med Clin 8 (2013) 29–41
http://dx.doi.org/10.1016/j.jsmc.2012.11.007
1556-407X/13/$ – see front matter © 2013 Elsevier Inc. All rights reserved.

genioglossus,[3,17,18] intrinsic palatal,[19] posterior cricoarytenoid, and even pharyngeal constrictor muscles[20] are responsible for maintaining airway patency. These muscles are in turn controlled by central and peripheral mechanoreceptor and chemoreceptor mechanisms,[21–24] which respond to changes in intraluminal pressure, airflow, temperature, lung volume, and systemic oxygen and carbon dioxide tension to regulate airway patency.[18,25–27] Disturbances in either structural or neural control, seen during sleep and anesthesia, can lead to airflow obstruction or complete occlusion of the airway.

Modeling the Upper Airway as a Simple Collapsible Conduit

Despite the complexities of upper airway structural and neuromuscular control, its susceptibility to collapse and obstruction is determined by factors governing the patency of a simple collapsible tube or Starling resistor.[28] The Starling resistor model is a collapsible tube with rigid proximal and distal ends flanking a collapsible region exposed to a variable level of surrounding tissue pressure (**Fig. 1**). The surrounding pressure (P_{CRIT}) is constant and when the pressure within the collapsible tube is less than the P_{CRIT}, the tube collapses. Conversely, when intraluminal pressure is greater than P_{CRIT}, the tube reopens. Whenever intraluminal pressure decreases to the level of P_{CRIT}, the airway is prone to collapse, leading us to define this intraluminal pressure as the critical pressure (P_{CRIT}).

The nonflow-limited condition (no airflow obstruction)

The Starling resistor can accurately describe the effects of airway pressures on airflow and the

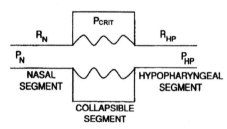

Fig. 1. The Starling resistor: a model for the upper airway, comprising a collapsible tube inside a chamber that has a static pressure (P_{CRIT}) inside. P_{CRIT} controls the collapsibility of the pharynx, which is flanked by rigid segments upstream in the nose and downstream in the hypopharynx. R_N, upstream nasal resistance; P_{HP}, hypopharyngeal pressure; R_{HP}, downstream hypopharyngeal resistance. (*From* Schwartz AR, Smith PL, Wise RA, et al. Effect of positive nasal pressure on upper airway pressure-flow relationships. J Appl Physiol 1989:1626–34; with permission.)

degree of upper airway obstruction in normal individuals as well as in those with snoring or OSA.[13,29,30] The critical pressure relative to pressures upstream and downstream to the collapsible site determines the degree of upper airway obstruction as follows. When pressures upstream (P_{US}) and downstream (P_{DS}) to the collapsible site are greater than the P_{CRIT}, the airway remains completely patent. In the absence of collapse, the airway behaves as a rigid tube, and flow is determined by the difference in pressure between the upstream and downstream ends and the resistance across the entire conduit, as expressed by the equation for inspiratory flow (V_I):

$$V_I = (P_{US} - P_{DS})/R \qquad (1)$$

where R is the combined resistance upstream and downstream to the collapsible site.

The flow-limited condition

The upper airway collapses and limits flow on inspiration as the downstream tracheal pressure becomes lower than P_{CRIT}. Specifically, as tracheal pressure decreases, inspiratory airflow increases to a maximal level ($V_I$max) and plateaus thereafter, becoming independent of further decreases in tracheal pressure (**Fig. 2**; right panel). This pattern is often associated with snoring during inspiration, which is caused by vibratory collapse and reopening of the upper airway as flow oscillates around a maximal level. Nonetheless, the flow-limited upper airway does not occlude, indicating that tracheal suction pressures cannot account for the development of complete obstruction, as might occur in patients with OSA.

Complete occlusion (a special case of flow limitation)

To occlude the upper airway completely, the pressure upstream to the collapsible (flow-limiting) site must be lower than a critical tissue pressure surrounding that site. This condition can be obtained experimentally by decreasing the upstream (nasal) pressure in normal individuals during sleep to subatmospheric levels less than a critical pressure. As upstream pressure is decreased progressively, the individual initially flow limits during inspiration if the upstream pressure remains greater than P_{CRIT}, even although downstream pressures are lower than P_{CRIT} during inspiration. Under these circumstances, maximal inspiratory airflow ($V_I$max) can be described by the relationship:

$$V_I max = (P_{US} - P_{CRIT})/R_{US} \qquad (2)$$

where P_{CRIT} replaces the downstream pressure in equation 1 as the effective downstream pressure

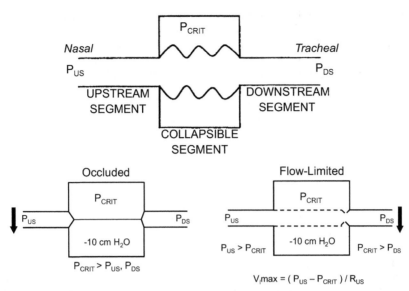

Fig. 2. Mechanisms of upper airway obstruction and the effects of decreasing upstream and downstream pressures. Pharyngeal collapsibility is determined by the surrounding pressure (P_{CRIT}). As pressure within the chamber of the Starling resistor changes, so does the collapsibility of the tube. When upstream pressure is lower than P_{CRIT}, complete occlusion of the tube occurs (*left panel*). When downstream pressure is decreased below P_{CRIT}, flow-limited breathing occurs (*right panel*). Under these circumstances, the level of maximal inspiratory airflow (VI max) is determined by the upstream and critical pressures and upstream nasal resistance as described in the equation at the lower right. (*Adapted from* Gold AR, Schwartz AR. The pharyngeal critical pressure. The whys and hows of using nasal continuous positive airway pressure diagnostically. Chest. 1996;110(4):1077–88; with permission.)

to flow and R_{US} is the resistance of the segment upstream to the site of collapse. As nasal pressure is decreased experimentally, maximal inspiratory airflow decreases progressively and airflow ceases once P_{US} is lower than P_{CRIT}. Under these circumstances, the upper airway occludes and recurrent obstructive apneas ensue during sleep (see **Fig. 2**, left panel).[12,13] These observations indicate that the upper airway occludes and obstructive apneas occur only under conditions of inspiratory airflow limitation whenever P_{CRIT} exceeds upstream pressure at the nose.

These experimental findings highlight that P_{CRIT} is a measure of pharyngeal collapsibility, and remains the major determinant of the severity of airway obstruction. Clinical risk factors, medications, and postural maneuvers can increase the susceptibility to upper airway obstruction by increasing pharyngeal collapsibility (P_{CRIT}). When the critical pressure is higher than atmospheric nasal pressure, obstructive apneic episodes are observed repeatedly in patients with OSA. Investigators have shown that quantitative differences in critical pressures, reflecting differences in pharyngeal collapsibility, distinguish among groups with varying degrees of upper airway obstruction clinically between health (normal breathing) and disease (OSA).[13,29,30] These findings lend credence to the concept that

alterations in pharyngeal collapsibility (P_{CRIT}), rather than airway resistance or compliance, determine the degree of airflow obstruction during sleep and anesthesia. An important corollary is that snoring, a marker for the flow-limited condition, represents an intermediate degree of upper airway obstruction in susceptible patients who are at risk for the development of complete occlusion. Under these conditions, airway patency can be restored only by increasing upstream pressure (eg, nasal continuous positive airway pressure [CPAP]) or by decreasing P_{CRIT} (eg, decreasing pharyngeal collapsibility with postural maneuvers).

In general, increases in pharyngeal collapsibility result from alterations in airway structures and anatomy as well as disturbances in neuromuscular control. In normal individuals, as mechanical loads are applied to the airway, airflow obstruction elicits compensatory increases in pharyngeal neuromuscular activity, which can help to restore airway patency. Current evidence supports the notion that combined defects in structural and neuromuscular control play a role in the pathogenesis of OSA.[3] Initially, structural loads on the pharynx predispose to upper airway collapse, leading to airflow obstruction during sleep. Neuromuscular responses to airflow obstruction can compensate for the load and protect against the development of OSA.[31–33] If these compensatory responses are inadequate or patients arouse from sleep before airway patency is restored, OSA ensues.[33] Studies in humans and animals have evaluated upper airway neuromechanical control mechanisms that predispose to airway obstruction or protect airway patency and have suggested that these physiologic characteristics mediate effects of sleep apnea risk factors (age, weight, sex) on the individual's susceptibility to this disorder.[21]

STRUCTURAL/MECHANICAL LOADS

Mechanical loads on the airway have been shown to cause airway collapse. By decreasing or eliminating the neuromuscular control of airway musculature, one can isolate the structural components necessary for maintaining airway patency. Isono and colleagues[25–27] administered total neuromuscular blockade under general anesthesia, thereby evaluating the passive pharynx, showing that intrinsic differences in the airway predispose patients to airway obstruction independently of neuromuscular control (**Fig. 3**). Also, by decreasing neuromuscular involvement, the mechanical load of the airway can be evaluated by calculating the P_{CRIT} during passive states of airflow. To determine the passive P_{CRIT}, nasal pressure in a CPAP mask can be increased initially to abolish inspiratory flow limitation. Electromyographic (EMG) activity in the genioglossal muscle (EMG_{GG}) decreases to low levels during sleep, confirming a hypotonic state for the upper airway muscles. Nasal pressure can then be decreased abruptly during sleep until airflow reaches zero (active P_{CRIT}). Holding pressures were statistically

lower in patients without OSA than in those with the diagnosis of OSA (9 vs 5.7 cm H_2O; P = .0007). The P_{CRIT} was also increased to levels causing severe airflow obstruction during sleep, suggesting that mechanical load contributes to the development of airway collapse in patients with OSA.[32] Patients, both adults and children, diagnosed with OSA have been shown to have a more collapsible airway compared with patients without OSA matched in body mass index (BMI, calculated as weight in kilograms divided by the square of height in meters) and age.[26] These findings suggest that structural loads predispose patients to upper airway obstruction independent of neuromuscular processes.

NEUROMUSCULAR CONTROL

Neuromuscular control for the maintenance of airway patency has been studied extensively. Neural involvement was originally described in rabbits in 1980, showing increases in EMG_{GG} to hypercapnic environments, which suggests that central neuromuscular factors contribute to airway patency.[18,34] During sleep, it has been shown that neuromuscular activity decreases in the genioglossal and tensor palatine muscles, leading to an increase in upper airway collapsibility.[22,35,36] The decrease in activity could be related to a withdrawal of direct wakefulness stimulation of the upper airway musculature, suggesting a central mechanism of airway control.[37] Neuromuscular control has also been evaluated in patients with OSA, monitoring EMG_{GG} during sleep. When compared with controls, patients with OSA had a diminished EMG_{GG} response during periods of

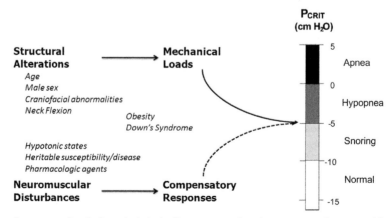

Fig. 3. Pharyngeal neuromechanical control, including structural and neuromuscular control in airway patency. Airway patency is determined by the sum of both the structural and neuromuscular determinants of airway collapsibility (P_{CRIT}). Risk factors for upper airway obstruction during sleep, sedation, analgesia, and anesthesia are shown to influence structural or neuromuscular control, leading to alterations in P_{CRIT} and increasing degrees of upper airway obstruction during sleep (see spectrum from normal breathing to obstructive apnea on right) and increasing perioperative risk.

induced airway obstruction, suggesting an inherited or acquired central mechanism increasing the propensity for airway collapse. In addition, neuromuscular response to the changes between active and passive P_{CRIT} was diminished in patients with OSA.[32,33] Considerable evidence has accumulated to suggest that both structural and neuromuscular factors contribute to the pathogenesis of OSA, leading to a 2-hit hypothesis for the cause of the disease (see **Fig. 3**).[3]

IMPACT OF CLINICAL RISK FACTORS ON PHARYNGEAL COLLAPSIBILITY

Demographic and clinical risk factors for sleep apnea have been evaluated for their effect on pharyngeal collapsibility, including sex, age, body weight, craniofacial anatomy, and body position. These attributes may determine the mechanical loads on the pharynx, neuromuscular control, or both, thus influencing airway patency. Similar mechanisms could also make patients with these characteristics prone to develop pharyngeal collapse during altered states of consciousness (**Box 1**).

Male gender is a risk factor for worsening airway collapse, men having an approximately 2 cm H_2O greater increase in passive P_{CRIT} than premenopausal women. Using techniques to eliminate neuromuscular effects of airway patency, investigators have shown that this increase in pharyngeal collapsibility in men compared with women is independent of BMI, age, and sleep apnea severity. These findings suggest that mechanical loads on the airway such as differences in fat distribution in the airway, pharyngeal length, or other soft tissue structures may play a role in maintaining airway patency during sleep.[1]

Age has also been shown to affect passive mechanical loads (passive P_{CRIT}). Although men are 3 times more likely to have OSA than women,[41] Kirkness and colleagues showed that passive P_{CRIT} was higher in women after menopause (age >51 years), reaching a prevalence similar to men. Suggested mechanisms responsible for this increased risk may involve perimenopausal hormonal changes. Data to support this hypothesis include a study that found that women who took hormone replacement therapy may be protected from the development of these changes. In addition, passive P_{CRIT} varies throughout the menstrual cycle, with decreases in the early compared with the later portion of the cycle, suggesting hormonal influences on pharyngeal collapsibility.[42] No changes in P_{CRIT} were observed in men as they age.[1] However, there is an age-related decrease in genioglossus activity, as a response to negative airway pressures.[34]

Box 1
Perioperative assessment, signs, and symptoms of OSA (American Society of Anesthesiologists [ASA] Task Force)[38–40]

A. Physical Characteristics Increasing Risk for OSA

　1. BMI 35 kg/m^2 or greater

　2. Neck circumference more than 43.18 cm (17 in) for men; more than 40.64 cm (16 in) for women

　3. Tonsils nearly touching or touching in the midline

　4. Craniofacial abnormalities affecting the airway

　5. Anatomic nasal obstruction

B. Patient History of Apparent Airway Obstruction During Sleep

　1. Frequent snoring

　2. Observed pauses in breathing during sleep

　3. Awakens from sleep with choking sensation

　4. Frequent arousals from sleep

C. Patient Somnolence

　1. Frequent somnolence or fatigue despite adequate sleep

　2. Falls asleep easily in nonstimulating environments (reading, watching TV, driving a car)

If a patient shows or reports 2 or more of the above categories, it is likely that the patient has OSA.

Adapted from Gross JB, Bachenberg KL Benumof JL, et al. American Society of Anesthesiologists Task Force on Perioperative Management. Practice guidelines for the perioperative management of patients with obstructive sleep apnea; a report by the American Society of Anesthesiologists Task Force on Perioperative Management of patients with obstructive sleep apnea. Anesthesiology 2006;104(5);1081–93, with permission; and *Data from* Refs.[38–40]

When evaluating children, there seems to be no change in P_{CRIT} in infants compared with school-aged children, despite differences in upper airway length.[43] Changes in P_{CRIT} do increase from pubertal children to adulthood, suggesting that changes to airway structure or function begin in the adolescent years. Changes in P_{CRIT} have not been shown to relate to hormonal changes during this age group, with further studies required to identify adolescent airway structure and function.[43] In the murine model, a greater increase in P_{CRIT} occurs in older mice that are obese compared with young obese mice, suggesting that these changes occur from aging as well.[44] Genioglossus activity has been shown to decrease with age, and in humans, airway collapse with aging has been shown to occur independent of obesity.[34,44,45]

In addition to demographic and morphologic characteristics, patient positioning affects airway patency in both mice and human individuals. In children and adults, the lateral decubitus position has been shown to increase airway diameter and reduce obstruction.[46,47] Neck flexion has been shown to significantly decrease the oropharyngeal opening. Conversely, neck extension significantly increased maximum airway size and decreased the closing pressures of the oropharynx.[48,49] By measuring the P_{CRIT} during neck rotation, flexion, and extension, one can further assess the effects of posture on airway patency. Investigators have shown that the P_{CRIT} decreases with neck extension and when patients sleep in the lateral decubitus compared with supine position. In contrast, no change was noted during neck rotation.[50,51] Thus, head position during sleep or after anesthesia may influence airway patency.

Craniofacial structure and airway anatomy also play a role in upper airway collapse. Many children with craniofacial abnormalities suffer from OSA, with associated risk factors of structural and neuromuscular causes, including hypotonia, fat deposition in the neck, midface hypoplasia, and abnormal autonomic function. Syndromes associated with craniofacial abnormalities include Down, Apert, Crouzon, Pfeiffer, and Rubinstein-Taybi syndromes, cleft palate, Pierre-Robin sequence, and hemifacial microsomia. Approximately 50% of patients who have a craniofacial abnormality also suffer from OSA. Patients with Down syndrome also have neuromuscular factors that contribute to developing OSA, including hypotonia and obesity.[7] In adults, cephalometric measurements have been shown to correlate to the success of mandibular advancement splints (MAS), which are used to improve airway patency. MAS produce a shorter soft palate and increased

cranial base angulation, improving symptoms of OSA.[52] Kushida and colleagues[53] developed a morphometric model for adults that used palatal height, maxillary and mandibular intermolar distances, the overjet (extension of the upper incisional teeth to the lower teeth when the mouth is closed normally), BMI, and neck circumference to predict whether patients in an ambulatory center had sleep-disordered breathing. However, these results have not been reproduced and these parameters have not been studied to be predictive of OSA severity in children.

With the exponential increase in obesity in the United States, multiple studies have evaluated its effects on airway collapsibility and sleep apnea. Investigators have shown that obesity, an independent risk factor for sleep apnea, leads to increases in passive P_{CRIT}, reflecting increased anatomic loading of pharyngeal structures as well as neuromuscular alterations in both human and murine models.[3,44,54] Airway obstruction may be caused by adipose deposition around upper airway structures and by concomitant decreases in resting lung volumes. The latter increases the passive P_{CRIT} when caudal traction on upper airway structures decreases at lower lung volumes.[3,55,56] Male pattern central adiposity is associated with further increases in passive P_{CRIT} compared with similarly obese women with a peripheral or gynecoid pattern of fat distribution. Women are further protected from developing upper airway obstruction during sleep because their active neuromuscular responses are generally better preserved than their male counterparts. Thus, differences in fat distribution as well as active neuromuscular responses protect premenopausal women from developing sleep apnea compared with men and postmenopausal women.

Current evidence suggests that neural effects also affect upper airway control in obese patients. The cause for such effects may be related to increased levels of inflammatory cytokines, specifically tumor necrosis factor α, which mediates somnogenesis centrally.[3] Furthermore, treatments like CPAP and etanercept have been shown to alleviate sleep apnea, presumably by decreasing these circulating cytokines. These findings suggest that these humoral effects may play an integral role in the pathogenesis of the disease.[57,58] To further investigate the neuromechanical modulation of upper airway collapsibility by obesity, a mouse model for measuring the active and passive upper airway properties has been studied. Pressures were manipulated at the nose in anesthetized lean and obese C57BL6 mice to derive active and passive components of upper airway function. Responses were examined in wild-type and leptin-deficient mice. Leptin, a recognized satiety factor produced by adipose tissue, feeds back to increase ventilatory responses and regulates body composition and the distribution of adiposity. Both obesity and leptin deficiency in these mice lead to marked increases in passive P_{CRIT}, producing a structural predisposition to airway collapse.[54] In a mouse model of upper airway obstruction, it was found that leptin deficiency was associated with marked reductions in active upper airway responses, which failed to protect or restore upper airway patency, and that these responses were restored by leptin administration. The findings suggested that obesity imposes structural loads on the upper airway, whereas neurohumoral effects of leptin mitigate these loads and preserve upper airway patency. These findings were also noted in mice as age increased, suggesting that compensatory mechanisms to maintain airway patency diminish over time.[44]

PHARMACOLOGIC MODULATION OF PHARYNGEAL COLLAPSIBILITY

When moving through states of consciousness, both at the onset of sleep and anesthesia, neuromechanical control of a patient's airway becomes markedly decreased, causing muscle relaxation. Different stages of consciousness produce varying effects on airway collapse, with mild sedation having less of an effect, allowing some regulation of normal airway reflexes to remain intact.[59] In contrast, deep sedation and general anesthesia have greater impact, increasing the propensity for airway obstruction and collapse. Patients with OSA have an increased vulnerability to airway collapse during sedation and anesthesia, requiring anesthesiologists to become familiar with the effects of anesthetic medications within this patient population.

Increasing levels of sedation and anesthesia can compromise upper airway patency, although the precise mechanisms remain unclear. Sedation with benzodiazepines can increase the propensity for upper airway obstruction.[11,60–62] Decreases in airflow may be caused not only by central nervous system depression but by the presence of γ-aminobutyric acid receptors on motor neurons that innervate the pharyngeal musculature.[63] Studies in which patients were administered slowly escalating propofol infusions, which caused an initial paradoxic increase in genioglossus activity[59] in the minimally sedated state, suggest a drug-induced disinhibition of muscle activity. Thereafter, patients showed a sudden sharp decrease in EMG_{GG} activity and increase in pharyngeal collapsibility, which

coincided with loss of consciousness, pointing to marked state-dependent changes in upper airway neuromotor control.[60] These findings suggest that sedation caused a loss of compensatory responses for maintaining airway patency (P_{CRIT}, see **Fig. 3**).

Analgesic medications can also produce deleterious effects on airway patency. To a greater or lesser degree, all opioids depress ventilatory and pharyngeal neuromotor drive, leading to reductions in airway patency (see **Fig. 3**). In addition to these baseline effects, pediatric patients with OSA have been shown to have an increased sensitivity to opioids, perhaps resulting from recurrent nocturnal hypoxic episodes, which can alter opiate-receptor expression. μ-Opioid receptors have been shown to be in abundance in the respiratory centers of the nucleus solitarius located in the medulla. During states of hypoxia, opioid peptides are released into this location in the brain. In developing animals exposed to repeated hypoxic episodes, the hyperventilatory response is attenuated to these peptides,[64] suggesting that children exposed to intermittent hypoxia, as observed in severe OSA, have an altered response to opioid medications.[65–67] Although opioid receptors in the nucleus tractus solitarius play an important role in ventilatory control, opioid receptors have also been found in the motor nucleus of the hypoglossal nerve, potentially modulating activity of the genioglossus, a major pharyngeal dilator muscle.[68–71] Hence, activation of the opioid receptors in nerves that control airway musculature may further interfere with maintaining airway patency, causing increases in airway collapsibility (P_{CRIT}) (see **Fig. 3**).

Anesthetic agents can abolish neuromuscular activity of the pharyngeal dilators, and the depth of anesthesia has been shown to correlate with disturbances in airway collapsibility. Although the mechanisms are not well understood, isoflurane and propofol have been shown to decrease upper airway muscle activity and increase pharyngeal collapsibility.[8,9,72,73] The observed variation in airway collapsibility with varying anesthetic depth has been postulated to be the consequence of dose-related depression of inspiratory input from respiratory neurons arising from the pontomedullary central pattern generator as well as negative pressure reflexes triggered by mechanoreceptors located in the larynx. These reflexes affect both the hypoglossal nerve and the pharyngeal dilator muscle activity that are instrumental in maintaining airway patency.[59] Eastwood and colleagues[9] showed that general anesthesia eliminated neuromuscular activity throughout most stages of anesthesia. Decreasing the depth of isoflurane anesthesia, without completely eliminating the anesthetic, did improve airway stability, but the EMG_{GG} activity remained unchanged at all levels of anesthesia, making an increase in neuromuscular activity an unlikely cause for this observed improvement in airway stability. After anesthesia had ceased, EMG_{GG} activity returned to normal. Isoflurane was also shown to inhibit genioglossus activity during complete upper airway collapse, which can trigger powerful negative pressure reflexes to this muscle during sleep and wakefulness (see **Fig. 3**).[63,74]

In contrast to propofol and inhalation anesthetics, dexmedetomidine, a centrally acting α_2 agonist that has sedative properties paralleling natural nonrapid eye movement sleep, does not produce significant respiratory depression.[75,76] The agent acts directly at the locus coeruleus and has been shown to have minimal to no impact on the patient's ability to maintain spontaneous ventilation. Dexmedetomidine, used as an anesthetic in patients with OSA, results in fewer episodes of oxygen desaturation compared with that observed in children anesthetized with propofol. Its beneficial effect seems to be even more pronounced in children diagnosed with severe OSA.[77,78]

Perioperative Management of Patients with OSA

Because patients with OSA have increased susceptibility for airway collapse in the perioperative period, careful attention must be paid by the anesthesiologist to provide the safest and most optimal care. Most patients with OSA do not carry a formal diagnosis, so vigorous screening efforts are required to identify those who may be at risk for airway and respiratory complications perioperatively. Patients with OSA are more likely to present challenges during mask ventilation and tracheal intubation than their counterparts who do not have OSA and may suffer from a variety of cardiopulmonary comorbidities.

The type of medications used for sedation and anesthesia also play a role, with varying effects on airway collapsibility and duration and rate of recovery of medication effects. Appropriate monitoring in the postoperative period, including pain management, airway and ventilation support, as well as the need for inhospital observation, must also be determined.

In 1996, the ASA convened a task force to address issues related to the identification and perioperative management of patients at risk for OSA.[79] Ideally, patients with OSA should be identified before the day of surgery, thereby allowing time to optimize management and mobilize

resources for managing a difficult airway or providing prolonged postoperative monitoring. For patients who have not yet undergone formal testing to detect the presence of OSA, clinical signs and symptoms can be assessed to determine the patient's risk of having the disorder. The patient's physical characteristics, their report of experiencing daytime somnolence, or admission of loud snoring suggest that the patient has a propensity for OSA (see **Box 1**). In addition, any sign or symptom that suggests that it may be difficult to ventilate the patient or intubate the trachea should alert the provider to the possibility that the patient is at risk for OSA.[80] The gold-standard test for detecting the presence of OSA is the overnight polysomnogram. Time-consuming and labor-intensive, this test measures several physiologic variables while the patient sleeps in a laboratory. Electroencephalography, eye movement, EMG activity, and vital signs including oxygen saturation, heart rate/rhythm (electrocardiography [EKG]), respiratory airflow, and temperature are used to determine the presence and severity of the disorder. Several investigators have attempted to create a clinical prediction model based on demographic data and symptoms to aid in the identification of patients with OSA. Recent publications studying the screening assessment STOP-BANG questionnaire (**Table 1**) have shown the tool to be sensitive for detecting the presence of OSA, although this questionnaire lacks specificity. When studied in populations seen either at a sleep disorder clinic or in a preoperative setting, application of the tool resulted in several false-positive results.[68,69] Frequently, when surgery is deemed urgent or emergent, there is insufficient time to obtain

Table 1 STOP-BANG questionnaire as published by Chung and colleagues. The STOP-BANG questionnaire has a high sensitivity for detecting patients with OSA with lower specificity. This may be a useful screening tool to diagnose patients suspected of having OSA	
STOP Questionnaire	**BANG**
Snoring	BMI >35 kg/m²
Tiredness	Age >50 y
Observed you stop breathing	Neck circumference >40 cm (>15.7 in)
Blood pressure	Gender male

High risk: yes to ≥3 items → refer for sleep testing.

From Chung F, Subramanyam R, Liao P, et al. High STOP-Bang score indicates a high probability of obstructive sleep apnoea. Br J Anaesth 2012;108(5):774; with permission.

a formal sleep study. Under these circumstances, surveillance for clinical predictors can alert perioperative providers that the patient is at risk for obstructive episodes and potential perioperative adverse events.

Patients presenting for ambulatory surgery with a formal diagnosis of OSA should have their disease treated with appropriate levels of CPAP before their surgery date. Patients who are at risk for OSA, but have not yet received a diagnosis, may not be suitable for outpatient surgery. Those patients with comorbid diseases (including hypertension, chronic obstructive pulmonary disease, arrhythmias, heart failure, cerebrovascular disease, and metabolic syndrome) that are not well controlled may require further testing. Postponement of surgery as well as a change of venue to an inpatient facility should be considered.[38] For children presenting for adenotonsillectomy, it has been recommended that all children obtain a polysomnogram to evaluate the severity of obstructive apnea before intervention.[81] However, neither sleep apnea risk factors nor polysomnography results have been shown to conclusively predict perioperative respiratory complications. It is not well understood which patients with predisposing structural alterations experience airway obstruction once neuromuscular compensatory responses have been depressed by anesthesia (see **Fig. 3**).

Intraoperative management, including medication selection and anesthetic technique, can influence postoperative airway dynamics. There is no evidence to support the superiority of a particular anesthetic agent over another (other than halothane,[73] which is not regularly used in practice in the United States) in the patient at risk for airway obstruction. Patients with OSA have an increased vulnerability to airway compromise and sensitivity to anesthesia; however, there is still a paucity of studies evaluating outcomes based on anesthetic technique, extubation criteria, and monitoring protocols for patients with OSA. Perioperative guidelines are primarily based on consensus of expert opinion. It has been suggested that when feasible, regional anesthesia (spinal, epidural, peripheral nerve block) is preferred over general anesthesia in patients with severe OSA. If regional anesthesia is impossible or impractical, the comparative effectiveness of inhalational and intravenous general anesthetics remains largely unexplored. Sedation can be separated into mild, moderate, and deep sedation, defined by the arousability of the patient. In addition to visual surveillance for adequate respiration, the ASA recommends end-tidal carbon dioxide monitoring for patients receiving moderate and deep sedation. If possible, sedation should be altogether avoided if local anesthesia and peripheral nerve blockade are sufficient for patient comfort. When moderate or deep sedation is required, especially for procedures involving the airway, general anesthesia with a secured airway is recommended.[79] Nonopioid techniques or minimal opioid dosing has also been suggested, especially in pediatric patients with OSA, because of an increased sensitivity to the medications.[38,65] If regional anesthesia with local anesthetics is inappropriate for the surgical intervention, alternatives to opioid medications for pain management should be considered. Recommendations for extubation include awake, fully reversed neuromuscular blockade, and semiupright positioning. Intraoperative anesthetics and analgesics induce varying degrees of disturbances in pharyngeal neuromuscular control, leading to variable increases in collapsibility (P_{CRIT}, see **Fig. 3**). Further study is required to assess which, if any, may be superior and lead to a lower risk of postoperative airway collapse.

Postoperative management of patients with OSA requires appropriate monitoring for respiratory depression and arrhythmias, as well as analgesia sedation mismatch, which are all potential perioperative complications.[82] Data are limited evaluating the efficacy of different postoperative monitoring techniques for patients with OSA. Current standard monitoring includes continuous EKG, pulse oximetry, and noninvasive blood pressure measurements. All of these modalities are late indicators of a respiratory embarrassment. However, end-tidal carbon dioxide and intranasal airflow monitoring may have usefulness in the postoperative setting, alerting providers to current or impending airway obstruction. It is also recommended that patients should not be recovered in the supine position. In addition, patients who require supplemental oxygen to maintain adequate oxygenation may still be at risk for hypoventilation, and detection of hypercarbia may be delayed while saturations are maintained. Patients being treated with CPAP or noninvasive positive pressure ventilation (NIPPV) preoperatively should have these treatment modalities reinstituted in the immediate postoperative period. In addition, patients receiving parenteral opioid medications postoperatively should be monitored with continuous pulse oximetry at a minimum. The use of patient-controlled analgesia should also be avoided, unless patients are closely monitored. Basal rate infusion of opioid medications is contraindicated. Determination of the optimal setting in which to monitor patients with OSA as well as the duration of monitoring postoperatively require further study. Ideally, the setting would confer a high level of patient safety, be cost-effective, and conserve valuable and potentially scarce resources. It remains unclear how much contribution the severity of OSA, preoperative compliance of CPAP or NIPPV, type of surgery, intraoperative techniques and complications, comorbid diseases, and requirement of opioids influence outcome.

FUTURE RESEARCH AREA

Future research is needed to enhance the safe care of patients with OSA in the perioperative period. Investigations evaluating preoperative risk factors, physiologic data recorded on polysomnography, types of surgery, and anesthetic techniques as they relate to postoperative respiratory complications should be conducted. Several changes can be made by clinicians to improve patient care. First, the patient should be treated with their home CPAP immediately after surgery to prevent upper airway obstruction and provide ventilatory support. For those without previous CPAP/NIPPV devices, monitoring should be improved in the immediate postoperative period. Snoring is a worrisome sign, indicating inspiratory flow limitation, which can lead to complete airway obstruction and death. Current monitors, including EKG and pulse oximetry, may alert providers long after an obstruction episode has occurred. Delays in intervention may be catastrophic, especially in patients whose airways are difficult to maintain. Heightened awareness of the importance of OSA in the perioperative period has led to several promising tools for identification of patients at risk and devices to monitor for adverse events. Among these, the measurement of tidal airflow as an adjuvant to routine postoperative monitoring may aid in alerting health care providers immediately to the development of inspiratory airflow limitation, in which case immediate intervention to stabilize the airway is indicated.[1] The cost and efficacy of this and other devices have yet to be determined.

SUMMARY

The optimal perioperative management of the patient with, or at risk for, OSA requires a multidisciplinary approach. Further studies are needed to facilitate a better understanding of the factors that place a patient with OSA at risk for adverse outcome and of the methods and duration of monitoring that confer optimal patient safety.

REFERENCES

1. Kirkness JP, Schwartz AR, Schneider H, et al. Contribution of male sex, age, and obesity to mechanical instability of the upper airway during sleep. J Appl Physiol 2008;104(6):1618–24.
2. Schwartz AR, Patil SP, Laffan AM, et al. Obesity and obstructive sleep apnea: pathogenic mechanisms and therapeutic approaches. Proc Am Thorac Soc 2008;5(2):185–92.
3. Schwartz AR, Patil SP, Squier S, et al. Obesity and upper airway control during sleep. J Appl Physiol 2010;108(2):430–5.
4. Marcus CL, Keens TG, Bautista DB, et al. Obstructive sleep apnea in children with Down syndrome. Pediatrics 1991;88(1):132–9.
5. Rosen D. Management of obstructive sleep apnea associated with Down syndrome and other craniofacial dysmorphologies. Curr Opin Pulm Med 2011; 17(6):431–6.
6. Watanabe T, Isono S, Tanaka A, et al. Contribution of body habitus and craniofacial characteristics to segmental closing pressures of the passive pharynx in patients with sleep-disordered breathing. Am J Respir Crit Care Med 2002;165(2):260–5.
7. Lam DJ, Jensen CC, Mueller BA, et al. Pediatric sleep apnea and craniofacial anomalies: a population-based case-control study. Laryngoscope 2010;120(10):2098–105.
8. Eastwood PR, Platt PR, Shepherd K, et al. Collapsibility of the upper airway at different concentrations of propofol anesthesia. Anesthesiology 2005;103(3):470–7.
9. Eastwood PR, Szollosi I, Platt PR, et al. Collapsibility of the upper airway during anesthesia with isoflurane. Anesthesiology 2002;97(4):786–93.
10. Eastwood PR, Szollosi I, Platt PR, et al. Comparison of upper airway collapse during general anaesthesia and sleep. Lancet 2002;359(9313):1207–9.
11. Montravers P, Dureuil B, Desmonts JM. Effects of i.v. midazolam on upper airway resistance. Br J Anaesth 1992;68(1):27–31.
12. King ED, O'Donnell CP, Smith PL, et al. A model of obstructive sleep apnea in normal humans. Role of the upper airway. Am J Respir Crit Care Med 2000;161(6):1979–84.
13. Schwartz AR, Smith PL, Wise RA, et al. Induction of upper airway occlusion in sleeping individuals with subatmospheric nasal pressure. J Appl Physiol 1988;64(2):535–42.
14. Randall DA, Hoffer ME. Complications of tonsillectomy and adenoidectomy. Otolaryngol Head Neck Surg 1998;118(1):61–8.
15. Smetana GW. Postoperative pulmonary complications: an update on risk assessment and reduction. Cleve Clin J Med 2009;76(Suppl 4):S60–5.
16. Rama AN. Sites of obstruction in obstructive sleep apnea. Chest 2002;122(4):1139–47.
17. Remmers JE, deGroot WJ, Sauerland EK, et al. Pathogenesis of upper airway occlusion during sleep. J Appl Physiol 1978;44(6):931–8.

18. Brouillette RT, Thach BT. Control of genioglossus muscle inspiratory activity. J Appl Physiol 1980; 49(5):801–8.

19. Tangel DJ, Mezzanotte WS, White DP. Respiratory-related control of palatoglossus and levator palatini muscle activity. J Appl Physiol 1995;78(2):680–8.

20. Kuna ST, Vanoye CR. Mechanical effects of pharyngeal constrictor activation on pharyngeal airway function. J Appl Physiol 1999;86(1):411–7.

21. Chin CH, Kirkness JP, Patil SP, et al. Compensatory responses to upper airway obstruction in obese apneic men and women. J Appl Physiol 2012; 112(3):403–10.

22. Seelagy MM, Schwartz AR, Russ DB, et al. Reflex modulation of airflow dynamics through the upper airway. J Appl Physiol 1994;76(6):2692–700.

23. Strohl KP, Hensley MJ, Hallett M, et al. Activation of upper airway muscles before onset of inspiration in normal humans. J Appl Physiol 1980;49(4):638–42.

24. Mathew OP, Abu-Osba YK, Thach BT. Influence of upper airway pressure changes on genioglossus muscle respiratory activity. J Appl Physiol 1982; 52(2):438–44.

25. Isono S, Shimada A, Utsugi M, et al. Comparison of static mechanical properties of the passive pharynx between normal children and children with sleep-disordered breathing. Am J Respir Crit Care Med 1998;157(4 Pt 1):1204–12.

26. Isono S, Remmers JE, Tanaka A, et al. Anatomy of pharynx in patients with obstructive sleep apnea and in normal subjects. J Appl Physiol 1997;82(4): 1319–26.

27. Isono S. Developmental changes of pharyngeal airway patency: implications for pediatric anesthesia. Paediatr Anaesth 2006;16(2):109–22.

28. Gold AR, Schwartz AR. The pharyngeal critical pressure. The whys and hows of using nasal continuous positive airway pressure diagnostically. Chest 1996; 110(4):1077–88.

29. Smith PL, Wise RA, Gold AR, et al. Upper airway pressure-flow relationships in obstructive sleep apnea. J Appl Physiol 1988;64(2):789–95.

30. Gleadhill IC, Schwartz AR, Schubert N, et al. Upper airway collapsibility in snorers and in patients with obstructive hypopnea and apnea. Am Rev Respir Dis 1991;143(6):1300–3.

31. Wellman A, Jordan AS, Malhotra A, et al. Ventilatory control and airway anatomy in obstructive sleep apnea. Am J Respir Crit Care Med 2004;170(11): 1225–32.

32. Patil SP, Schneider H, Marx JJ, et al. Neuromechanical control of upper airway patency during sleep. J Appl Physiol 2007;102(2):547–56.

33. McGinley BM, Schwartz AR, Schneider H, et al. Upper airway neuromuscular compensation during sleep is defective in obstructive sleep apnea. J Appl Physiol 2008;105(1):197–205.

34. Malhotra A, Huang Y, Fogel R, et al. Aging influences on pharyngeal anatomy and physiology: the predisposition to pharyngeal collapse. Am J Med 2006;119(1):72.e9–72.e14.

35. Schwartz AR, Thut DC, Brower RG, et al. Modulation of maximal inspiratory airflow by neuromuscular activity: effect of CO_2. J Appl Physiol 1993;74(4): 1597–605.

36. Rowley JA, Williams BC, Smith PL, et al. Neuromuscular activity and upper airway collapsibility. Mechanisms of action in the decerebrate cat. Am J Respir Crit Care Med 1997;156(2 Pt 1):515–21.

37. Lo YL, Jordan AS, Malhotra A, et al. Influence of wakefulness on pharyngeal airway muscle activity. Thorax 2007;62(9):799–805.

38. Joshi GP, Ankichetty SP, Gan TJ, et al. Society for ambulatory anesthesia consensus statement on preoperative selection of adult patients with obstructive sleep apnea scheduled for ambulatory surgery. Anesth Analg 2012;115(5):1060–8.

39. Stierer TL, Wright C, George A, et al. Risk assessment of obstructive sleep apnea in a population of patients undergoing ambulatory surgery. J Clin Sleep Med 2010;6(5):467–72.

40. Stearns JD, Stierer TL. Peri-operative identification of patients at risk for obstructive sleep apnea. Semin Anesth Perioperat Med Pain 2007;26(2):73–82.

41. Young T, Palta M, Dempsey J, et al. The occurrence of sleep-disordered breathing among middle-aged adults. N Engl J Med 1993;328(17):1230–5.

42. Ayuse T, Hoshino Y, Kurata S, et al. The effect of gender on compensatory neuromuscular response to upper airway obstruction in normal subjects under midazolam general anesthesia. Anesth Analg 2009;109(4):1209–18.

43. Bandla P, Huang J, Karamessinis L, et al. Puberty and upper airway dynamics during sleep. Sleep 2008;31(4):534–41.

44. Polotsky M, Elsayed-Ahmed AS, Pichard L, et al. Effect of age and weight on upper airway function in a mouse model. J Appl Physiol 2011;111(3):696–703.

45. Ray AD, Ogasa T, Magalang UJ, et al. Aging increases upper airway collapsibility in Fischer 344 rats. J Appl Physiol 2008;105(5):1471–6.

46. Litman RS, Wake N, Chan LM, et al. Effect of lateral positioning on upper airway size and morphology in sedated children. Anesthesiology 2005;103(3):484–8.

47. Penzel T, Möller M, Becker HF, et al. Effect of sleep position and sleep stage on the collapsibility of the upper airways in patients with sleep apnea. Sleep 2001;24(1):90–5.

48. Isono S, Tanaka A, Tagaito Y, et al. Influences of head positions and bite opening on collapsibility of the passive pharynx. J Appl Physiol 2004;97(1):339–46.

49. Liistro G, Stănescu D, Dooms G, et al. Head position modifies upper airway resistance in men. J Appl Physiol 1988;64(3):1285–8.

50. Walsh JH, Maddison KJ, Platt PR, et al. Influence of head extension, flexion, and rotation on collapsibility of the passive upper airway. Sleep 2008;31(10):1440–7.

51. Boudewyns A, Schwartz AR, Van de Heyning PH. Upper airway collapsibility: measurement techniques and therapeutic implications. Acta Otorhinolaryngol Belg 2002;56(2):121–5.

52. Ng AT, Darendeliler MA, Petocz P, et al. Cephalometry and prediction of oral appliance treatment outcome. Sleep Breath 2012;16(1):47–58.

53. Kushida CA, Efron B, Guilleminault C. A predictive morphometric model for the obstructive sleep apnea syndrome. Ann Intern Med 1997;127(8 Pt 1):581–7.

54. Polotsky M, Elsayed-Ahmed AS, Pichard LE, et al. Effects of leptin and obesity on the upper airway. J Appl Physiol 2012;112(10):1637–43.

55. Heinzer RC, Stanchina ML, Malhotra A, et al. Effect of increased lung volume on sleep disordered breathing in patients with sleep apnoea. Thorax 2006;61(5):435–9.

56. Jordan AS, White DP, Owens RL, et al. The effect of increased genioglossus activity and end-expiratory lung volume on pharyngeal collapse. J Appl Physiol 2010;109(2):469–75.

57. Vgontzas AN, Zoumakis E, Bixler EO, et al. Selective effects of CPAP on sleep apnoea-associated manifestations. Eur J Clin Invest 2008;38(8):585–95.

58. Arias MA, García-Río F, Alonso-Fernández A, et al. CPAP decreases plasma levels of soluble tumour necrosis factor-alpha receptor 1 in obstructive sleep apnoea. Eur Respir J 2008;32(4):1009–15.

59. Hillman DR, Walsh JH, Maddison KJ, et al. Evolution of changes in upper airway collapsibility during slow induction of anesthesia with propofol. Anesthesiology 2009;111(1):63–71.

60. Norton JR, Ward DS, Karan S, et al. Differences between midazolam and propofol sedation on upper airway collapsibility using dynamic negative airway pressure. Anesthesiology 2006;104(6):1155–64.

61. Drummond GB. Comparison of sedation with midazolam and ketamine: effects on airway muscle activity. Br J Anaesth 1996;76(5):663–7.

62. Genta PR, Eckert DJ, Gregorio MG, et al. Critical closing pressure during midazolam-induced sleep. J Appl Physiol 2011;111(5):1315–22.

63. Horner RL, Innes JA, Murphy K, et al. Evidence for reflex upper airway dilator muscle activation by sudden negative airway pressure in man. J Physiol 1991;436:15–29.

64. Laferrière A, Liu JK, Moss IR. Neurokinin-1 versus mu-opioid receptor binding in rat nucleus tractus solitarius after single and recurrent intermittent hypoxia. Brain Res Bull 2003;59(4):307–13.

65. Brown KA, Laferrière A, Lakheeram I, et al. Recurrent hypoxemia in children is associated with increased analgesic sensitivity to opiates. Anesthesiology 2006;105(4):665–9.

66. Moss IR, Brown KA, Laferrière A. Recurrent hypoxia in rats during development increases subsequent respiratory sensitivity to fentanyl. Anesthesiology 2006;105(4):715–8.

67. Rabbitts JA, Groenewald CB, Dietz NM, et al. Perioperative opioid requirements are decreased in hypoxic children living at altitude. Paediatr Anaesth 2010;20(12):1078–83.

68. Farney RJ, Walker BS, Farney RM, et al. The STOP-Bang equivalent model and prediction of severity of obstructive sleep apnea: relation to polysomnographic measurements of the apnea/hypopnea index. J Clin Sleep Med 2011;7(5):459–465B.

69. Chung F, Subramanyam R, Liao P, et al. High STOP-Bang score indicates a high probability of obstructive sleep apnoea. Br J Anaesth 2012; 108(5):768–75.

70. Richardson KA, Gatti PJ. Genioglossal hypoglossal muscle motoneurons are contacted by nerve terminals containing delta opioid receptor but not mu opioid receptor-like immunoreactivity in the cat: a dual labeling electron microscopic study. Brain Res 2005;1032(1–2):23–9.

71. Hajiha M, DuBord MA, Liu H, et al. Opioid receptor mechanisms at the hypoglossal motor pool and effects on tongue muscle activity in vivo. J Physiol 2009;587(Pt 11):2677–92.

72. Eikermann M, Malhotra A, Fassbender P, et al. Differential effects of isoflurane and propofol on upper airway dilator muscle activity and breathing. Anesthesiology 2008;108(5):897–906.

73. Litman RS, McDonough JM, Marcus CL, et al. Upper airway collapsibility in anesthetized children. Anesth Analg 2006;102(3):750–4.

74. Wheatley JR, Tangel DJ, Mezzanotte WS, et al. Influence of sleep on response to negative airway pressure of tensor palatini muscle and retropalatal airway. J Appl Physiol 1993;75(5):2117–24.

75. Nelson LE, Lu J, Guo T, et al. The alpha2-adrenoceptor agonist dexmedetomidine converges on an endogenous sleep-promoting pathway to exert its sedative effects. Anesthesiology 2003;98(2):428–36.

76. Hsu YW, Cortinez LI, Robertson KM, et al. Dexmedetomidine pharmacodynamics: part I: crossover comparison of the respiratory effects of dexmedetomidine and remifentanil in healthy volunteers. Anesthesiology 2004;101(5):1066–76.

77. Mahmoud M, Gunter J, Donnelly LF, et al. A comparison of dexmedetomidine with propofol for magnetic resonance imaging sleep studies in children. Anesth Analg 2009;109(3):745–53.

78. Mahmoud M, Radhakrishman R, Gunter J, et al. Effect of increasing depth of dexmedetomidine anesthesia on upper airway morphology in children. Paediatr Anaesth 2010;20(6):506–15.

79. Gross JB, Bachenberg KL, Benumof JL, et al. Practice guidelines for the perioperative management of

patients with obstructive sleep apnea: a report by the American Society of Anesthesiologists Task Force on Perioperative Management of patients with obstructive sleep apnea. Anesthesiology 2006;104(5):1081–93 [quiz: 1117–8].

80. Hillman DR, Platt PR, Eastwood PR. Anesthesia, sleep, and upper airway collapsibility. Anesthesiol Clin 2010;28(3):443–55.

81. Marcus CL, Brooks LJ, Draper KA, et al. Diagnosis and management of childhood obstructive sleep apnea syndrome. Pediatrics 2012;130(3): 576–84.

82. Kaw R, Chung F, Pasupuleti V, et al. Meta-analysis of the association between obstructive sleep apnoea and postoperative outcome. Br J Anaesth 2012; 109(6):897–906.

Medical Sedation and Sleep Apnea

Mithri R. Junna, MD[a], Bernardo J. Selim, MD[b],
Timothy I. Morgenthaler, MD[b],*

KEYWORDS

- Obstructive sleep apnea • Sleep-disordered breathing • Sleep architecture • Sedation • Hypnotics
- Benzodiazepines • Non-benzodiazepine GABA receptor agonists • Opioids

KEY POINTS

- Although there is continued caution about the use of benzodiazepines in patients with obstructive sleep apnea (OSA), there is scant clinical evidence supporting significant worsening of sleep-related breathing.
- Nonbenzodiazepine receptor agonists seem to be relatively well tolerated by most patients with OSA and, in selected cases, may show promise as a component of therapy for OSA.
- Opioids exert their effects on respiration by reducing the ventilatory rate and tidal volume, decreasing chemoresponsiveness to hypercapnia/hypoxia, and decreasing upper airway muscle tone.
- Chronic opioid therapy may lead to irregular breathing patterns, OSA and central sleep apnea, and sleep-related hypoxia.
- There is a need for a better understanding of the pharmacologic interaction and clinical impact of hypnosedatives and opioids in patients with OSA.

INTRODUCTION

Obstructive sleep apnea (OSA) is the most common form of sleep-disordered breathing (SDB) and a highly prevalent disorder in the community, reaching up to 2% of middle-aged women and 4% of middle-aged men.[1] It is estimated that approximately 1 out of 4 American adults in the general population are at risk for OSA.[2] This prevalence is even higher in referral populations, such as primary care practices and inpatient practices, whereby the risk for OSA in middle-aged patients approximates 23% to 32%.[3,4]

It is calculated that approximately 2.5% of North American adults use prescription hypnotics, and a projected 201.9 million opioid prescriptions were dispensed in the United States in 2009.[5,6]

Considering the likely overlap of patients at risk for OSA and those prescribed opioids or hypnosedating agents, understanding the impact of such commonly prescribed medications on manifestations of OSA is of great importance. Understanding the effects of these medications and, in particular, the possible deleterious effects on patients with OSA would be necessary to make an informed decision that takes into account both goals and risks when prescribing these substances. Considering that 93% of women and 82% men with moderate to severe OSA remain undiagnosed, careful screening of patients at high risk for OSA is essential.[7] Several methods for OSA risk stratification have already been published, and this material is beyond the scope of this review.[8–10] The goal of this review article is

Disclosures: nil.
Conflicts of interest: nil.
[a] Department of Neurology, Mayo Clinic Center for Sleep Medicine, Mayo Clinic, 200 First Street Southwest, Rochester, MN 55905, USA; [b] Division of Pulmonary and Critical Care Medicine, Mayo Clinic Center for Sleep Medicine, Mayo Clinic, 200 First Street Southwest, Rochester, MN 55905, USA
* Corresponding author.
E-mail address: tmorgenthaler@mayo.edu

Sleep Med Clin 8 (2013) 43–58
http://dx.doi.org/10.1016/j.jsmc.2012.11.012

to characterize the effects of these medications in patients with OSA. In particular, the authors review the pharmacology relevant to the regulation of SDB and provide a systematic review of the medical literature evaluating the effects of benzodiazepines (BDZ), non-BDZ ligand-gated ion channel γ-aminobutyric acid (GABA)$_A$ receptor agonists, and opioids on the clinical manifestations of OSA.

PATHOPHYSIOLOGIC MECHANISMS OF OSA

OSA is characterized by a repetitive intermittent reduction of airflow associated with collapse at the level of the pharynx and ongoing ventilatory effort during sleep. This action results in either complete (apnea) and/or partial (hypopnea) cessation of airflow. Occasional obstructive apneas and hypopneas during sleep are common, but when the frequency of such events increases beyond 5 per hour of sleep, both symptoms and pathologic consequences of OSA begin to manifest. The

pathophysiology behind OSA is complex. The interaction of local pharyngeal anatomy and reflex loops within the central respiratory control system may predispose certain individuals to develop OSA (**Table 1**).

Physiologically, upper airway (UA) patency and stability are the result of a continuous balance between collapsing and expanding forces. While awake, patients with OSA have smaller cross-sectional areas of UA (circular or elliptical shape) and higher critical closure pressures (P$_{crit}$) than patients without OSA, predisposing the airway to collapse.[11,12] During wakefulness, the stability and opening of the UA is achieved by increased genioglossus muscle tone.[13] When falling asleep, collapse of the UA in patients with OSA is the result of the complex interaction of a decline in UA dilating muscle tone, impaired responses to local stimuli (reflex response to mechanoreceptors sensing intrapharyngeal pressures), ventilatory overshoot associated with high loop gain of the respiratory control system, and a concomitant

Table 1
Pathophysiology in patients with OSA in comparison with normal subjects

Normal Subjects	Patients with OSA
Differences in anatomy and function of upper airways	

1. In awake patients
   a. Large cross-sectional area; geometric configuration: elliptical shape (long axis in lateral dimension)
   b. Normal compliance
   c. Low pressure at which UA collapses (negative P$_{crit}$)
   d. Normal muscle tone of genioglossus
 2. During transition or superficial sleep
   a. Low airway instability, uncommon apneas or hypopneas
 3. In slow-wave sleep
   a. Recovery of UA dilator muscle activity and respiratory stability
	1. In awake patients
	   a. Small cross-sectional area; change in geometric configuration: circular or elliptical (long axis A-P dimension)
	   b. High compliance
	   c. High pressure at which UA collapses (positive P$_{crit}$)
	   d. High muscle tone of genioglossus
	 2. During transition or superficial sleep
	   a. High airway instability, increase in apneas or hypopneas
	 3. In slow-wave sleep
	   a. Tendency toward recovery of UA dilator muscle activity and improved respiratory stability

Modulators of UA muscle tone	
Brisk pharyngeal dilator reflexes and normal mechanoreceptor and chemoreceptor sensitivity	Impaired genioglossus reflex responsiveness to local baroreceptors: higher negative intrapharyngeal pressures needed for response
Arousal threshold	
Normal arousal response to airway occlusion	Impaired arousal response to airway occlusion
Stability of the respiratory control system	
Normal respiratory response and loop gain	Increased respiratory response and elevated loop gain
Lung volume changes	
Normal UA stability to low lung volumes	Increased tendency of UA to collapse at low lung volumes (below FRC)

Abbreviations: A-P, anterior-posterior; FRC, functional residual capacity; P$_{crit}$, critical collapsing pressures.

increase of the arousal threshold that might otherwise terminate the collapse.[14–17] The pharmacologic agents covered by this review affect various aspects of this pathophysiology in ways generally deleterious but at times salutary to ventilation during sleep.[18–20]

BDZ GABA_A RECEPTOR AGONISTS
Relevant Pharmacology

The varied therapeutic indications for BDZ result from exploiting their hypnotic, anxiolytic, anticonvulsant, antispasmodic, and amnestic effects. These effects are mediated by the agonistic action of BDZ on various GABA_A receptor subtypes. Which effects predominate with a given BDZ depend in large part on which subunits are most affected and in which part of the nervous system the receptors are located. The pharmacology of GABA_A receptors and their subtypes is well worked out. In brief, the GABA_A receptor is comprised of 5 subunits, most typically 2 α, 2 β, and 1 γ. Each of these subunits is further differentiated into subtypes (α_{1-6}, β_{1-3}, and γ_{1-3}), shown in **Fig. 1**. Nonselective or classic BDZ tend to bind at the interface of the α and β subunits (see **Fig. 1**), which depending on the subtype of subunits present, may produce any of the spectrum of BDZ effects. BDZ with a high affinity for α_1 subunits tend to promote significant hypnotic effects, whereas α_2 receptor stimulation causes anxiety reduction, antispasmodic activity, cognitive blunting, and motor incoordination (**Fig. 2**). Concerns for ventilatory control arise from both sedation, which may blunt ventilatory drive, and antispasmodic activity, which may reduce muscle tone. The receptors may be upregulated with chronic exposure, and tolerance and withdrawal may be anticipated with chronic use.

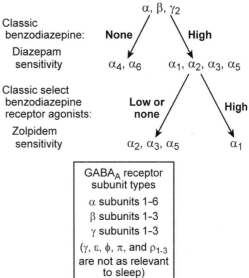

Sensitivity of the GABA_A/Benzodiazepine Receptors

α, β, γ_2

Classic benzodiazepine: Diazepam sensitivity — **None** → α_4, α_6 / **High** → α_1, α_2, α_3, α_5

Classic select benzodiazepine receptor agonists: Zolpidem sensitivity — **Low or none** → α_2, α_3, α_5 / **High** → α_1

GABA_A receptor subunit types
α subunits 1–6
β subunits 1–3
γ subunits 1–3
(γ, ε, ϕ, π, and ρ_{1-3} are not as relevant to sleep)

Fig. 2. Subunit specificity and actions of the GABA_A receptors. (*Courtesy of* The Mayo Foundation for Medical Education and Research; with permission.)

In addition to their varying effects, BDZ agents have diverse pharmacokinetics and may be roughly divided into those with short-, intermediate-, and long-acting compounds. The duration of action depends on the half-life, shown in **Table 2**. Diazepam and chlordiazepoxide are metabolized into desmethyldiazepam, a partial agonist with a very long half-life. For the most part, the ventilatory effects of these agents are not differentiated according to half-life, although any observed effects may be prolonged with longer-acting agents.

Effects of BDZ on Sleep Apnea Syndromes

Although the literature is replete with admonitions to avoid BDZ in patients with OSA, much of this advice is based on scant data, often involving older long-acting and/or nonselective BDZ and much are extrapolated from animal studies. The general effects of BDZ on sleep are summarized in **Table 3** and are based on solid human polysomnographic studies. The actions of BDZ on the respiratory system depend on pharmacokinetic variables, such as dose, route, persistence of active drug and/or metabolite in the body (elimination half-life), and major metabolic breakdown pathways (conjugation vs oxidation). BDZ have been associated with the reduction of UA muscle tone with increased UA resistance as well as blunting of the ventilatory response to hypoxia.[21–23] Although some studies show BDZ increasing

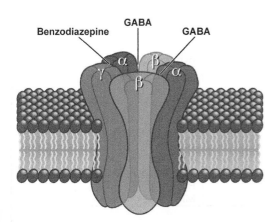

Fig. 1. GABA_A receptor. The receptor is pentameric. The GABA and BDZ binding sites are labeled. Other substances of interest that interact with the GABA_A receptor include alcohol and propofol.

Table 2
GABA$_A$ receptor agonists

Drug	Dosage	Onset	Half-Life (Hours)	Studied in OSA
Non-BDZ GABA$_A$ receptor agonists				
Zaleplon (Sonata)	5–10 mg	Fast	1.0–1.5	−
Zolpidem (Ambien)	2.5–10.0 mg	Fast	1.5–4.0	+
Eszopiclone (Lunesta)	1–3 mg	Fast	5–6	+
Zopiclone	3.75–7.5 mg	Fast	5–6	+
BDZ GABA$_A$ receptor agonists				
Triazolam (Halcion)	0.125–0.25 mg	Fast	2–5	+
Temazepam (Restoril)	7.5–30.0 mg	Moderate	8–12	+
Estazolam (Prosom)	1–2 mg	Moderate	12–20	−
Oxazepam (Serax)	10–25 mg	Moderate	5–15	−
Alprazolam (Xanax)	0.25–1.0 mg	Fast	12–20	−
Lorazepam (Ativan)	0.5–2.0 mg	Moderate	10–22	−
Clonazepam (Klonopin)	0.5–2.0 mg	Slow	22–38	−
Quazepam (Doral)	7.5–15.0 mg	Fast	50–200	−
Flurazepam (Dalmane)	15–30 mg	Fast	50–200	+
Midazolam (Versed)	0.1 mg/kg	Fast	2–6	+

Abbreviations: +, substance has been studied in humans with OSA; −, substance has not been studied in humans with OSA.

the arousal threshold and worsening oxygen saturation, others do not.[24–26] Contrary to BDZ, GABAergic non-BDZ receptor agonists (non–BDZ-RA) agents, especially those stimulating α1 subunits, have fewer muscle relaxant effects.[27] In animal models, the use of sedative-hypnotics may show complex effects. For example, loraze-pam (BDZ) and zolpidem (non-BDZ) have dual

Table 3
Effects of sedatives, hypnotics, and opioids on sleep architecture according to polysomnographic studies

Drug Subclasses	Effects on Sleep Architecture	Potentially Important Effects in OSA
BDZ	↓ Sleep latency ↑ Sleep efficiency ↓ Arousals ↑ N2 sleep ↓ Slow-wave sleep	↓ UA muscle tone ↓ UA reflex response to stretch ↑ Arousal threshold ↓ Ventilatory response to hypoxia ↓ Ventilatory response to hyperpnea (increased Pa$_{CO_2}$)
Non-BDZ	↓ Sleep latency ↑ Sleep efficiency ↓ Arousals ↑ N2 sleep No change in slow-wave or REM sleep	↑ Arousal threshold
Opioids	↓ Sleep latency ↓ Sleep efficiency ↑ N2 sleep ↓ Slow-wave sleep ↓ REM	↓ UA muscle tone ↓ Arousal threshold ↓ Ventilatory response to hypoxia ↑ Hypercapnia ↓ Minute ventilation
Melatonin receptor agonists	↓ Sleep latency ↑ Sleep efficiency	

Abbreviations: N2 sleep, stage N2 sleep; Pa$_{CO_2}$, arterial carbon dioxide tension; REM, rapid eye movement; UA, upper airway.

and opposing effects on genioglossus motor neuron output, with inhibitory effects at the hypoglossal nucleus (type I and II GABA$_A$ receptor), and excitatory effects via premotor input.[28] The *potential* adverse effects of BDZ on the regulation of breathing in sleep (based mostly on animal experiments) are summarized in **Table 4**, but clinical studies in humans do not provide such a neat picture. Only in some cases have the effects of BDZ on patients with OSA been studied (**Table 4**). The authors next summarize the findings of these studies.

Flurazepam

The authors found no studies directly assessing the effects of flurazepam on muscle tone or ventilation control; they found only 2 articles that directly addressed the effect of flurazepam on OSA, and they had opposite results. The oldest article was a single case report in which the administration of 30 mg of flurazepam to a patient with insomnia caused a marked increase in the apnea/hypopnea index (AHI) with increased daytime sleepiness.[29] This patient had not been formally assessed for OSA but had a history of loud snoring and excessive daytime sleepiness. Curiously, he had a baseline polysomnogram as part of a research study that did not show OSA. Cessation of flurazepam resolved daytime symptoms and AHI elevations. In another case series that specifically excluded those with a clinical history OSA, the aim was to evaluate the safety of midazolam versus flurazepam. Patients using flurazepam showed no significant increase in AHI. Thus, based only on very scant data, it seems that some patients might show susceptibility to flurazepam, but the magnitude of the risk cannot be assessed from the available data.

Midazolam

Several case series indicate that midazolam, used in clinical doses of about 0.1 mg/kg intravenously (IV), can increase airway resistance and result in a decline in arterial oxygen saturation (SaO$_2$). Both decreases in UA tone[30] and suppression of ventilatory drive have been implicated.[30–34] Flumazenil, a GABA$_A$ antagonist, inhibits this effect of midazolam. These fairly predictable effects are being exploited in the developing field of sleep endoscopy, wherein heavy sedation is used to induce a sleeplike state during which the site and extent of UA collapse can be directly visualized. This technique is beyond the scope of this review but may show promise for both diagnostic and therapeutic purposes.[35–37] Apart from that, midazolam has been frequently used for attended sedation during endoscopy (often in combination with fentanyl) and has been associated anecdotally with the onset of unexpected respiratory emergencies. Counterbalancing these anecdotal reports are findings from a case series of 553 patients undergoing endoscopy using midazolam and fentanyl in which having OSA did not increase the risk of cardiorespiratory complications.[38] Again, although certain susceptible individuals may have particularly significant adverse respiratory responses to midazolam, predictive risk factors are not yet available. In the meanwhile, guidelines for attended sedation during endoscopy ought to be followed to enhance patient safety.[39]

Nitrazepam

Nitrazepam is not frequently used in the United States. One polysomnographic study evaluated the effect on SDB of nitrazepam 5 or 10 mg given to patients with mild to moderate OSA. Nitrazepam did not have a consistent effect on either the apnea frequency or oxygenation, but some patients did experience notable worsening. The analysis did not suggest factors that were predictive of worsening SDB; but clearly, not all patients were adversely affected. Importantly, the total sleep time increased only with the higher dose of nitrazepam.

Temazepam

Temazepam was studied and found beneficial to the apnea index in patients with altitude and heart failure–associated central sleep apnea (CSA).[40,41] However, the authors found 2 polysomnographic studies of 10 to 30 mg of temazepam in patients with OSA. Interestingly, in patients with mild to moderate OSA, there was little or no improvement in sleep parameters. In patients with mild to moderate OSA, there was no significant increase in AHI or oxyhemoglobin saturation for the group as a whole.[42] However, patients who had higher ventilatory central chemosensitivity had worse respiratory depression following temazepam. When elderly patients with OSA and concurrent insomnia were randomized to either temazepam 15 to 30 mg or nonpharmacologic treatment of their insomnia, there was no increase in the respiratory disturbance index as a result of temazepam. However, again, there was little polysomnographic improvement with temazepam, calling into question the efficacy.[26]

Triazolam

The authors identified 2 prospective placebo-controlled polysomnographic studies addressing the effect of triazolam on sleep and breathing in patients with mild to moderate OSA. The results were a bit conflicting. Bonnet and colleagues found that triazolam decreased the AHI without

Table 4
Hypnotic and sedative medications studied in patients with OSA

Study	Drug	Intervention	Safety	Effectiveness
Rosenberg et al,[27] 2007	Eszopiclone	DBCT eszopiclone 3 mg in patients with AHI 10–40	No significant differences in total arousals, respiratory arousals, duration of apnea and hypopnea episodes, or oxygen saturation were noted.	Improved sleep maintenance and efficiency
Eckert et al,[52] 2011	Eszopiclone	Eszopiclone 3 mg vs placebo to patients with OSA without marked O_2 desaturations	Eszopiclone increased the arousal threshold and lowered the AHI in patients with OSA without marked overnight hypoxemia. Reductions in the AHI occurred in the absence of respiratory event prolongation or increased hypoxemia.	Increased TST, decreased AI
Schönhofer and Köhler,[87] 1996	Flumazenil	Flumazenil given to men with severe OSA	There were no adverse effects.	No improvement in AHI
Montravers,[32] 1992	Midazolam	Midazolam 0.1 mg/kg administered IV to healthy individuals	There was marked increase in airway resistance with reduction in central apneas.	Sedation was achieved; not a PSG study
Oshima,[88] 1999	Midazolam	Flumazenil given to normal subjects whose airway resistance had increased with midazolam	There were no problems with midazolam; 2 subjects developed obstructive apneas and 4 developed snoring.	Flumazenil reverses increased airway resistance of midazolam
Rishi et al,[89] 2010	Mixed	BDZ in patients with atypical antipsychotic use	When corrected for weight, age, and so forth, no increased AHI in patients taking BDZ. However, there was a slight increased risk of OSA and increased AHI in patients taking atypical antipsychotic vs not.	Not assessed
Höijer et al,[90] 1994	Nitrazepam	Nitrazepam 5 or 10 mg tablets give to 14 patients with AHI 10–30	Nitrazepam had no consistent effect on AHI or oxygenation in these patients. Some patients experienced significant worsening but not predictably.	Total sleep time increased only with higher doses of nitrazepam

Study	Drug	Description	Findings
Wang et al,[42] 2011	Temazepam	Temazepam 10 mg given to patients with mild to moderate OSA	There was no significant difference between placebo and temazepam in AHI or oxygenation. However, patients with OSA with higher awake central chemosensitivity had worse respiratory depression during sleep with the use of a mild CNS depressant (temazepam).	No real differences other than REM suppression after temazepam administration
Camacho and Morin,[26] 1995	Temazepam	Elderly patients with mild OSA and insomnia were randomized to either Temazepam 15–30 mg or nonpharmacologic treatment	There was no increase in the RDI between those receiving 15–30 mg of temazepam compared with nonpharmacologic therapy.	No real temazepam effect compared with nonpharmacologic treatment group
Bonnet,[43] 1990	Triazolam	Placebo, triazolam 0.125, 0.25 mg given to patients with CSA	There was a decrease in AHI and CAI and no change in oxygenation.	Improved TST, AI with active drug
Berry et al,[25] 1995	Triazolam	Triazolam 0.25 mg vs placebo to patients with OSA	There was no significant increase in AHI (but trend); there was longer apneas, slightly deeper desaturation. The arousal threshold was higher.	Decreased WASO, increased TST
Berry and Patel,[48] 2006	Zolpidem	Zolpidem 10 mg administered to patients undergoing CPAP titration	There was no difference in levels of CPAP ultimately prescribed.	Slight decrease in sleep latency and arousal frequency
Steens et al,[46] 1993	Zolpidem	Zolpidem 5 mg, 10 mg, and triazolam 0.25 mg were administered to mild-moderate COPD patients with insomnia	There were no real changes in oxygenation or AHI between drugs.	All 3 drug conditions improved TST, WASO, and sleep efficiency
Lofaso et al,[51] 1997	Zopiclone	Zopiclone 7.5 mg vs placebo in patients with mild OSA	There was no change in AHI or oxygenation.	No change in AI, TST, or sleep architecture
Kryger,[55] 2007	Ramelteon	Ramelteon 16 mg vs placebo in patients with moderate OSA	AHI and oxygen saturation were not significantly altered by ramelteon.	No significant effects on sleep parameters or subjective sleep assessment
Gooneratne et al,[56] 2010	Ramelteon	Ramelteon vs placebo treatment of elderly patients with insomnia and OSA on APAP	AHI was not different between the groups. APAP adherence and PSQI were also not different.	Ramelteon did result in a modest, but significant, improvement in SOL compared with placebo; no other differences noted

Abbreviations: AHI, apnea hypopnea index; AI, apnea index; APAP, autotitrating positive airway pressure; BDZ, benzodiazepine; CAI, central apnea index; CNS, central nervous system; COPD, chronic obstructive pulmonary disease; CPAP, continuous positive airway pressure; CSA, central sleep apnea; DBCT, double blind controlled trial; IV, intravenous; OSA, obstructive sleep apnea; PSG, polysomnogram; PSQI, Pittsburg sleep quality index; RDI, respiratory disturbance index; REM, rapid eye movement; TST, total sleep time.

a change in oxygenation, whereas Berry and colleagues[25,43] found no significant change in AHI but slightly deeper oxyhemoglobin desaturation. With these limited data, it would seem that this shorter-acting benzodiazepine may have some margin of safety in patients with OSA or with risk factors for OSA. Triazolam also may have limited usefulness in the treatment of primary CSA.[44] However, in some countries, triazolam has been removed from the market because of other worrisome side effects.[45]

NON-BDZ GABA$_A$ RA HYPNOTICS
Relevant Pharmacology

Several agents have been developed that selectively bind to the α_1 subtype GABA$_A$ subunit. These non–BDZ-RA preferentially cause sedation and less prominent muscle relaxation and anxiolysis promoted by nonselective BDZ (see **Fig. 2**). These agents include zolpidem, zaleplon, zopiclone, and eszopiclone. Because of the selectivity of their pharmacologic targets, non–BDZ-RA have generally been associated with a more favorable side-effect profile than the nonselective BDZ. However, because they do not cross-react with the other subunits and subtypes, care must be taken in the use of these agents. For example, the substitution of a non–BDZ-RA for BDZ in patients chronically using BDZ will likely lead to withdrawal responses.

These agents all show rapid onset and short to intermediate durations of action. Perhaps unique among them is zaleplon, which has a very short half-life. Because of this, it is approved for use in both sleep-onset insomnia and in sleep-maintenance insomnia taken in the middle of the night should awakening occur. In this setting, there is little carryover sedation or cognitive impairment.

Effects of Non-BDZ GABA$_A$ RA on Sleep Apnea Syndromes

Realizing that non–BDZ-RA have little effect on subunits or subtypes that affect muscle relaxation, researchers quickly assessed their safety and usefulness in respiratory disorders, including OSA.

Zolpidem

Zolpidem has been studied both for its effect on sleep and breathing in patients with OSA and for its effect on continuous positive airway pressure (CPAP) efficacy in patients with OSA. The effect on AHI is only indirectly assessed in 2 studies that evaluated the safety and effect of zolpidem on patients with chronic obstructive pulmonary disease (COPD), some of whom had elevations in the AHI at baseline. In both studies, zolpidem 5 to 10 mg had little significant effect on either

oxygenation or AHI.[46,47] In a more direct study of the effect of zolpidem on patients with OSA, Berry and colleagues[49] evaluated the effect of zolpidem on patients undergoing CPAP titration. In a placebo-controlled study, they found no significant difference in the CPAP that controlled SDB, suggesting that the usual dose of zolpidem has little effect on muscle tone (a finding that was not unexpected). In the authors' sleep center, they have used zolpidem as an aid to sleep during polysomnography with confidence that it does not significantly affect AHI or oxygenation. However, the authors may be reevaluating this usage in light of the recent association of zolpidem with an increased risk of falling, opting instead for perhaps one of the other non–BDZ-RA.[49]

Zaleplon

The authors were unable to find any polysomnographic studies that directly assessed the effect of zaleplon on sleep and breathing in OSA. Park and colleagues[50] have published data suggesting that zaleplon had no significant effect on sleep or subsequent CPAP adherence.

Zopiclone and eszopiclone

Zopiclone is a cyclopyrrolone non–BDZ-RA with a rapid onset and an intermediate duration of effect. In the United States, zopiclone is not commercially available; but its active stereo-isomer, eszopiclone, is marketed as Lunesta. In polysomnographic studies of normal persons, zopiclone generally preserves slow-wave sleep and does not impair daytime performance. It has been studied in patients with COPD and had no significant effect on ventilatory control parameters. In one study by Lofaso and colleagues,[51] zopiclone 7.5 mg at bedtime showed no real changes in either sleep architecture or sleep breathing parameters compared with placebo in patients with mild OSA. Eszopiclone has been studied in patients with mild to severe OSA. Rosenberg and colleagues[27] evaluated the effect of eszopiclone 3 mg in patients with an initial AHI of 1 to 40. They found no significant influence over the duration or frequency of SDB events, no change in oxygen saturation, and no change in total arousals. Sleep maintenance and efficiency did improve. In a novel study evaluating the effect of eszopiclone on the AHI of patients thought to have a low arousal threshold as contributors to their OSA, eszopiclone led to a significant decrease in AHI.[52] This study is the first published clinical trial seeking to directly pharmacologically combat the contribution of arousals to ventilatory instability, an approach that seems promising. Additional studies document the lack of adverse effects and potentially beneficial effects on subsequent CPAP adherence in patients with OSA treated with eszopiclone.[53,54]

Novel Hypnotics

Ramelteon

Ramelteon is an MT1/MT2 melatonin RA hypnotic agent. It has been assessed for safety in patients with moderately severe OSA in a randomized blinded placebo-controlled trial. Ramelteon 16 mg did not alter the AHI or oxygen saturation.[55] However, it also had no measurable effects on sleep architecture or continuity. In another trial looking at the effect of ramelteon on patients with autotitrating positive airway pressure (APAP) treated OSA and comorbid insomnia, ramelteon did not result in significant changes in AHI or oxygen saturation; but again, there were no notable improvements in Pittsburg Sleep Quality Index (PSQI), Epworth Sleepiness Scale (ESS), or polysomnographic measures of sleep with the exception of a modest improvement in sleep onset latency (SOL).[56] It seems that ramelteon is safe but not very efficacious in patients with OSA.

Although several other agents are in use off label to promote sleep, such as tricyclic antidepressants, antihistaminics, and antipsychotics, these are not approved hypnotics or sedatives, are rarely studied in patients with OSA, and are beyond the scope of this review.

Summary Regarding Hypnotics and Sedative Medications in Patients with OSA

The individual pharmacologic actions of many benzodiazepine GABA$_A$ agonists, especially those that are less selective, tend to reduce muscle tone, decrease ventilatory responsiveness to hypoxemia and hypercapnia, and increase the arousal threshold. Each of these would seem to make this class of agents undesirable and dangerous in patients with a predisposition toward or documented OSA. Consistent with this elementary understanding, there are case reports of marked worsening of OSA after the administration of these agents. However, the now prevalent admonitions against usage may be overstated in view of scant clinical evidence that often shows limited or no worsening of sleep-related breathing in patients with OSA, or in some cases marginal improvements in SDB. (A possibly notable exception is the rather consistently unpropitious effects of midazolam on patients with predilection toward OSA.)

In contrast to the effects of BDZ, non–BDZ-RA seem to be relatively well tolerated by most patients with OSA and, in some cases, may prove to be an adjunct to therapy for cases of patients with OSA where raising the arousal threshold may help stabilize ventilation.

These, at times paradoxic or surprising effects of GABA$_A$ RA likely reflect the more complex underlying mechanisms involved in the perpetuation of airway collapse in OSA. The current understanding implicates not only muscle tone and anatomic considerations but also dynamic ventilatory control and how it is modulated by sleep state. In any given patient, different mechanisms may predominate, leaving the response to interventions at any given point difficult to predict.

One theme common to the earlier discussion is that none of these agents prove highly effective in improving subjective or objective measures of sleep continuity or architecture. From a safety and efficacy viewpoint, certainly nonpharmacologic approaches should be considered when confronted with patients with OSA who have concurrent insomnia. If transient hypnosedation is needed, one may be most prudent to try one of the non–BDZ-RA drugs.

OPIOIDS

The quantity of opioid prescriptions in the United States has grown exceedingly in recent years. In 1990, it is estimated that more than 2.2 million grams of morphine, 3273 g of fentanyl, and 118 455 g of hydromorphone were used medically. Subsequent follow-up measures suggested that the use of morphine had increased by 59%, fentanyl by more than 1000%, and hydromorphone by 19%.[57] Only meperidine use declined over this interval.[58] In the authors' sleep practice, they see clear increases in the proportion of patients presenting for evaluation who are treated with chronic opioid medications. In the inpatient arena, opioids are commonly encountered components of acute and comfort care. It is, therefore, important that we explore how opioids and SDB interact. Conceptually, the authors consider the general pharmacology of opioids, then review the acute and/or chronic effects on SDB for each agent studied.

Relevant Pharmacology

Opioids are naturally occurring and synthetic agents that bind to a class of four G protein-coupled receptors in the central and peripheral nervous systems and respiratory and gastrointestinal tracts, leading to decreased neuronal excitability.[59] These receptors fall into four classes, including δ, μ, nociception/orphanin, and the κ receptor.[60] Opioid medications, mimicking endogenous ligands (endorphins, enkephalins, dynorphins, and so forth), act through these receptors at different levels of the peripheral and central nervous systems. Each receptor has at least one endogenous ligand; these receptors mediate pain, respiration, and stress.[61] Nearly all receptor types influence analgesia, with the possible exception of nociception/orphanin receptors, which may instead lead to hyperalgesia. Ligands that stimulate μ and κ receptors particularly suppress central respiratory pattern generation, resulting in decreases in the respiratory rate and tidal volume.[62–64] Both naturally occurring and synthetic opioids may exhibit preferential receptor affinity and may act as agonists, mixed agonists/antagonists, or antagonists.

Effects of Opioids on Sleep Apnea Syndromes

The effects of opioids on respiration share common pathophysiological pathways with OSA,

resulting in potential additive adverse consequences. Most studies of opioid effects are either mechanistic ones performed on isolated chemosensitive neural areas, such as the brainstem or carotid bodies of animals, or more systemic administration to awake, sleeping, or anesthetized animals or humans. Animal research, supported by limited work in humans, describes opioids acting on medullary respiratory neurons with the suppression of respiration rate and respiratory drive (pre-Bötzinger complex), central chemoreceptors' response to hypercapnia, peripheral response to hypoxemia (glomus cell of carotid body), and depression of the arousal system, as seen in **Fig. 3**.[63,65–67] In animal models, μ-opioid receptors and δ- receptors in the motor neuron of the hypoglossal nerve induce suppression of hypoglossal muscle activity with a resultant tendency toward collapse of UA.[68]

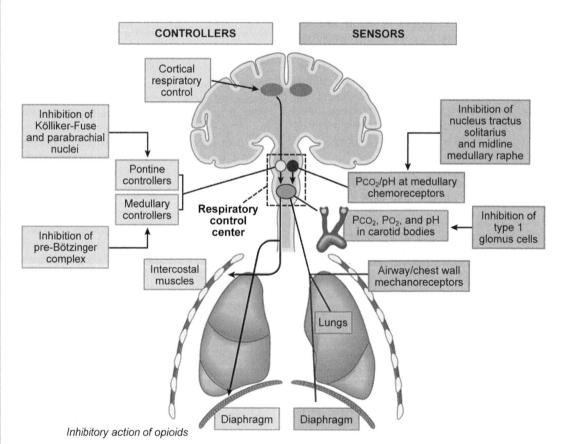

Inhibitory action of opioids

Fig. 3. Opioid effects in the respiratory system. Control of ventilation is achieved by a feedback control system. Central nervous system controllers (*right*) include oscillators in the medulla like the pre-Bötzinger complex, retrotrapezoid, and parafacial respiratory group modulated by the pontine Kölliker-Fuse nucleus, the complex, and the locus coeruleus, as well as sensory input from the medullary chemoreceptors, the carotid bodies, and mechanoreceptors from the airway and chest wall. The medullary respiratory controllers integrate these inputs to produce the efferent signals (*left*) that integrate the respiratory muscle activity. Opioids exert influence at multiple levels, as is shown in the periphery of the diagram. (*Courtesy of* The Mayo Foundation for Medical Education and Research; with permission.)

The effects of opioid agonists on respiration when systemically administered in animals and humans show more marked variation. For example, in goats or cats, opioids may increase tidal volume and respiratory rate, whereas in humans, they most often lead to ventilatory depression. Generally, in humans, opioids tend to decrease hypoxic and hypercapnic ventilatory responsiveness.[63] Opioid agonists (particularly fentanyl, see later discussion) tend to decrease UA muscle tone and the compensatory response to resistive loading.[69,70] In addition, some agents have been associated with an increased rigidity of accessory respiratory muscles, further limiting ventilation.[71]

These influences clearly suggest that opioids may increase susceptibility to SDB. At lower doses, respiratory depression occurs secondary to a decrease in tidal volume, and at higher doses, secondary to a decrease in respiratory rate.[64,71] A decreased ventilatory response to hypercapnia/hypoxia also occurs.[72] This decrease can lead to ataxic/Biot breathing respiration associated with the development of central sleep apneas, OSA, periodic or cluster breathing patterns, and sleep-related hypoxia, as seen in **Fig. 4**.[73,74] Given that the effect of opioids on human ventilatory control is influenced by dose and ligand specificity, a review of clinical data for specific agents is warranted. A clear dose-response effect has been shown in the tendency of opioids to induce SDB (**Fig. 5**).

Opioid agonists also influence sleep. The general effects of opioids on sleep are summarized in

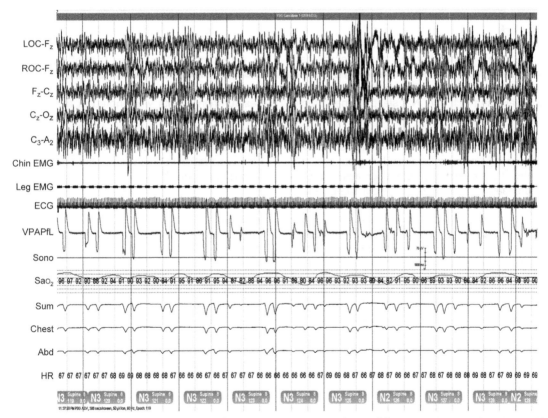

Fig. 4. Opioids and ataxic breathing. This polysomnogram segment obtained from a patient on chronic opioid medications shows 300 seconds of non–rapid-eye-movement sleep (stages are shown at bottom). Each heavy vertical line demarks 30 seconds. The airflow signal from a bilevel positive airway pressure unit, (labeled VPAPfL) shows an ataxic or irregular breathing pattern with clustering. Note that most apneas here are central, but there is no clear period. Not discernible from this level of scrutiny, most of these apneas are not associated with arousals, despite the clear oxyhemoglobin desaturation (see signal labeled SaO2). Chin electromyogram (EMG) and leg EMG represent submental and pretibial EMGs. The electrocardiogram (ECG) shows sinus rhythm. Sono is a snoring microphone and is unremarkable. Abdominal (Abd) and chest (chest) respiratory impedance plethysmography signals demonstrate changes in circumference at those levels, usually taken to represent muscular effort. The arithmetic summation of deflection of Abd and chest signals (the Sum signal) parallels tidal volume when calibrated. C3-A2, central electroencephalogram montage; Cz-Oz, occipital electroencephalogram montage; EEG, electroencephalogram; Fz-Cz, frontal electroencephalogram montage; HR, pulse rate (as read from the pulse oximeter); LOC-Fz, left electro-oculograms; ROC-Fz, right electro-oculograms.

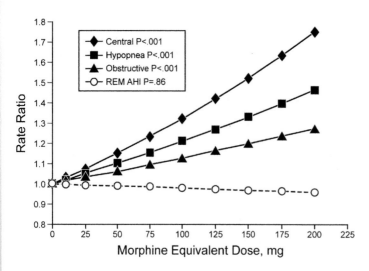

Fig. 5. Rate of apneas as a function of opioid dose. The AHI increases as a function of morphine-equivalent dosing in a population of chronic opioid users. The disordered breathing events included central apneas, obstructive apneas, and hypopneas during rapid eye movement (REM) sleep. (*From* Walker J, Farney R, Rhondeau S, et al. Chronic opioid use is a risk factor for the development of central sleep apnea and ataxic breathing. J Clin Sleep Med 2007;3: 455–61; with permission.)

Table 3. Polysomnographic effects on sleep during acute opioid administration include decreases in slow-wave and rapid eye movement (REM) sleep with decreased sleep efficiency and increases in arousals and N1 and N2 sleep. Other studies have shown a decrease in slow-wave sleep with increased N2 sleep and no change in sleep efficiency or total sleep time in patients receiving either morphine or methadone during polysomnography.[75] During chronic opioid administration, the decreases in slow-wave and REM sleep tend to normalize with improvement in sleep efficiency.[72] A randomized controlled trial of 19 patients who received either saline or remifentanil infusion during a sleep study demonstrated increased N1 sleep with decreased sleep efficiency and REM sleep in the group that received remifentanil.[76]

General Considerations Regarding Opioids

Opioids have in case series been associated with increased SDB when administered acutely. Based on anesthesia literature, patients with OSA managed with opioid-based analgesia have increased extubation complications, increased paradoxic breathing patterns, and pronounced oxygen desaturations.[77–79] Contrary to acute administration, opioids administered chronically lead to a dose-dependent higher rate of OSA, central sleep apnea during non-REM (NREM) sleep associated with ataxic/Biot respiration, and hypoxemia but rarely significant hypercapnia.[73,80–82] In fact, patients with OSA with chronic opioid use have a decreased respiratory effort during the apneic event in comparison with matched patients with OSA not on opioids.[83] The authors next review individual agents and their relationship with sleep apnea in particular.

Morphine and tramadol

In a randomized controlled trial of 66 children receiving either tramadol or morphine postoperatively following adenotonsillectomy for OSA, fewer desaturation events were noted in the tramadol group when compared with the morphine group at 3 hours, with statistically significant findings at 2 hours. No statistically significant differences in pain or sedation scores were noted up to 6 hours following surgery.[84]

Remifentanil

In a randomized controlled trial of 19 patients with moderate OSA receiving either a saline or remifentanil infusion, a decrease in obstructive apnea rate (presumably secondary to the decrease in REM sleep) and an increase in the central apnea rate were found in the remifentanil group.[76]

Methadone

A case series of methadone users showed a high prevalence of central sleep apnea and OSA.[82] There has been a case report of reversal of SDB, including obstructive hypoventilation and both central and obstructive apneas and hypopneas, with discontinuation of methadone.[85]

Multiple opioids

In a review of 22 patients with sleep apnea who had been receiving opioid medications for at least 6 months, the average AHI was noted to be 66.6 ± 37.3 with both obstructive and central components.[86] A study of 140 patients receiving chronic opioid therapy in the form of methadone, oxycodone, hydrocodone, morphine, hydromorphone, and tramadol found 75% of patients to have an elevated AHI, with 39% described as OSA, 4%

as "indeterminate" sleep apnea, 24% as central sleep apnea, 8% as "mixed sleep apnea" (which the authors take to mean complex sleep apnea syndrome), and 25% with no sleep apnea.[81] A direct relationship between the total daily dose of opioid and the AHI was found only among methadone users and not among other opioid users.

Summary Regarding Opioid Medications in Patients with OSA

Opioids exert their effects on respiration by reducing the ventilatory rate and tidal volume, decreasing chemoresponsiveness to hypercapnia/hypoxia, and decreasing UA muscle tone. Such effects can lead to irregular breathing patterns, OSA and central sleep apnea, and sleep-related hypoxia. Furthermore, opioids have been shown to reduce slow-wave sleep and increase N2 sleep. There are very limited studies demonstrating the effects of opioids on OSA. Tramadol has been shown to produce less desaturations events when compared with morphine during administration in children following adenotonsillectomy for OSA. Remifentanil has been shown to decrease OSA (likely because of a decrease in REM sleep during acute administration) and increase central sleep apnea when compared with saline in postoperative patients. Large studies of patients being administered chronic opioid therapy have demonstrated both central sleep apnea and OSA and, furthermore, a direct relationship between opiate dosage and AHI.

REFERENCES

1. Young T, Palta M, Dempsey J, et al. The occurrence of sleep-disordered breathing among middle-aged adults. N Engl J Med 1993;328(17):1230–5.
2. Hiestand DM, Britz P, Goldman M, et al. Prevalence of symptoms and risk of sleep apnea in the US population: results from the national sleep foundation sleep in America 2005 poll. Chest 2006;130(3):780–6.
3. Finkel KJ, Searleman AC, Tymkew H, et al. Prevalence of undiagnosed obstructive sleep apnea among adult surgical patients in an academic medical center. Sleep Med 2009;10(7):753–8.
4. Netzer NC, Hoegel JJ, Loube D, et al. Prevalence of symptoms and risk of sleep apnea in primary care. Chest 2003;124(4):1406–14.
5. Wysowski DK, Baum C. Outpatient use of prescription sedative-hypnotic drugs in the United States, 1970 through 1989. Arch Intern Med 1991;151(9):1779–83.
6. Volkow ND, McLellan TA, Cotto JH, et al. Characteristics of opioid prescriptions in 2009. JAMA 2011;305(13):1299–301.
7. Young T, Evans L, Finn L, et al. Estimation of the clinically diagnosed proportion of sleep apnea syndrome in middle-aged men and women. Sleep 1997;20(9):705–6.
8. Netzer NC, Stoohs RA, Netzer CM, et al. Using the Berlin Questionnaire to identify patients at risk for the sleep apnea syndrome. Ann Intern Med 1999;131(7):485–91.
9. Chung SA, Yuan H, Chung F. A systemic review of obstructive sleep apnea and its implications for anesthesiologists. Anesth Analg 2008;107(5):1543–63.
10. Chung F, Elsaid H. Screening for obstructive sleep apnea before surgery: why is it important? Curr Opin Anaesthesiol 2009;22(3):405–11.
11. Schwab RJ, Gupta KB, Gefter WB, et al. Upper airway and soft tissue anatomy in normal subjects and patients with sleep-disordered breathing. Significance of the lateral pharyngeal walls. Am J Respir Crit Care Med 1995;152(5 Pt 1):1673–89.
12. Isono S, Remmers JE, Tanaka A, et al. Anatomy of pharynx in patients with obstructive sleep apnea and in normal subjects. J Appl Physiol 1997;82(4):1319–26.
13. Mezzanotte WS, Tangel DJ, White DP. Waking genioglossal electromyogram in sleep apnea patients versus normal controls (a neuromuscular compensatory mechanism). J Clin Invest 1992;89(5):1571–9.
14. Mezzanotte WS, Tangel DJ, White DP. Influence of sleep onset on upper-airway muscle activity in apnea patients versus normal controls. Am J Respir Crit Care Med 1996;153(6 Pt 1):1880–7.
15. Eckert DJ, McEvoy RD, George KE, et al. Genioglossus reflex inhibition to upper-airway negative-pressure stimuli during wakefulness and sleep in healthy males. J Physiol 2007;581(Pt 3):1193–205.
16. Berry RB, Kouchi KG, Der DE, et al. Sleep apnea impairs the arousal response to airway occlusion. Chest 1996;109(6):1490–6.
17. Wellman A, Jordan AS, Malhotra A, et al. Ventilatory control and airway anatomy in obstructive sleep apnea. Am J Respir Crit Care Med 2004;170(11):1225–32.
18. Younes M. Role of arousals in the pathogenesis of obstructive sleep apnea. Am J Respir Crit Care Med 2004;169(5):623–33.
19. Jordan AS, Wellman A, Heinzer RC, et al. Mechanisms used to restore ventilation after partial upper airway collapse during sleep in humans. Thorax 2007;62(10):861–7.
20. Jordan AS, Eckert DJ, Wellman A, et al. Termination of respiratory events with and without cortical arousal in obstructive sleep apnea. Am J Respir Crit Care Med 2011;184(10):1183–91.
21. Bonora M, St John WM, Bledsoe TA. Differential elevation by protriptyline and depression by diazepam of upper airway respiratory motor activity. Am Rev Respir Dis 1985;131(1):41–5.

22. Leiter JC, Knuth SL, Krol RC, et al. The effect of diaz-epam on genioglossal muscle activity in normal human subjects. Am Rev Respir Dis 1985;132(2):216–9.

23. Hanly P, Powles P. Hypnotics should never be used in patients with sleep apnea. J Psychosom Res 1993;37(Suppl 1):59–65.

24. Hedemark LL, Kronenberg RS. Flurazepam attenu-ates the arousal response to CO_2 during sleep in normal subjects. Am Rev Respir Dis 1983;128(6): 980–3.

25. Berry RB, Kouchi K, Bower J, et al. Triazolam in patients with obstructive sleep apnea. Am J Respir Crit Care Med 1995;151(2 Pt 1):450–4.

26. Camacho ME, Morin CM. The effect of temazepam on respiration in elderly insomniacs with mild sleep apnea. Sleep 1995;18(8):644–5.

27. Rosenberg R, Roach JM, Scharf M, et al. A pilot study evaluating acute use of eszopiclone in patients with mild to moderate obstructive sleep apnea syndrome. Sleep Med 2007;8(5):464–70.

28. Park E, Younes M, Liu H, et al. Systemic vs. central administration of common hypnotics reveals oppos-ing effects on genioglossus muscle activity in rats. Sleep 2008;31(3):355–65.

29. Mendelson WB, Garnett D, Gillin JC. Flurazepam-induced sleep apnea syndrome in a patient with insomnia and mild sleep-related respiratory changes. J Nerv Ment Dis 1981;169(4):261–4.

30. Drummond GB. Comparison of sedation with mida-zolam and ketamine: effects on airway muscle activity. Br J Anaesth 1996;76(5):663–7.

31. Nozaki-Taguchi N, Isono S, Nishino T, et al. Upper airway obstruction during midazolam sedation: modi-fication by nasal CPAP. Can J Anaesth 1995;42(8): 685–90.

32. Montravers P, Dureuil B, Desmonts JM. Effects of i.v. midazolam on upper airway resistance. Br J Anaesth 1992;68(1):27–31.

33. Molliex S, Dureuil B, Montravers P, et al. Effects of midazolam on respiratory muscles in humans. Anesth Analg 1993;77(3):592–7.

34. Montravers P, Dureuil B, Molliex S, et al. Effects of intravenous midazolam on the work of breathing. Anesth Analg 1994;79(3):558–62.

35. Ravesloot MJ, de Vries N. One hundred consecutive patients undergoing drug-induced sleep endos-copy: results and evaluation. Laryngoscope 2011; 121(12):2710–6.

36. Genta PR, Eckert DJ, Gregorio MG, et al. Critical closing pressure during midazolam-induced sleep. J Appl Physiol 2011;111(5):1315–22.

37. Gregório MG, Jacomelli M, Inoue D, et al. Com-parison of full versus short induced-sleep poly-somnography for the diagnosis of sleep apnea. Laryngoscope 2011;121(5):1098–103.

38. Mador MJ, Nadler J, Mreyoud A, et al. Do patients at risk of sleep apnea have an increased risk of cardio-respiratory complications during endoscopy proce-dures? Sleep Breath 2012;16(3):609–15.

39. Thomson A, Andrew G, Jones DB. Optimal sedation for gastrointestinal endoscopy: review and recom-mendations. J Gastroenterol Hepatol 2010;25(3): 469–78.

40. Nickol AH, Leverment J, Richards P, et al. Temaze-pam at high altitude reduces periodic breathing without impairing next-day performance: a random-ized cross-over double-blind study. J Sleep Res 2006;15(4):445–54.

41. Guilleminault C, Clerk A, Labanowski M, et al. Car-diac failure and benzodiazepines. Sleep 1993;16(6): 524–8.

42. Wang D, Marshall NS, Duffin J, et al. Phenotyping interindividual variability in obstructive sleep apnoea response to temazepam using ventilatory chemore-flexes during wakefulness. J Sleep Res 2011;20(4): 526–32.

43. Bonnet MH, Dexter JR, Arand DL. The effect of tria-zolam on arousal and respiration in central sleep apnea patients. Sleep 1990;13(1):31–41.

44. Aurora RN, Chowdhuri S, Ramar K, et al. The treatment of central sleep apnea syndromes in adults: practice parameters with an evidence-based literature review and meta-analyses. Sleep 2012;35(1):17–40.

45. Abraham J. Transnational industrial power, the medical profession and the regulatory state: adverse drug reactions and the crisis over the safety of Halcin in the Netherlands and the UK. Soc Sci Med 2002;55(9):1671–90.

46. Steens RD, Pouliot Z, Millar TW, et al. Effects of zol-pidem and triazolam on sleep and respiration in mild to moderate chronic obstructive pulmonary disease. Sleep 1993;16(4):318–26.

47. Rhodes SP, Parry P, Hanning CD. A comparison of the effects of zolpidem and placebo on respiration and oxygen saturation during sleep in the healthy elderly. Br J Clin Pharmacol 1990;30(6):817–24.

48. Berry RB, Patel PB. Effect of zolpidem on the effi-cacy of continuous positive airway pressure as treat-ment for obstructive sleep apnea. Sleep 2006;29(8): 1052–6.

49. Kolla BP, Lovely JK, Mansukhani MP, et al. Zolpidem is independently associated with in-creased risk of inpatient falls. J Hosp Med 2013; 8:1–6. http://dx.doi.org/10.1002/jhm.1985.

50. Park JG, Olson EJ, Morgenthaler TI. Impact of zale-plon on continuous positive airway pressure therapy compliance. J Clin Sleep Med 2013, in press.

51. Lofaso F, Goldenberg F, Thebault C, et al. Effect of zopiclone on sleep, night-time ventilation, and day-time vigilance in upper airway resistance syndrome. Eur Respir J 1997;10(11):2573–7.

52. Eckert DJ, Owens RL, Kehlmann GB, et al. Eszopi-clone increases the respiratory arousal threshold and lowers the apnoea/hypopnoea index in obstructive

sleep apnoea patients with a low arousal threshold. Clin Sci (Lond) 2011;120(12):505–14.

53. Lettieri CJ, Quast TN, Eliasson AH, et al. Eszopiclone improves overnight polysomnography and continuous positive airway pressure titration: a prospective, randomized, placebo-controlled trial. Sleep 2008;31(9):1310–6.

54. Lettieri CJ, Shah AA, Holley AB, et al. Effects of a short course of eszopiclone on continuous positive airway pressure adherence: a randomized trial. Ann Intern Med 2009;151(10):696–702.

55. Kryger M, Wang-Weigand S, Roth T. Safety of ramelteon in individuals with mild to moderate obstructive sleep apnea. Sleep Breath 2007;11(3):159–64.

56. Gooneratne NS, Gehrman P, Gurubhagavatula I, et al. Effectiveness of ramelteon for insomnia symptoms in older adults with obstructive sleep apnea: a randomized placebo-controlled pilot study. J Clin Sleep Med 2010;6(6):572–80.

57. Gilson AM, Ryan KM, Joranson DE, et al. A reassessment of trends in the medical use and abuse of opioid analgesics and implications for diversion control: 1997-2002. J Pain Symptom Manage 2004;28(2):176–88.

58. Joranson DE, Ryan KM, Gilson AM, et al. Trends in medical use and abuse of opioid analgesics. JAMA 2000;283(13):1710–4.

59. Atweh SF, Kuhar MJ. Distribution and physiological significance of opioid receptors in the brain. Br Med Bull 1983;39(1):47–52.

60. Meunier JC, Mollereau C, Toll L, et al. Isolation and structure of the endogenous agonist of opioid receptor-like ORL1 receptor. Nature 1995;377(6549):532–5.

61. Hughes J, Smith TW, Kosterlitz HW, et al. Identification of two related pentapeptides from the brain with potent opiate agonist activity. Nature 1975;258(5536):577–80.

62. Bouillon T, Bruhn J, Roepcke H, et al. Opioid-induced respiratory depression is associated with increased tidal volume variability. Eur J Anaesthesiol 2003;20(2):127–33.

63. Weil JV, McCullough RE, Kline JS, et al. Diminished ventilatory response to hypoxia and hypercapnia after morphine in normal man. N Engl J Med 1975;292(21):1103–6.

64. Leino K, Mildh L, Lertola K, et al. Time course of changes in breathing pattern in morphine- and oxycodone-induced respiratory depression. Anaesthesia 1999;54(9):835–40.

65. Mellen NM, Janczewski WA, Bocchiaro CM, et al. Opioid-induced quantal slowing reveals dual networks for respiratory rhythm generation. Neuron 2003;37(5):821–6.

66. Zhang Z, Xu F, Zhang C, et al. Activation of opioid mu receptors in caudal medullary raphe region

67. Pokorski M, Lahiri S. Effects of naloxone on carotid body chemoreception and ventilation in the cat. J Appl Physiol 1981;51(6):1533–8.

68. Hajiha M, DuBord MA, Liu H, et al. Opioid receptor mechanisms at the hypoglossal motor pool and effects on tongue muscle activity in vivo. J Physiol 2009;587(Pt 11):2677–92.

69. Santiago TV, Edelman NH. Opioids and breathing. J Appl Physiol 1985;59(6):1675–85.

70. Drummond GB. Comparison of decreases in ventilation caused by enflurane and fentanyl during anaesthesia. Br J Anaesth 1983;55(9):825–35.

71. Lalley PM. Opioidergic and dopaminergic modulation of respiration. Respir Physiol Neurobiol 2008;164(1–2):160–7.

72. Wang D, Teichtahl H. Opioids, sleep architecture and sleep-disordered breathing. Sleep Med Rev 2007;11(1):35–46.

73. Walker JM, Farney RJ, Rhondeau SM, et al. Chronic opioid use is a risk factor for the development of central sleep apnea and ataxic breathing [Erratum appears in J Clin Sleep Med 2007;3(6):table of contents]. J Clin Sleep Med 2007;3(5):455–61.

74. Yue HJ, Guilleminault C. Opioid medication and sleep-disordered breathing. Med Clin North Am 2010;94(3):435–46.

75. Dimsdale JE, Norman D, DeJardin D, et al. The effect of opioids on sleep architecture. J Clin Sleep Med 2007;3(1):33–6.

76. Bernards CM, Knowlton SL, Schmidt DF, et al. Respiratory and sleep effects of remifentanil in volunteers with moderate obstructive sleep apnea. Anesthesiology 2009;110(1):41–9.

77. Catley DM, Thornton C, Jordan C, et al. Pronounced, episodic oxygen desaturation in the postoperative period: its association with ventilatory pattern and analgesic regimen. Anesthesiology 1985;63(1):20–8.

78. Esclamado RM, Glenn MG, McCulloch TM, et al. Perioperative complications and risk factors in the surgical treatment of obstructive sleep apnea syndrome. Laryngoscope 1989;99(11):1125–9.

79. Ostermeier AM, Roizen MF, Hautkappe M, et al. Three sudden postoperative respiratory arrests associated with epidural opioids in patients with sleep apnea. Anesth Analg 1997;85(2):452–60.

80. Mogri M, Desai H, Webster L, et al. Hypoxemia in patients on chronic opiate therapy with and without sleep apnea. Sleep Breath 2009;13(1):49–57.

81. Webster LR, Choi Y, Desai H, et al. Sleep-disordered breathing and chronic opioid therapy. Pain Med 2008;9(4):425–32.

82. Wang D, Teichtahl H, Drummer O, et al. Central sleep apnea in stable methadone maintenance treatment patients. Chest 2005;128(3):1348–56.

inhibits the ventilatory response to hypercapnia in anesthetized rats. Anesthesiology 2007;107(2):288–97.

83. Guilleminault C, Cao M, Yue HJ, et al. Obstructive sleep apnea and chronic opioid use. Lung 2010; 188(6):459–68.

84. Hullett BJ, Chambers NA, Pascoe EM, et al. Tramadol vs morphine during adenotonsillectomy for obstructive sleep apnea in children. Paediatr Anaesth 2006;16(6):648–53.

85. Ramar K. Reversal of sleep-disordered breathing with opioid withdrawal. Pain Pract 2009;9(5):394–8.

86. Farney RJ, Walker JM, Boyle KM, et al. Adaptive servoventilation (ASV) in patients with sleep disordered breathing associated with chronic opioid medications for non-malignant pain. J Clin Sleep Med 2008;4(4):311–9.

87. Schönhofer B, Köhler D. Benzodiazepine receptor antagonist (flumazenil) does not affect sleep-related breathing disorders. Eur Respir J 1996;9(9):1816–20.

88. Oshima T, Masaki Y, Toyooka H. Flumazenil antagonizes midazolam-induced airway narrowing during nasal breathing in humans. Br J Anaesth 1999; 82(5):698–702.

89. Rishi MA, Shetty M, Wolff A, et al. Atypical antipsychotic medications are independently associated with severe obstructive sleep apnea. Clin Neuropharmacol 2010;33(3):109–13.

90. Höijer U, Hedner J, Ejnell H, et al. Nitrazepam in patients with sleep apnoea: a double-blind placebo-controlled study. Eur Respir J 1994;7(11):2011–5.

Pathophysiologic Considerations of Perioperative Respiratory Managements of Obese Patients with Obstructive Sleep Apnea

Shiroh Isono, MD

KEYWORDS

- Obstructive sleep apnea • Obesity • Perioperative respiratory management
- Postoperative respiratory complications

KEY POINTS

- Anesthesia and surgical interventions increase the severity of obstructive sleep apnea, possibly by further reducing the lung volume and producing upper airway swelling.
- Strategies for maintaining pharyngeal airway patency by improving lung volume and upper airway anatomic imbalance may therefore decrease the incidence of adverse postoperative respiratory complications in obese patients with obstructive sleep apnea.
- These speculations need further extensive collaborative investigations between anesthesiologists and sleep physicians.

Anesthesia and surgical interventions significantly alter the structures and neural control of the respiratory system, resulting in respiratory depression to some extent in any postoperative subject (**Fig. 1**). The respiratory depression leads to pathologic hypoxemia, possibly increasing postoperative morbidity and mortality when subjects have risk factors for the respiratory complications. Among the risk factors, obesity and obstructive sleep apnea (OSA) make it difficult for anesthesiologists and other related medical personnel, including sleep physicians, to achieve safe and appropriate perioperative airway management of these patients. Obesity and OSA are independent risk factors for a combination of impossible mask ventilation and difficult tracheal intubation during anesthesia induction, possibly leading to a fatal outcome.[1] Impaired oxygenation is commonly encountered in anesthetized and mechanically ventilated patients with obesity.[2] Obesity is a significant independent risk factor for respiratory complications such as upper airway obstruction and hypoxemia immediately after surgery.[3] Furthermore, morbid obesity and OSA are identified as independent risk factors for increased postoperative mortality, particularly in male

This work was completed at the Department of Anesthesiology, Graduate School of Medicine, Chiba University.
Funding: This study was supported by grant-in-aid no. 24390363 from the Ministry of Education, Culture, Sports, Science and Technology, Tokyo, Japan.
Department of Anesthesiology, Graduate School of Medicine, Chiba University, 1-8-1 Inohana-cho, Chuo-ku, Chiba 260-8670, Japan
E-mail address: shirohisono@yahoo.co.jp

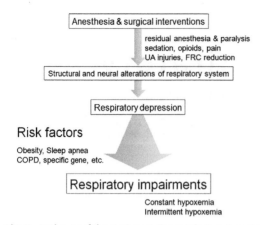

Fig. 1. Pathway of the perioperative respiratory impairments. COPD, chronic obstructive pulmonary disease; FRC, functional residual capacity; UA, upper airway.

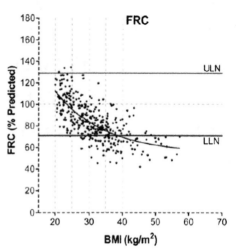

Fig. 2. Relationship between BMI and FRC with an exponential regression line [FRC = 231.9 exp ($-0.070 \times$ BMI) 55.2, r^2 = 0.49], in 373 individuals of both genders with normal FEV_1/FVC (forced expiratory volume in 1 second/forced vital capacity). LLN, lower limit of normal; ULN, upper limit of normal. (*From* Jones RL, Nzekwu MM. The effects of body mass index on lung volumes. Chest 2006;130:832; with permission.)

patients.[4,5] This article discusses pathophysiologic considerations in the perioperative respiratory management of obese patients with OSA.

THE BURDEN OF OBESITY ON RESPIRATORY FUNCTIONS: THE IMPORTANCE OF FAT DISTRIBUTION

Obesity is a burden on various respiratory functions. In particular, fat deposition in 2 distinct regions, the abdomen and upper airways, significantly influences oxygenation and upper airway patency. Body mass index (BMI) is a global expression of obesity and does not indicate fat distribution. BMI is a significant but weak variable predicting impairments of various respiratory functions. Fat distribution in these regions can be easily assessed clinically by waist/hip ratio and neck circumference, which is significantly associated with oxygenation[6] and development of OSA.[7]

LUNG FUNCTION IN OBESE PATIENTS

Obesity significantly impairs lung function.[8] Both total lung capacity and vital capacity decrease with increasing BMI, but are maintained at more than 80% of predicted values even in morbidly obese patients. In contrast, functional residual capacity (FRC) significantly and progressively decreases with increasing BMI and is less than 70% of a predicted value when BMI exceeds 35 kg/m² (Fig. 2). FRC reduction is mainly caused by reduction of expiratory reserve volume and not reserve volume, indicating involvement of alveolar atelectasis. Diffusion capacity is not impaired by obesity alone and constant hypoxemia in obese patients is usually caused by FRC reduction if ventilation is maintained.

PERIOPERATIVE CONSTANT HYPOXEMIA IN OBESE PATIENTS

Induction of general anesthesia produces alveolar atelectasis at dependent lung regions within a few minutes and decreases FRC by approximately 500 mL, corresponding with 17% of awake FRC in nonobese subjects.[9] Hypoxemia during mechanical ventilation in anesthetized and paralyzed patients is attributed to FRC reduction[10] (Fig. 3). This phenomenon is more common and persistent in morbidly obese patients. In patients with BMIs of 51 ± 10 kg/m², Damia and colleagues[11] showed significant FRC reduction by 1.20 ± 0.72 L, which corresponds with 50% of the awake FRC value. The FRC reduction continues more than 24 hours after cessation of general anesthesia in patients undergoing major abdominal surgery[12] and in obese patients undergoing even minor surgery.[13] To prevent or reverse the FRC reduction in obese patients, application of positive end-expiratory pressure (PEEP) alone is not enough and a combination of lung recruitment maneuver (40 cm H_2O for 40 seconds) and application of high PEEP (10 cm H_2O) is necessary.[14] Reversed Trendelenburg position, beach chair position, or sitting position improves both lung volume and oxygenation, but pneumoperitoneum offsets the beneficial effects of these maneuvers and techniques.[15] Use of nasal continuous positive airway pressure (CPAP) immediately after

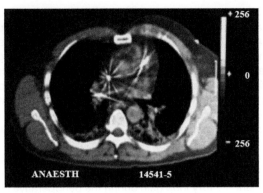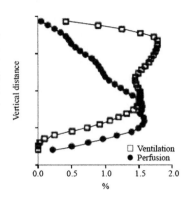

Fig. 3. Transverse computed tomography scan showing pulmonary atelectasis at the dependent parts of both lungs (*left panel*) and corresponding vertical distributions of ventilation and lung blood flow (*right panel*) in an anesthetized subject. The mismatch between the ventilation and perfusion caused by the atelectasis is the main mechanism of the postoperative constant hypoxemia. (*Reprinted* by permission of Edizioni Minerva Medica from Minerva Anestesiologica 2002 May;68(5):332–6.)

surgery improves oxygenation and decreases the incidence of postoperative reintubation.[16]

OBESITY AND OSA

Longitudinal epidemiologic studies show that weight gain increases OSA frequency in both men and women, and weight loss improves OSA severity more in men than in women.[17] However, cross-sectional studies show that larger neck circumference as an indicator of fat deposition around the pharyngeal airway, and larger waist/hip ratio as an indicator of abdominal fat deposition differentiate OSA and non-OSA better than BMI.[7] Fat deposition at different locations increases pharyngeal collapsibility differently.

FAT DEPOSITION AROUND THE PHARYNGEAL AIRWAY: UPPER AIRWAY ANATOMIC IMBALANCE

The pharyngeal airway is surrounded by soft tissue such as the tongue, soft palate, and tonsils, and is enclosed by bony structures such as the mandible, maxilla, and cervical spines. Based on the structural feature, we proposed that anatomic imbalance caused by either an excessive amount of soft tissue or smaller bony enclosure size can result in narrowing of the pharyngeal airway space and development of OSA (the anatomic balance theory; **Fig. 4**).[18] The tongue is larger in patients with OSA than in subjects with size-matched bony enclosures and without OSA, which supports the anatomic balance theory.[19] OSA can be caused by a small increase in fat deposition around the pharyngeal airway in patients with smaller craniofacial size. The anatomic imbalance can be clinically indicated by larger neck circumference,[20] higher Mallampati class,[21]

and excessive submandibular soft tissue.[22] In addition to excessive perioperative fluid administration and direct surgical procedures on the upper airway region, the Trendelenburg or prone positions can produce marked swelling of the upper airway soft tissue, further impairing the upper airway anatomic balance during the perioperative period.

POSTOPERATIVE LUNG VOLUME REDUCTION AND INTERMITTENT EPISODIC HYPOXEMIA

In addition to development of constant hypoxemia, postoperative FRC reduction possibly contributes to worsening of OSA severity because the lung volume reduction increases pharyngeal

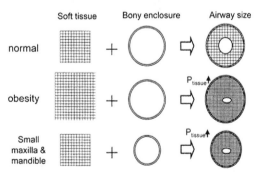

Fig. 4. Interaction between soft tissue around the pharyngeal airway and craniofacial bony enclosure (anatomic balance theory). P_{tissue}, tissue pressure. (*Reprinted* with permission of the American Thoracic Society. Copyright © 2013 American Thoracic Society. Watanabe T, Isono S, Tanaka A, et al. Contribution of body habitus and craniofacial characteristics to segmental closing pressures of the passive pharynx in patients with sleep-disordered breathing. American Journal of Respiratory and Critical Care Med 2002;165:260–5. Official journal of the American Thoracic Society.)

collapsibility and breathing instability.[23] Although the lung does not directly connect to the pharyngeal airway, the trachea is displaced caudally with increasing lung volume, increasing longitudinal tension of the pharyngeal airway wall. A change of lung volume of 0.7 L resulted in an average change of closing pressure of 2 cm H_2O in patients with OSA, and the effect was greater in obese patients with OSA.[24] A 1-L increase in the lung volume during sleep decreased OSA frequency by approximately one-third in obese patients with OSA.[25] The effect of lung volume on pharyngeal collapsibility was more prominent in men than in women.[26] Although speculative at present, lung volume increase or prevention of lung volume reduction during the perioperative period may be beneficial for obese male patients with OSA.

POSSIBLE CHANGES OF LOOP GAIN OF THE RESPIRATORY CONTROL SYSTEM DURING THE PERIOPERATIVE PERIOD

Recent evidence suggests that any increase in the loop gain of negative feedback to the respiratory system promotes respiratory instability leading to central and/or obstructive periodic breathing.[27] In patients with OSA with similar pharyngeal collapsibility, the loop gain obtained during sleep was significantly associated with OSA severity.[28] Although various mechanisms may be involved in the increased loop gain in obese patients with OSA, increased visceral fat possibly increases the gain. A low lung volume associated with abdominal obesity accelerates changes of alveolar carbon dioxide concentration increasing plant gain of the respiratory loop gain. Hypercapnic ventilatory response, which increases controller gain of the respiratory loop gain, is reported to be associated with levels of circulating leptin, which is predominantly secreted from visceral fat.[29] Although the respiratory loop gain during the perioperative period has not been assessed, reversal and maintenance of lung volume by optimizing body position and applying CPAP may stabilize breathing during postoperative nights. Residual anesthetics and opioids for postoperative pain can depress the hypercapnic ventilatory and arousal responses, possibly decreasing the controller gain, and therefore may be beneficial if not excessive. Higher leptin levels in obese patients with OSA were independent of obesity and were reversed by short-term CPAP,[30] suggesting the importance of preoperative CPAP for stabilizing breathing as well as for getting used to the device. More importantly, oxygen administration, which reduces the respiratory loop gain, is reported to decrease the Apnea-Hypopnea Index in patients with OSA with higher loop gain,[31]

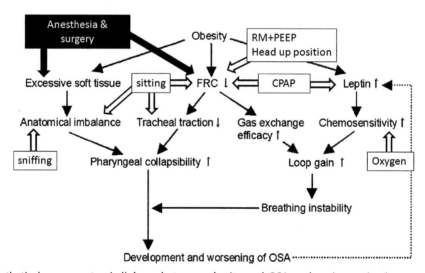

Fig. 5. Hypothetical neuroanatomic linkage between obesity and OSA and perioperative interventions to the pathways. Anatomic imbalance of the pharyngeal airway, lung volume reduction, and breathing instability may significantly contribute to development and deterioration of OSA in obese persons (*thin arrows*). Anesthesia and surgical interventions further increase OSA by further reducing FRC and producing upper airway swelling (*thick closed arrows*). CPAP application, oxygen administration, sniffing position with an appropriate pillow, and sitting position can prevent or improve OSA (*thick open arrows*). RM, Recruitment maneuver. (*Modified from* Isono S. Obstructive sleep apnea of obese adults: pathophysiology and perioperative airway management. Anesthesiology 2009;110:908–21; with permission.)

suggesting an advantage of postoperative oxygen therapy, particularly in patients with CPAP intolerance.

AIRWAY MANAGEMENT STRATEGIES DURING THE PERIOPERATIVE PERIOD

The pathophysiologic considerations discussed earlier suggest that obesity-related postoperative respiratory complications such as constant hypoxemia and intermittent hypoxemia can be reduced by (1) increasing or maintaining lung volume, (2) improving anatomic imbalance, and (3) controlling the respiratory loop gain (**Fig. 5**).[32] Among the possible strategies clinically available and applicable, CPAP is effective but has poor compliance, particularly in patients with OSA who have no experience of wearing the CPAP mask. The sniffing position, using an appropriately placed pillow, improves anatomic balance and pharyngeal airway patency.[33] If patients are hemodynamically stable, the sitting posture is a comfortable and effective position for improving oxygenation and pharyngeal airway patency because it improves anatomic balance by displacing soft tissue outside the bony enclosure, and increases longitudinal pharyngeal wall tension by increasing lung volume (**Fig. 6**).[34] Furthermore, in patients with CPAP intolerance, oxygen therapy reduces the respiratory loop gain and improves the OSA severity.[28]

In conclusion, anesthesia and surgical interventions increase the severity of OSA, possibly by further reducing the lung volume and producing upper airway swelling. Strategies for maintaining pharyngeal airway patency by improving lung volume and upper airway anatomic imbalance may therefore decrease the incidence of adverse postoperative respiratory complications in obese patients with OSA. These strategies are speculative and need further extensive collaborative investigation between anesthesiologists and sleep physicians.

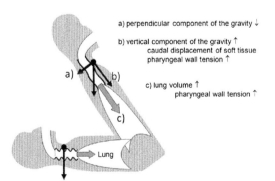

Fig. 6. Possible mechanisms of pharyngeal airway patency improvement in the sitting position. (*From* Tagaito Y, Isono S, Tanaka A, et al. Sitting posture decreases collapsibility of the passive pharynx in anesthetized paralyzed patients with obstructive sleep apnea. Anesthesiology 2010;113:812–8; with permission.)

Labels in figure:
a) perpendicular component of the gravity ↓
b) vertical component of the gravity ↑
caudal displacement of soft tissue
pharyngeal wall tension ↑
c) lung volume ↑
pharyngeal wall tension ↑
Lung

REFERENCES

1. Kheterpal S, Martin L, Shanks AM, et al. Prediction and outcomes of impossible mask ventilation: a review of 50,000 anesthetics. Anesthesiology 2009;110:891–7.
2. Aldenkortt M, Lysakowski C, Elia N, et al. Ventilation strategies in obese patients undergoing surgery: a quantitative systematic review and meta-analysis. Br J Anaesth 2012;109:493–502.
3. Asai T, Koga K, Vaughan RS. Respiratory complications associated with tracheal intubation and extubation. Br J Anaesth 1998;80:767–75.
4. Flancbaum L, Belsley S. Factors affecting morbidity and mortality of Roux-en-Y gastric bypass for clinically severe obesity: an analysis of 1,000 consecutive open cases by a single surgeon. J Gastrointest Surg 2007;11:500–7.
5. Longitudinal Assessment of Bariatric Surgery (LABS) Consortium, Flum DR, Belle SH, King WC, et al. Perioperative safety in the longitudinal assessment of bariatric surgery. N Engl J Med 2009;361:445–54.
6. Zavorsky GS, Christou NV, Kim do J, et al. Preoperative gender differences in pulmonary gas exchange in morbidly obese subjects. Obes Surg 2008;18:1587–98.
7. Grunstein R, Wilcox I, Yang TS, et al. Snoring and sleep apnoea in men: association with central obesity and hypertension. Int J Obes Relat Metab Disord 1993;17:533–40.
8. Jones RL, Nzekwu MM. The effects of body mass index on lung volumes. Chest 2006;130:827–33.
9. Hedenstierna G, Strandberg A, Brismar B, et al. Functional residual capacity, thoracoabdominal dimensions, and central blood volume during general anesthesia with muscle paralysis and mechanical ventilation. Anesthesiology 1985;62:247–54.
10. Hedenstierna G. Airway closure, atelectasis and gas exchange during anaesthesia. Minerva Anestesiol 2002;68:332–6.
11. Damia G, Mascheroni D, Croci M, et al. Perioperative changes in functional residual capacity in morbidly obese patients. Br J Anaesth 1988;60:574–8.
12. Ford GT, Whitelaw WA, Rosenal TW, et al. Diaphragm function after upper abdominal surgery in humans. Am Rev Respir Dis 1983;127:431–6.
13. Eichenberger A, Proietti S, Wicky S, et al. Morbid obesity and postoperative pulmonary atelectasis: an underestimated problem. Anesth Analg 2002;95:1788–92.
14. Futier E, Constantin JM, Pelosi P, et al. Noninvasive ventilation and alveolar recruitment maneuver

improve respiratory function during and after intubation of morbidly obese patients: a randomized controlled study. Anesthesiology 2011;114:1354–63.

15. Valenza F, Vagginelli F, Tiby A, et al. Effects of the beach chair position, positive end-expiratory pressure, and pneumoperitoneum on respiratory function in morbidly obese patients during anesthesia and paralysis. Anesthesiology 2007;107:725–32.

16. Squadrone V, Coha M, Cerutti E, et al, Piedmont Intensive Care Units Network (PICUN). Continuous positive airway pressure for treatment of postoperative hypoxemia: a randomized controlled trial. JAMA 2005;293:589–95.

17. Newman AB, Foster G, Givelber R, et al. Progression and regression of sleep-disordered breathing with changes in weight: the Sleep Heart Health Study. Arch Intern Med 2005;165:2408–13.

18. Watanabe T, Isono S, Tanaka A, et al. Contribution of body habitus and craniofacial characteristics to segmental closing pressures of the passive pharynx in patients with sleep-disordered breathing. Am J Respir Crit Care Med 2002;165:260–5.

19. Tsuiki S, Isono S, Ishikawa T, et al. Anatomical balance of the upper airway and obstructive sleep apnea. Anesthesiology 2008;108:1009–15.

20. Flemons WW, Whitelaw WA, Brant R, et al. Likelihood ratios for a sleep apnea clinical prediction rule. Am J Respir Crit Care Med 1994;150:1279–85.

21. Nuckton TJ, Glidden DV, Browner WS, et al. Physical examination: Mallampati score as an independent predictor of obstructive sleep apnea. Sleep 2006; 29:903–8.

22. Tsai WH, Remmers JE, Brant R, et al. A decision rule for diagnostic testing in obstructive sleep apnea. Am J Respir Crit Care Med 2003;167:1427–32.

23. Isono S, Sha M, Suzukawa M, et al. Preoperative nocturnal desaturations as a risk factor for late postoperative nocturnal desaturations. Br J Anaesth 1998;80:602–5.

24. Tagaito Y, Isono S, Remmers JE, et al. Lung volume and collapsibility of the passive pharynx in patients with sleep-disordered breathing. J Appl Physiol 2007;103:1379–85.

25. Heinzer RC, Stanchina ML, Malhotra A, et al. Effect of increased lung volume on sleep disordered breathing in patients with sleep apnoea. Thorax 2006;61:435–9.

26. Squier SB, Patil SP, Schneider H, et al. Effect of end-expiratory lung volume on upper airway collapsibility in sleeping men and women. J Appl Physiol 2010; 109:977–85.

27. Younes M, Ostrowski M, Thompson W, et al. Chemical control stability in patients with obstructive sleep apnea. Am J Respir Crit Care Med 2001; 163:1181–90.

28. Wellman A, Jordan AS, Malhotra A, et al. Ventilatory control and airway anatomy in obstructive sleep apnea. Am J Respir Crit Care Med 2004;170: 1225–32.

29. Makinodan K, Yoshikawa M, Fukuoka A, et al. Effect of serum leptin levels on hypercapnic ventilatory response in obstructive sleep apnea. Respiration 2008;75:257–64.

30. Chin K, Shimizu K, Nakamura T, et al. Changes in intra-abdominal visceral fat and serum leptin levels in patients with obstructive sleep apnea syndrome following nasal continuous positive airway pressure therapy. Circulation 1999;100:706–12.

31. Wellman A, Malhotra A, Jordan AS, et al. Effect of oxygen in obstructive sleep apnea: role of loop gain. Respir Physiol Neurobiol 2008;162:144–51.

32. Isono S. Obstructive sleep apnea of obese adults: pathophysiology and perioperative airway management. Anesthesiology 2009;110:908–21.

33. Isono S, Tanaka A, Ishikawa T, et al. Sniffing position improves pharyngeal airway patency in anesthetized patients with obstructive sleep apnea. Anesthesiology 2005;103:489–94.

34. Tagaito Y, Isono S, Tanaka A, et al. Sitting posture decreases collapsibility of the passive pharynx in anesthetized paralyzed patients with obstructive sleep apnea. Anesthesiology 2010;113:812–8.

A Screening Tool of Obstructive Sleep Apnea
STOP-Bang Questionnaire

Yiliang Yang, MD, PhD[a], Frances Chung, MBBS, FRCPC[b],*

KEYWORDS

• STOP-Bang questionnaire • Obstructive sleep apnea • Surgical patient • Sensitivity • Specificity
• Screening tool

KEY POINTS

• The STOP-Bang questionnaire is a concise and easy-to use screening tool to identify patients with obstructive sleep apnea (OSA).
• A STOP-Bang score of 0 to 2 identifies patients with low risk of OSA; a STOP-Bang score of 3 to 4 identifies patients at intermediate risk of OSA; and a STOP-Bang score of 5 to 8 identifies patients at high risk of OSA.

Preoperative screening, evaluation, and optimization of the patient's medical condition before surgery are important components of safe practice. Obstructive sleep apnea (OSA) is a common disorder (2%–26% of the population) that is caused by repetitive partial or complete obstruction of the upper airway, characterized by episodes of breathing cessation during sleep. Patients with OSA may pose significant problems in the perioperative period. Some studies showed that OSA is associated with an increase in postoperative complications and is an independent risk factor for increased morbidity and mortality.[1–3] Therefore, it is imperative to have an early diagnosis of OSA.

OSA is characterized by repetitive narrowing and closure of the upper airway during sleep. Sleep apnea should be suspected in the patient with the signs and symptoms shown in **Table 1**.[4] In addition, epidemiologic and clinical evidences strongly suggest that there are many predisposing conditions and risk factors associated with OSA, such as sex, aging, obesity, menopausal status, ethnic origin, alcohol, and smoking.[5]

It has been estimated that 82% of men and 92% of women with moderate to severe sleep apnea have not been diagnosed.[6,7] The diagnosis of OSA is established by an overnight sleep study (polysomnography [PSG]). Although PSG is the gold standard for the identification of patients with OSA, it is expensive, requiring highly trained personnel and sophisticated equipment. The limited availability of PSG has created demand to use clinical features to screen patients for possible OSA.

Simpler strategies are needed in the diagnostic clinical pathway for OSA. A screening tool is necessary to stratify patients based on their clinical symptoms, their physical examinations, and their risk factors, to ascertain patients at high risk and in urgent need of PSG or further treatment and patients at low risk who may not need PSG. The use of preoperative screening tools helps to identify patients with undiagnosed OSA.

There have been numerous efforts to devise alternative clinical methods of predicting OSA, which are broadly classified as questionnaires and clinical prediction models. A clinical model

[a] Department of Anesthesia, Toronto Western Hospital, University Health Network, University of Toronto, 399 Bathurst Street, Toronto, Ontario M5T 2S8, Canada; [b] Department of Anesthesia, Toronto Western Hospital, University Health Network, University of Toronto, Room 405, 2McL, 399 Bathurst Street, Toronto, Ontario M5T 2S8, Canada
* Corresponding author.
E-mail address: Frances.Chung@uhn.ca

Sleep Med Clin 8 (2013) 65–72
http://dx.doi.org/10.1016/j.jsmc.2012.11.004
1556-407X/13/$ – see front matter © 2013 Elsevier Inc. All rights reserved.

Table 1
Symptoms and signs of OSA

Diurnal Symptoms of OSA	Nocturnal Symptoms of OSA
Daytime sleepiness; memory and concentration dysfunction; sexual dysfunction; gastroesophageal reflux; behavioral irritability (irritability, depression, chronic fatigue, delirium); road traffic accident	Heavy persistent snoring, worse in supine position or after alcohol or sedatives; apnea with limb movement, witnessed by bed partner; sudden awakening with noisy breathing; accidents related to sleepiness; nocturnal sweating; wake up with dry mouth; nocturnal epilepsy; nocturia

Signs Associated with OSA

Edematous soft palate or uvula
Long soft palate and uvula
Decreased oropharyngeal dimensions
Nasal obstruction
Maxillary hypoplasia
Retrognathia
Central adiposity and increased neck circumference
Hypertension and other cardiovascular consequences

From Chung F, Elsaid H. Screening for obstructive sleep apnea before surgery: why is it important? Curr Opin Anaesthesiol 2009;22:406; with permission.

combines elements of history and physical examination, with or without additional measurements and investigations (radiology or oximetry). A questionnaire is defined as a set of questions, with no additional physical measurement involved. Clinical models designed for OSA screening usually require specific technology, such as cephalometry and morphometry or the assistance of a computer. Despite high test accuracy, these models may not be suitable for clinical practice because they are cumbersome in routine evaluation.

Most of predictive models, based on the different combinations of witnessed apneas, snoring, gasping, body mass index (BMI, calculated as weight in kilograms divided by the square of height in meters), age, sex, and hypertension, were developed and validated in patients from sleep centers. They may not apply to the patients in general because there are basic differences between the study population in sleep laboratories and the general population.

Several questionnaire-based screening tools for OSA are available,[8] such as the STOP-Bang questionnaires,[9] the snoring questionnaire,[10] the sleep questionnaire,[11] the Berlin questionnaire,[12] the sleep apnea clinical score,[13] the sleep apnea scale of the sleep disorders questionnaire,[14] the American Society of Anesthesiologists (ASA) checklist,[15] the perioperative sleep apnea prediction score,[16] and the Epworth Sleepiness Scale.[17]

The Berlin questionnaire is a widely used screening tool for OSA with 10 questions and was developed for a primary care population.[12] It consists of 5 items on snoring, 3 items on excessive daytime sleepiness, 1 item on sleepiness while driving, and 1 item enquiring about a history of hypertension. The ASA checklist was developed by the ASA taskforce on OSA and comprises 14 items categorized into physical characteristics, history of apparent airway obstruction during sleep, and complaints of somnolence.[15]

The STOP-Bang questionnaire comprises 8 items on snoring, tiredness/sleepiness, observed apnea, hypertension, BMI, age, neck circumference, and gender (**Table 2**). The linear scale and the simple acronym make the STOP-Bang practical in the preoperative setting to identify patients with a high risk of OSA.[9]

This article reviews the STOP-Bang questionnaire and its validation in the different population.

DEVELOPMENT OF STOP-BANG QUESTIONNAIRE

The STOP-Bang questionnaire was developed and validated in surgical patients.[9] The Berlin questionnaire was condensed and modified into a shorter 4-item OSA screening questionnaire (STOP). The STOP questionnaire contains 4 questions: S, "Do you snore loudly, loud enough to be heard through a closed door?"; T, "Do you feel tired or fatigued during the daytime almost every day?"; O, "Has anyone observed that you stop breathing during sleep?"; and P, "Do you have

Table 2
STOP-Bang questionnaire

	Question	Answer	Answer
S	Snoring: do you snore loudly (louder than talking or loud enough to be heard through closed doors)?	Yes	No
T	Tired: do you often feel tired, fatigued, or sleepy during daytime?	Yes	No
O	Observed: has anyone observed you stop breathing during your sleep?	Yes	No
P	Blood pressure: do you have or are you being treated for high blood pressure?	Yes	No
B	BMI: >35 kg/m^2?	Yes	No
A	Age: >50 y?	Yes	No
N	Neck circumference: neck circumference >40 cm?	Yes	No
G	Gender: male?	Yes	No

STOP-Bang score 0–2, low risk of OSA.
STOP-Bang score 3–4, intermediate risk of OSA.
STOP-Bang score 5–8, high risk of OSA.
    Modified from Chung F, Yegneswaran B, Liao P, et al. STOP questionnaire a tool to screen obstructive sleep apnea. Anesthesiology 2008;108:812–21 and Chung F, Subramanyam R, Liao P, et al. High STOP-Bang score indicates a high probability of obstructive sleep apnoea. Br J Anaesth 2012;108:768–75.

a history of high blood pressure with or without treatment?". In order to keep the questionnaire concise and easy to use, the questions were designed in a yes/no format. The sensitivity of the STOP questionnaire with apnea-hypopnea index (AHI) greater than 15 and greater than 30 as cutoffs was 74% and 80% and the specificity 53% and 49%, respectively.

When incorporating 4 additional variables with the acronym Bang (B, BMI >35 kg/m^2; A, age older than 50 years; N, neck circumference >40 cm; G, male gender), the STOP-Bang questionnaire (see **Table 2**) improved the sensitivity to 93% and 100% at the cutoffs of AHI >15 and AHI >30, respectively.[9] The specificity of the STOP-Bang was 43% and 37%. By incorporating BMI, age, neck circumference, and male gender (Bang) into the STOP questionnaire, the STOP-Bang model reached a very high level of sensitivity and negative predictive value (NPV), especially for patients with moderate and severe OSA. If the patient is ranked as a low risk of OSA by the STOP-Bang scoring model, one can be highly confident about excluding the possibility that the patient has moderate to severe sleep apnea.

We have shown that there was no significant difference in the predictive parameters of the Berlin questionnaire, the ASA checklist, and the STOP questionnaire. All the questionnaires showed a moderately high level of sensitivity for OSA screening (**Table 3**).[4] The sensitivities of the Berlin questionnaire, the ASA checklist, and STOP questionnaire were similar: 69% to 87%, 72% to 87%, and 66% to 80% at different AHI cutoffs.[18]

Table 3
Predictive parameters of STOP, STOP-Bang, Berlin, and ASA questionnaires

	STOP	STOP-Bang	Berlin	ASA
AHI >5				
Sensitivity (%)	65.6	83.6	68.9	72.1
Specificity (%)	60.0	56.4	56.4	38.2
PPV (%)	78.4	81.0	77.9	72.1
NPV (%)	44.0	60.8	44.9	38.2
Odds ratio	2.857	6.587	2.855	1.559
AHI >15				
Sensitivity (%)	74.3	92.9	78.6	78.6
Specificity (%)	53.3	43.0	50.5	37.4
PPV (%)	51.0	51.6	50.9	45.1
NPV (%)	76.0	90.2	78.3	72.7
Odds ratio	3.293	9.803	3.736	2.189
AHI >30				
Sensitivity (%)	79.5	100	87.2	87.2
Specificity (%)	48.6	37.0	46.4	36.2
PPV (%)	30.4	31.0	31.5	27.9
NPV (%)	89.3	100	92.8	90.9
Odds ratio	3.656	>999.999	5.881	3.862

Abbreviation: PPV, positive predictive value.
    Data are presented as mean.
    From Chung F, Elsaid H. Screening for obstructive sleep apnea before surgery: why is it important? Curr Opin Anaesthesiol 2009;22:408; with permission.

A recent meta-analysis of clinical screening tests for OSA identified 26 different clinical prediction tests, with 8 in the form of questionnaires, and 18 algorithms, regression models, or neural networks.[8] As a preoperative screening test, the summary recommendation was based on ease of use, false-negative rate, and test accuracy. The STOP-Bang questionnaire was a user-friendly and excellent method to predict severe OSA (AHI >30), with a high diagnostic odds ratio.

In a study of 1426 patients who were referred to the Sleep Disorder Center, Farney and colleagues[19] evaluated the possibility of using the STOP-Bang model to identify OSA. These investigators concluded that the STOP-Bang questionnaire can be used to estimate the probabilities of no OSA or mild, moderate, or severe OSA. There is a greater probability of more severe OSA with a higher cumulative score of the known risk factors as reflected by the STOP-Bang score. With any score greater than 4, the probability of having severe OSA increases continuously. With a score of 8, the probability of severe OSA was 81.9%.

Chung and colleagues[20] also evaluated the association between the STOP-Bang score and the probability of OSA in 746 surgical patients. With an increase in the STOP-Bang score, there was a corresponding increase in the predicted probability, odds ratio, and specificity for having OSA, moderate/severe OSA, and severe OSA. For detecting severe OSA, the odds ratio of a STOP-Bang score of 5 was 10 and the odds ratio of a STOP-Bang score of 7 and 8 was 15.[20] As the STOP-Bang score increased from 0 to 2 to 7 and 8, the probability of having moderate/severe OSA was increased from 18% to 60% and severe OSA from 4% to 38%, respectively.

The association between the STOP-Bang score and the probability of OSA would provide the perioperative care team with a useful tool to stratify patients for unrecognized OSA and triage patients for urgent diagnosis and treatment. Because a STOP-Bang score of 3 or greater showed a very high sensitivity and NPV for identifying moderate/severe OSA, score 3 as cutoff may be good for a surgical population with high OSA prevalence, such as bariatric surgical patients. Clinicians would be confident in ruling out the possibility of moderate/severe or severe OSA in patients with a STOP-Bang score of 0 to 2. On the other hand, a STOP-Bang score of 5 to 8 shows a high specificity to detect moderate and severe OSA (**Fig. 1**). For the general patient population, who have a low OSA prevalence, a high specificity may be useful to reduce the false-positive rate. The STOP-Bang score enables identification of those patients most in need of urgent evaluation and allows exclusion of patients from possible harm because of unrecognized sleep apnea.

A STOP-Bang score of 0 to 2 indicates a low risk of OSA. Patients with a score of 3 and 4 are at intermediate risk of OSA. A STOP-Bang score of 5 to 8 allows the team to identify patients with increased probability of moderate/severe OSA (see **Fig. 1**). The STOP-Bang score can help the health care team to stratify patients for unrecognized OSA, practice perioperative precautions, or triage patients for diagnosis and treatment.

VALIDATION OF STOP-BANG QUESTIONNAIRE

The STOP-Bang questionnaire has been used worldwide for screening patients with OSA. It has been validated in surgical patients,[21] the general population,[22,23] and patients referred to sleep clinics.[24]

In a study of patients in a sleep clinic setting, Silva and colleagues[22] found that the STOP-Bang

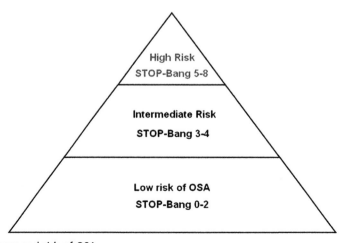

Fig. 1. STOP-Bang score and risk of OSA.

questionnaire had a higher sensitivity to predict moderate to severe (87.0%) and severe (70.4%) sleep-disordered breathing, whereas the 4-variable screening tool including sex, BMI, blood pressure, and snoring had a higher specificity to predict moderate to severe and severe sleep-disordered breathing (93.2% for both). In the community, a questionnaire with high specificity may be more useful in excluding low-risk patients and avoiding false-positive results, and it was suggested that sleep clinicians may prefer to use screening tools with high sensitivity, like the STOP-Bang questionnaire, to avoid missing cases, which may lead to adverse health consequences and increased health care costs.

Recently, the STOP-Bang questionnaire was studied in 319 Singaporean patients.[24] The sensitivity of STOP-Bang in identifying patients with AHI >15 and AHI >30 was 74.3% and 79.5%, respectively. It was easy to use, and 90% of patients were able to complete the questionnaire without any help. Because the Asian population is less obese, use of a BMI cutoff of 30 in the STOP-Bang tool may simplify its use without compromising its accuracy. In another study based on the Chinese population, the sensitivities of the STOP-Bang scoring model for AHI ≥ 5, ≥ 15 and ≥ 30 were 85.7%, 92.5%, and 100% and the NPVs were 48%, 80%, and 100%, respectively.[25]

USE OF STOP-BANG QUESTIONNAIRE IN BARIATRIC SURGICAL PATIENTS

OSA is a common comorbidity in morbidly obese patients. A retrospective study showed that the incidence of OSA in bariatric surgical patients is greater than 70%.[26] Thirty-eight percent of morbidly obese patients with significant sleep apnea were previously undiagnosed, despite showing clear symptoms of the disease.[27] To avoid the potential perils of undiagnosed sleep apnea during the perioperative period, patients who undergo bariatric surgery should be screened, tested, and treated for this comorbidity.

Gafsou and colleagues[28] used the STOP-Bang questionnaire as a screening tool for OSA in patients scheduled for bariatric surgery. Seventy-seven percent of patients were at high risk of OSA (STOP-Bang ≥ 3). The sensitivity and NPV of the STOP-Bang questionnaire were 96% and 93%, respectively, for predicting moderate to severe OSA (AHI >15). In the bariatric surgical patients, the STOP-Bang score ruled out a severe OSA diagnosis (AHI >30), with an NPV of 100% making it a valuable screening tool for OSA in obese patients scheduled for bariatric surgery.

In practice, the STOP-Bang questionnaire was reported as a screening tool for OSA in bariatric patients in 2 studies. In a retrospective observational study of outpatient laparoscopic gastric banding, Kurrek and colleagues[29] used the STOP-Bang questionnaire to identify patients at high risk of OSA. Eikermann and colleagues[30] also applied the STOP-Bang questionnaire to define clinical suspicion of OSA in morbidly obese patients scheduled for weight loss surgery.

USE OF STOP-BANG QUESTIONNAIRE IN PATIENTS UNDERGOING ENDOSCOPY

Among patients undergoing endoscopy, unrecognized OSA could predict sedation-related complications and the need for airway maneuvers.[31] The STOP-Bang questionnaire was used as an OSA screening tool to identify patients at high risk for OSA. Patients with a positive STOP-Bang score required more airway maneuvers and had more frequent airway-related sedation-related complications, including hypoxemia and apnea.

In a prospective cohort study of patients undergoing deep sedation for endoscopic procedures,[32] patients were divided into high risk and low risk for OSA by a STOP-Bang score 3 or greater. Patients with high risk for OSA were at a higher risk for hypoxemia during deep sedation. In deep sedation for colonoscopy in young and middle-aged outpatients, Deng and colleagues[33] found that the STOP questionnaire has high sensitivity, specificity, and NPV for hypoxemia. The STOP-Bang questionnaire complements the current approach to assessment before endoscopic procedures and helps the anesthesiologist to identify patients likely to encounter sedation-related complications, allowing an appropriate sedation strategy.

USE OF STOP-BANG QUESTIONNAIRE TO IDENTIFY UNDIAGNOSED OSA IN MEDICAL PATIENTS

Identification of OSA in cardiovascular patients is especially important, because untreated OSA may be accompanied by increased cardiovascular events and continuous positive airway pressure can attenuate this risk. During treatment of acute myocardial infarction, a large group of patients with OSA were underdiagnosed.[34] McCormack and colleagues[21] suggest that the high sensitivity of the STOP-Bang questionnaire makes it a potentially useful screening tool for sleep apnea in patients with acute myocardial infarction. The ease of bedside application can identify patients with undiagnosed OSA whose prognosis may be improved by treatment.

Dias and colleagues[35] reported that more than 40% of patients with multiple sclerosis presenting to an outpatient clinic were identified as high risk for OSA based on the STOP-Bang questionnaire. The investigators suggested that the STOP-BANG questionnaire offers clinicians an efficient and objective tool for improving detection of OSA risk in patients with multiple sclerosis.

Also, patients with severe mental illness are at high risk for OSA, and screening for OSA seems to be inadequate. The STOP-Bang score was used to classify those at high risk for OSA in patients with severe mental illness. The STOP-Bang screening may be beneficial, because OSA diagnosis and treatment may improve mental and physical health outcomes in patients with mental illness.[36]

SERUM BICARBONATE IMPROVES THE SPECIFICITY OF STOP-BANG QUESTIONNAIRE

The relative low specificity of the STOP-Bang questionnaire can be a disadvantage as a screening tool. A STOP-Bang score of 3 or greater yields a specificity of only 43% and 37% for moderate/severe OSA, respectively, suggesting a high false-positive rate.[9]

Ten to thirty-eight percent of patients with OSA have chronic daytime hypercapnia ($Paco_2$ [partial pressure of carbon dioxide, arterial] $\geq$45 mm Hg).[37] With increasing OSA severity (as measured by the AHI or the degree of nocturnal hypoxemia), the risk of chronic daytime hypercapnia may increase.[38] However, it is plausible that serum HCO_3^- level may increase in moderate/severe OSA without reaching overt chronic daytime hypercapnia.

A recent study by Chau and colleagues[39] evaluated the predictive parameters of the STOP-Bang questionnaire at various levels of serum HCO_3^- for screening patients with OSA. The combination of the STOP-Bang questionnaire with a higher serum HCO_3^- level improves the specificity for detecting OSA. By combining HCO_3^- level of 28 mmol/L or greater and STOP-Bang score of 3 or greater, the specificity for moderate/severe and severe OSA was 82% and 79%, respectively.

Serum HCO_3^- level is easily ordered in the preoperative clinic. Thus, it is an additional tool in the preoperative stratification of patients with unrecognized OSA. The higher the serum HCO_3^- level, the higher is the specificity for OSA with the STOP-Bang questionnaire.

STOP-BANG SCORE AND POSTOPERATIVE COMPLICATIONS

A retrospective cohort study by Liao and colleagues[2] reported that patients with OSA have a higher incidence of postoperative complications versus matched surgical patients without OSA. Memtsoudis and colleagues[3] found a 2-fold higher risk of pulmonary complications in patients with OSA after noncardiac surgery compared with matched controls without OSA. A recent meta-analysis by Kaw and colleagues[1] reported an increased risk of postoperative adverse events, transfer to an intensive care unit, and longer hospital stay in surgical patients with OSA.

However, most preoperative patients with OSA have not had their conditions diagnosed, raising the potential for a negative effect on postoperative outcome.[40] In a historical cohort study of 135 patients undergoing elective surgery, Vasu and colleagues[41] evaluated the association between STOP-Bang score and postoperative complication. A high-risk score for OSA on the STOP-Bang questionnaire is associated with an increased incidence of postoperative complications. Most patients with OSA are not diagnosed and may be at risk in the perioperative setting. The STOP-Bang questionnaire is a convenient and useful screening tool to reliably identify patients who are at increased risk for postoperative complications.

WHEN SHOULD SURGICAL PATIENTS BE REFERRED FOR FURTHER WORKUP?

When should preoperative patients with a high STOP-Bang score be referred? The Canadian Thoracic Society 2011 guideline for the diagnosis and treatment of sleep-disordered breathing gives recommendations about the assessment to initiate treatment of patients at risk of OSA to give a better outcome.[42] Patients with suspected severe obstructive sleep, a STOP-Bang score 5 to 8, and daytime somnolence, or patients working in safety-critical occupations, should be referred for consultation of sleep breathing disorder. Patients with comorbidities such as unstable ischemic heart disease, recent cerebrovascular disease, congestive heart failure, refractory systemic hypertension, obstructive/restrictive lung disease, pulmonary hypertension, and hypercapnic respiratory failure should also be referred for further evaluation.[42]

SUMMARY

The STOP-Bang questionnaire has been validated in medical and surgical patients and in different ethnic groups. A STOP-Bang score of 0 to 2 indicates a low risk of OSA; a STOP-Bang score of 3 to 4 indicates an intermediate risk of OSA; and a STOP-Bang score of 5 to 8 indicates a high risk of OSA; a STOP-Bang score of 3 or greater plus a high serum HCO_3^- level also increases the specificity for moderate/severe OSA. Further information is available at http://www.stopbang.ca/.

REFERENCES

1. Kaw R, Chung F, Pasupuleti V, et al. Meta-analysis of the association between obstructive sleep apnoea and postoperative outcome. Br J Anaesth 2012; 109(6):897–906.

2. Liao P, Yegneswaran B, Vairavanathan S, et al. Postoperative complications in patients with obstructive sleep apnea: a retrospective matched cohort study. Can J Anaesth 2009;56:819–28.

3. Memtsoudis S, Liu SS, Ma Y, et al. Perioperative pulmonary outcomes in patients with sleep apnea after noncardiac surgery. Anesth Analg 2011;112: 113–21.

4. Chung F, Elsaid H. Screening for obstructive sleep apnea before surgery: why is it important? Curr Opin Anaesthesiol 2009;22:405–11.

5. Punjabi NM. The epidemiology of adult obstructive sleep apnea. Proc Am Thorac Soc 2008;5:136–43.

6. Ancoli-Israel S, Kripke DF, Klauber MR, et al. Sleep-disordered breathing in community-dwelling elderly. Sleep 1991;14:486–95.

7. Young T, Evans L, Finn L, et al. Estimation of the clinically diagnosed proportion of sleep apnea syndrome in middle-aged men and women. Sleep 1997;20:705–6.

8. Ramachandran SK, Josephs LA. A meta-analysis of clinical screening tests for obstructive sleep apnea. Anesthesiology 2009;110:928–39.

9. Chung F, Yegneswaran B, Liao P, et al. STOP questionnaire: a tool to screen obstructive sleep apnea. Anesthesiology 2008;108:812–21.

10. Bliwise DL, Nekich JC, Dement WC. Relative validity of self-reported snoring as a symptom of sleep apnea in a sleep clinic population. Chest 1991;99: 600–8.

11. Haraldsson PO, Carenfelt C, Knutsson E, et al. Preliminary report: validity of symptom analysis and daytime polysomnography in diagnosis of sleep apnea. Sleep 1992;15:261–3.

12. Netzer NC, Stoohs RA, Netzer CM, et al. Using the Berlin Questionnaire to identify patients at risk for the sleep apnea syndrome. Ann Intern Med 1999; 131:485–91.

13. Flemons WW. Clinical practice. Obstructive sleep apnea. N Engl J Med 2002;347:498–504.

14. Weatherwax KJ, Lin X, Marzec ML, et al. Obstructive sleep apnea in epilepsy patients: the Sleep Apnea scale of the Sleep Disorders Questionnaire (SA-SDQ) is a useful screening instrument for obstructive sleep apnea in a disease-specific population. Sleep Med 2003;4:517–21.

15. Gross JB, Bachenberg KL, Benumof JL, et al. Practice guidelines for the perioperative management of patients with obstructive sleep apnea: a report by the American Society of Anesthesiologists Task Force on Perioperative Management of patients with obstructive sleep apnea. Anesthesiology 2006;104:1081–93.

16. Ramachandran SK, Kheterpal S, Consens F, et al. Derivation and validation of a simple perioperative sleep apnea prediction score. Anesth Analg 2010; 110:1007–15.

17. Johns MW. A new method for measuring daytime sleepiness: the Epworth sleepiness scale. Sleep 1991;14:540–5.

18. Chung F, Yegneswaran B, Liao P, et al. Validation of Berlin questionnaire and ASA checklist as screening tools for obstructive sleep apnea in surgical patients. Anesthesiology 2008;108:822–30.

19. Farney RJ, Walker BS, Farney RM, et al. The STOP-Bang equivalent model and prediction of severity of obstructive sleep apnea: relation to polysomnographic measurements of the apnea/hypopnea index. J Clin Sleep Med 2011;7:459–65.

20. Chung F, Subramanyam R, Liao P, et al. High STOP-Bang score indicates a high probability of obstructive sleep apnoea. Br J Anaesth 2012;108:768–75.

21. McCormack DJ, Pabla R, Babu MH, et al. Undiagnosed sleep apnoea syndrome in patients with acute myocardial infarction: potential importance of the STOP-BANG screening tool for clinical practice. Int J Cardiol 2012;155:342–3.

22. Silva GE, Vana KD, Goodwin JL, et al. Identification of patients with sleep disordered breathing: comparing the four-variable screening tool, STOP, STOP-Bang, and Epworth Sleepiness Scales. J Clin Sleep Med 2011;7:467–72.

23. Cruces-Artero C, Martin-Miguel MV, Herves-Beloso C, et al. Validation of the STOP and STOP BANG questionnaire in primary health care. J Sleep Res 2012;21(Suppl s1):226.

24. Ong TH, Raudha S, Fook-Chong S, et al. Simplifying STOP-BANG: use of a simple questionnaire to screen for OSA in an Asian population. Sleep Breath 2010;14:371–6.

25. Yu Y, Mei W, Cui Y. Primary evaluation of the simplified Chinese version of STOP-Bang scoring model in predicting obstructive sleep apnea hypopnea syndrome. Lin Chung Er Bi Yan Hou Tou Jing Wai Ke Za Zhi 2012;26:256–9.

26. Lopez PP, Stefan B, Schulman CI, et al. Prevalence of sleep apnea in morbidly obese patients who presented for weight loss surgery evaluation: more evidence for routine screening for obstructive sleep apnea before weight loss surgery. Am Surg 2008;74: 834–8.

27. Rasmussen JJ, Fuller WD, Ali MR. Sleep apnea syndrome is significantly underdiagnosed in

bariatric surgical patients. Surg Obes Relat Dis 2012;8:569–73.

28. Gafsou B, Marsac L, Fournier JL, et al. Validation of the STOP-Bang questionnaire as screening tools for obstructive sleep apnea in patients scheduled for bariatric surgery: 1AP3-5. Eur J Anaesthesiol 2010; 27(47):13.

29. Kurrek MM, Cobourn C, Wojtasik Z, et al. Morbidity in patients with or at high risk for obstructive sleep apnea after ambulatory laparoscopic gastric banding. Obes Surg 2011;21:1494–8.

30. Eikermann M, Garzon-Serrano J, Kwo J, et al. Do patients with obstructive sleep apnea have an increased risk of desaturation during induction of anesthesia for weight loss surgery? Open Respir Med J 2010;4:58–62.

31. Cote GA, Hovis CE, Hovis RM, et al. A screening instrument for sleep apnea predicts airway maneuvers in patients undergoing advanced endoscopic procedures. Clin Gastroenterol Hepatol 2010;8: 660–5.

32. Corso RM, Piraccini E, Agnoletti V, et al. Clinical use of the STOP-BANG questionnaire in patients undergoing sedation for endoscopic procedures. Minerva Anestesiol 2012;78:109–10.

33. Deng L, Li CL, Ge SJ, et al. Stop questionnaire to screen for hypoxemia in deep sedation for young and middle-aged colonoscopy. Dig Endosc 2012; 24:255–8.

34. Konecny T, Kuniyoshi FH, Orban M, et al. Underdiagnosis of sleep apnea in patients after acute myocardial infarction. J Am Coll Cardiol 2010;56: 742–3.

35. Dias RA, Hardin KA, Rose H, et al. Sleepiness, fatigue, and risk of obstructive sleep apnea using the STOP-BANG questionnaire in multiple sclerosis: a pilot study. Sleep Breath 2012;16(4):1255–65.

36. Alam A, Chengappa KN, Ghinassi F. Screening for obstructive sleep apnea among individuals with severe mental illness at a primary care clinic. Gen Hosp Psychiatry 2012;34(6):660–4.

37. Mokhlesi B. Obesity hypoventilation syndrome: a state-of-the-art review. Respir Care 2010;55: 1347–62.

38. Kaw R, Hernandez AV, Walker E, et al. Determinants of hypercapnia in obese patients with obstructive sleep apnea: a systematic review and metaanalysis of cohort studies. Chest 2009;136:787–96.

39. Chau EH, Liao P, Yang Y, et al. Serum bicarbonate level improves specificity of STOP-Bang screening for OSA[A039]. In: Anesthesiology 2011: American Society of Anesthesiologists Annual Meeting, October 15-19, 2011, Chicago (IL)..

40. Finkel KJ, Searleman AC, Tymkew H, et al. Prevalence of undiagnosed obstructive sleep apnea among adult surgical patients in an academic medical center. Sleep Med 2009;10:753–8.

41. Vasu TS, Doghramji K, Cavallazzi R, et al. Obstructive sleep apnea syndrome and postoperative complications: clinical use of the STOP-BANG questionnaire. Arch Otolaryngol Head Neck Surg 2010; 136:1020–4.

42. Fleetham J, Ayas N, Bradley D, et al. Canadian Thoracic Society 2011 guideline update: diagnosis and treatment of sleep disordered breathing. Can Respir J 2011;18:25–47.

Preoperative Evaluation of Obstructive Sleep Apnea
Home Sleep Testing Versus Laboratory Testing

Susheel P. Patil, MD, PhD

KEYWORDS

- Obstructive sleep apnea • Portable monitoring • Polysomnography • Preoperative evaluation

KEY POINTS

- Obstructive sleep apnea (OSA) is underdiagnosed and undertreated in the general and surgical populations.
- OSA can be diagnosed using portable monitoring (PM) pathways or in-laboratory polysomnography (PSG) pathways.
- Owing to differences in PM and PSG, clinicians need to be aware of the advantages and limitations of PM for OSA.
- When appropriately used, PM pathways have outcomes comparable to those for in-laboratory PSG pathways.
- Preoperative clinics may desire to establish pathways to identify OSA to minimize postoperative complications.

INTRODUCTION

Obstructive sleep apnea (OSA) is a highly prevalent condition affecting 24% of men and 9% of women,[1] associated with an increased risk for adverse cardiovascular,[2,3] metabolic,[4] neurocognitive outcomes,[5,6] and early mortality.[7,8] Patients with OSA are at increased risk for postoperative respiratory and cardiovascular complications, which can result in the need for increased levels of monitoring and longer hospitalizations.[9] The prevalence of OSA in surgical populations is estimated to be at least as high as in the general population, owing to obesity and other comorbid conditions.[10] Most patients at risk for OSA, however, remain undiagnosed or untreated,[11,12] thus placing the surgical patient with OSA at risk for postoperative complications. Timely identification of OSA and initiation of therapy

before surgery can therefore represent an important target in improving postoperative outcomes.

The diagnosis of OSA begins with identification of the at-risk patient based on the history and physical examination. Administration of simple questionnaires, which incorporate measures of obesity, the presence of obstructive breathing symptoms, the presence of comorbidities such as hypertension, and/or the presence of excessive daytime sleepiness can streamline identification of the at-risk patient in a busy preoperative clinic.[13–18] Once identified, diagnostic testing with attended, in-laboratory polysomnography (PSG) is traditionally performed to confirm the diagnosis and assess the severity of OSA. However, the use of unattended, limited-channel portable monitoring (PM) for the diagnosis of OSA has been growing because of the increased convenience of the

Disclosures: The author has no conflicts of interest.
Division of Pulmonary and Critical Care Medicine, Johns Hopkins School of Medicine, Johns Hopkins Sleep Disorders Center, 5501 Hopkins Bayview Circle, Room 4B.50, Baltimore, MD 21224, USA
E-mail address: spatil@jhmi.edu

Sleep Med Clin 8 (2013) 73–91
http://dx.doi.org/10.1016/j.jsmc.2012.12.003

patient sleeping at home and the potential cost savings. Both diagnostic approaches have advantages and limitations that should be considered. Although attended in-laboratory polysomnography is currently considered the gold standard for the diagnosis of OSA, its expense, labor requirements, and timely availability may limit the usefulness of the test when a patient needs to urgently have surgery. Conversely, although the technology for portable monitors can be comparable with that of in-laboratory polysomnography, problems may arise such as insufficient recordings due to sensor failure and false-negative tests. PM for OSA is also referred to as limited-channel testing (LCT) and home sleep testing (HST). For the purposes of this article, ambulatory testing for OSA is referred to as portable monitoring (PM). The article reviews the use of PM and in-laboratory PSG in the assessment of OSA.

DIFFERENCES BETWEEN PM RECORDERS AND PSG

The term PSG is used when a collection of physiologic signals are recorded during sleep. There are a host of physiologic measurements that can be recorded including, but not limited, to brainwave activity, eye movements, muscle activity, behaviors arising from sleep, cardiac rhythm, respiration, and gas exchange. PSG has been used to help characterize several sleep disorders such as sleep-disordered breathing (SDB), hypersomnias, insomnias, sleep-related movement disorders, circadian rhythm disorders, and parasomnias.[19] Furthermore, PSG can be used to assess the response to therapies for the various sleep disorders. By contrast, PM devices generally collect a limited subset of these physiologic signals, and as currently implemented have one specific goal: to determine the presence or absence of certain forms of SDB (eg, OSA, central sleep apnea, Cheyne-Stokes respiration) (**Fig. 1**). More complex PM devices that approach the diversity of information that a PSG study provides are available; however, such devices require more resources such as sending a sleep technologist to the home to set up the monitor. Furthermore, there are important differences in signal recordings and scoring between PM and PSG for the detection of SDB. Understanding these differences is important for the clinician who is reviewing sleep-study reports from these 2 diagnostic approaches.

Signal Collection

There are some important differences in signal acquisition between PSG and PM devices (**Table 1**). A PSG study requires a sleep technologist to apply sensors to the patient, whereas with a PM device the patient will generally self-apply the sensors in the home. Patients may be trained in the application of the sensors by having them come to a testing center for instruction, whereas in other cases the use of a CD or voice-automated system has been used to guide the patient. Self-application of sensors by the patient can potentially lead to incorrect application of sensors and thus may affect the quality of the collected data. In addition, the more complex the PM device, the greater is the potential for technical issues. Because PSG studies are continuously monitored, if sensors are dislodged or another technical issue arises, there is the opportunity to correct the fault and to maximize the collection of a quality recording. With a PM study, sensor dislodgment will not be corrected because the sleeping patient will be unaware of the fault

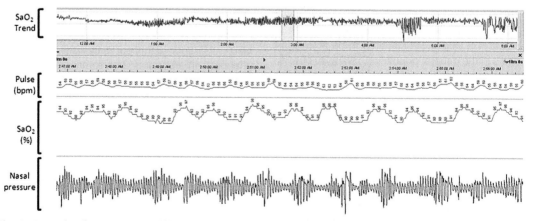

Fig. 1. Example of a type IV portable monitor recording, showing recurrent disordered breathing events with associated desaturations. The lack of respiratory efforts sensors makes differentiation between central and obstructive sleep apnea more difficult. bpm, beats per minute; SaO₂, arterial oxygen saturation.

Table 1
Differences between polysomnography and portable monitoring

	Polysomnography	Portable Monitor
Signal collection		
Setup	Technologist prepares patient for testing	Patient typically self-applies sensors or technologist comes to the home for setup
Sensor management	Technologist monitors and addresses sensor loss issues	Patient must be aware to address issues, unless PM system has a warning system
Technical support	Technologist immediately available in the laboratory	Patient can typically call a round-the-clock service that the laboratory or third-party vendor provides
Video monitoring	Standard with in-laboratory PSG	Not typical with PM devices
Signal acquisition	Use of standard sensors with standardization of amplifier, filtering and display of signals	Many PM devices use standard sensors; however, there are others that use unique sensors for detecting SDB
Scoring		
Sleep/wake	Standard feature	Not a standard feature, unless type 2 monitor used
Disordered breathing events	Apnea, hypopneas, and RERAs can be scored	Apneas and hypopneas can be scored
SDB severity	Expressed per hour of sleep (AHI or RDI)	Expressed per hour of recording time (REI)
Identification of types of disordered breathing (central/mixed/obstructive)	Standard with in-laboratory PSG	Only if the PM device selected can integrate respiratory effort signals
Automated scoring	Can be performed, but more commonly manual scoring performed by a sleep technologist	Often performed; however, systems should allow for manual review of scoring

Abbreviations: AHI, apnea-hypopnea index; PM, portable monitoring; PSG, polysomnography; RDI, respiratory disturbance index; REI, respiratory event index; RERA, respiratory effort–related arousals; SDB, sleep-disordered breathing.

(**Fig. 2**). Some PM systems attempt to correct this using a voice-activated system to inform the patient of sensor failure. Signals collected during PSG can be calibrated, and provide more quantitative information; with PM studies calibration of signals is usually not possible, which results in more qualitative information. PSG also provides the additional advantage of video monitoring to assess changes of body position, important in the assessment of OSA, which are not as easy to implement with PM. Some PM systems incorporate a body-position sensor to overcome this problem. PSG acquisition systems are also more open, allowing more customization and control of signal acquisition, which allows for more standardization of amplification, filtering, and display of the signals. PM devices, because of their proprietary nature, are often less transparent, and signal acquisition can be inadequately validated owing to attempts to provide a low-cost device.

Scoring and Interpretation

There are some important distinctions in the scoring and interpretation of a PSG study compared with a PM study (see **Table 1**). Scoring of sleep studies in the United States uses a rule set from a scoring manual developed by the American Academy of Sleep Medicine, which provides standards for acquisition, scoring, and reporting.[20] The same rule set is used in the scoring of both PSG and PM studies; however, because of the limited number of channels collected with PM studies, the rule set cannot be fully implemented.

The primary limitation of PM devices is that sleep/wake status cannot be determined owing

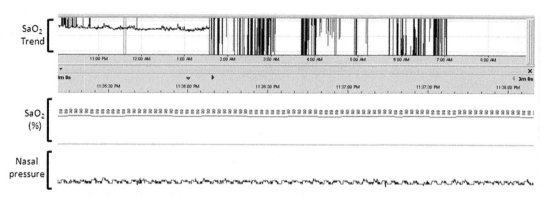

Fig. 2. Example of a type IV portable monitor recording with sensor dislodgment showing only an oximetry reading, with absence of airflow caused by dislodgement of the nasal cannula. Later in the night the oximeter was also lost, resulting in a study that was not useful. While this is a possibility during a polysomnography (PSG) recording, the presence of a technologist would ensure attempts to correct the sensor positioning.

to the lack of electroencephalography (EEG) in most systems. Assessment of sleep/wake status is important, as it is used to define the presence and severity of SDB during sleep. The severity of SDB is reported based on the presence of disordered breathing events as either an apnea-hypopnea index (AHI) or a respiratory disturbance index (RDI). The AHI is defined as the number of apneas and hypopneas per hour of sleep. The RDI, a more sensitive measure of disordered breathing, is defined as the number of hypopneas, apneas, and respiratory effort–related arousals (RERAs) per hour of sleep (**Table 2**). There are specific definitions used to define an apnea, hypopnea, and RERA (see **Table 2**). Two airflow signals are typically used to define the presence of disordered breathing events: a nasal pressure signal and an oronasal thermal sensor. The scoring of an apnea requires the presence of 2 airflow signals, and is independent of changes in oxyhemoglobin saturation or arousals from sleep. By contrast, the scoring of a hypopnea or RERA requires additional information from an oximetery signal and an EEG signal to detect arousal.

Because most PM devices do not assess the presence of arousals, only apneas and hypopneas can be scored. Furthermore, because most PM devices do not assess sleep state, the SDB severity is presented as the number of apneas and hypopneas per hour of recording time, sometimes referred to as a respiratory event index (REI).[21] If the recording time is significantly longer than the sleep time, this will result in a lower measured severity by PM than by PSG. Furthermore, if there is a loss of the oximeter signal during a PM study, hypopneas cannot be scored and the severity of SDB is based only on the apnea severity. There is also the possibility that disordered breathing events are scored during

wakefulness because of breath-holding maneuvers or breathing variability, and could falsely elevate the disordered-breathing count. In addition, some PM devices do not include an assessment of thoracoabdominal effort, which is required to determine the presence of obstructive, central, or mixed apneas. Because the treatment of obstructive versus central sleep apnea can be quite different, this can be an issue when considering the use of PM in a patient population at risk for central apnea, such as patients on narcotic medications or with congestive heart failure. Finally, many systems provide an automatic scoring algorithm of PM studies from which a sleep-study report can be generated. However, based on the foregoing discussion, review of the raw recording with overscoring by a sleep technologist is considered best practice to ensure as accurate a report as possible. Based on these considerations, a clinician must decide whether the information obtained from the PM device is usable, and place the results in the context of the patient's history.

TYPES OF PM DEVICES

PM devices have been present for 15 years or more, and the technology has steadily improved, with many devices having sensors and technical specifications similar to those of their PSG counterparts. The Sleep Heart Health Study demonstrated in a research setting that PM devices could be deployed on a large scale.[22] Because of the myriad number of devices and sensors, hierarchical classification schemes have been developed to help provide some level of comparison between devices regarding complexity and reimbursement issues. The reader is referred elsewhere for a detailed history of the decision by

Table 2
Description of sleep-disordered breathing events and parameters

	Event or Parameter	Description
Types of disordered breathing events	Apnea	A ≥90% decrease in peak amplitude from an oronasal thermistor signal from baseline for ≥10 s *Obstructive*: An apnea with continued or increasing respiratory effort *Central*: An apnea with an absence of respiratory effort *Mixed:* An apnea with initial absence of respiratory effort, followed by resumption of respiratory effort
	Hypopnea	**AASM definition**: A ≥30% decrease in peak amplitude from a nasal pressure signal from baseline for ≥10 s in association with a ≥3% oxygen desaturation or an arousal **CMS definition**: A ≥30% decrease in peak amplitude from a nasal pressure signal from baseline for ≥10 s in association with a ≥4% oxygen desaturation only *Obstructive*: During the hypopnea, either snoring, increased flattening of the nasal pressure signal, or thoracoabdominal paradox breathing is observed *Central*: During the hypopnea, there is an absence of all of the following: snoring, increased flattening of the nasal pressure signal, thoracoabdominal paradox breathing
	Respiratory effort–related arousals (RERA)	A sequence of breaths ≥10 s with flattening of the nasal pressure waveform or increasing effort associated with arousal when the breath sequence does not meet apnea or hypopnea criteria
Sleep-disordered breathing parameters	Apnea-hypopnea index (AHI)	(Apneas + hypopneas)/hour of sleep
	Respiratory disturbance index (RDI)	(Apneas + hypopneas + RERAs)/hour of sleep
	Respiratory event index (REI)	(Apneas + hypopneas)/hour of recording time Reported only for PM devices because of lack of sleep assessment

Abbreviations: AASM, American Academy of Sleep Medicine; CMS, Center for Medicare and Medicaid Services.

the Center of Medicare and Medicaid Services (CMS) in approving reimbursement for PM and the evolution of classification schemes.[23,24]

The classification scheme used by the CMS[25] is essentially a minor modification of the original American Sleep Disorders Association classification developed in 1994 (**Table 3**).[26] The scheme defines the testing as a type I, II, III, or IV study. Type I studies are attended by a sleep technologist in the sleep laboratory with at least 7 channels recorded, whereas types II to IV are considered to be unattended studies with differences in the number of sensors recorded. A type II study is essentially an unattended type I study but with at least

7 channels recorded. Type III and type IV studies have a minimum of 4 channels or 3 channels recorded, respectively. Although simple, the scheme does not help separate within each study type the diverse number of PM that are available with differing levels of complexity.

Unique, nontraditional sensors have been and will continue to be developed (**Table 4**). These nontraditional sensors may evaluate sleep or breathing without the use of EEG, electro-oculography (EOG), electromyography (EMG), nasal pressure, or thermal sensors. For example, actigraphy has been implemented in some PM monitors for the assessment of sleep time.[27]

Table 3
Definitions of sleep testing according to CMS

HCPSC Code[a]	Device Type	Location	Channel Specifications[b]
	Type I	In-laboratory	Minimum of 7 channels: EEG, EOG, EMG, ECG/heart rate, airflow, respiratory effort, and oxygen saturation
G0398	Type II	Unattended	Minimum of 7 channels: EEG, EOG, EMG, ECG/heart rate, airflow, respiratory effort, and oxygen saturation
G0399	Type III	Unattended	Minimum of 4 channels: 2 respiratory movement/airflow signals, 1 ECG/heart rate, 1 oxygen saturation
G0400	Type IV	Unattended	Minimum of 3 channels Some local carriers may require 1 channel to be airflow

Abbreviations: ECG, electrocardiogram; EEG, electroencephalogram; EMG, electromyogram; EOG, electro-oculogram.
[a] Most carriers now use established CPT codes rather than G-codes.
[b] For some local carriers, peripheral arterial tonometry can replace airflow in type II–IV studies.
Data from Novitas Solutions 2012. LCD 27350 – sleep disorders testing. Available at: https://www.novitas-solutions.com/policy/mac-ab/l27530-r11.html. Accessed November 30, 2012.

Although an improvement over using recording time, actigraphy can underestimate sleep time in patients with significant OSA, owing to the arousal-related movements that can occur.[28] Other PM systems have looked at novel methods of sleep-wake estimation using anterior tibialis EMG data,[29] energy expenditure,[30] and jaw movements.[31] Pulse transit time, a cardiovascular response, has been used as a measure of arousals and disordered breathing events.[32] Several different nontraditional approaches have also been used to detect disordered breathing events, one example of which is peripheral arterial tonometry (PAT), a marker of sympathetic activity (**Fig. 3**). With disordered breathing events, sympathetic activity increases, resulting in vasoconstriction that is detected by the device.[33] Other sensors include sound measurements[34,35] and end-tidal CO_2 for disordered breathing events,[36] and venous pulsations[37] for respiratory effort. Some of these approaches have been reasonably validated while others remain to be validated.[21] Furthermore, whether these sensors yield more useful information than current, standardized traditional approaches remains to be seen.

With the evolution in sensors, there has been growing recognition that the sleep-study classification scheme is outdated and difficult to use when comparing PM devices. In 2011, the AASM published a new classification scheme based on the collection and quality of key physiologic signals during a study that was named SCOPER (Sleep, Cardiovascular, Oximetry, Position, Effort, and Respiration).[21] Under this scheme, devices are classified based on the presence or absence of measures of key physiologic signals, with further classification within each category according to the type of sensor used (**Table 5**). In the AASM guideline, this classification was used to help evaluate the validity of currently available sensors relative to full, attended PSG. Whether this classification scheme is eventually adopted by the CMS remains to be determined; however, at the very least it serves a purpose in communicating the complexity and diversity of PM devices used.

Table 4
Traditional and nontraditional sensors used in the assessment of sleep and breathing

	Traditional	Nontraditional
Sleep	EEG; EOG; EMG	Actigraphy Anterior tibialis EMG Energy expenditure Jaw movement
Arousal	EEG; EOG; EMG	Pulse transit time Heart-rate variability
Disordered breathing events	Nasal pressure Thermal sensor	Peripheral arterial tone Breath sounds Tracheal sounds End-tidal CO_2 Cardiopulmonary coupling

Abbreviations: EEG, electroencephalogram; EMG, electromyogram EOG, electro-oculogram.

SELECTION OF PM DEVICES

Selection of a PM device in the assessment of OSA will depend on several factors including the goals of

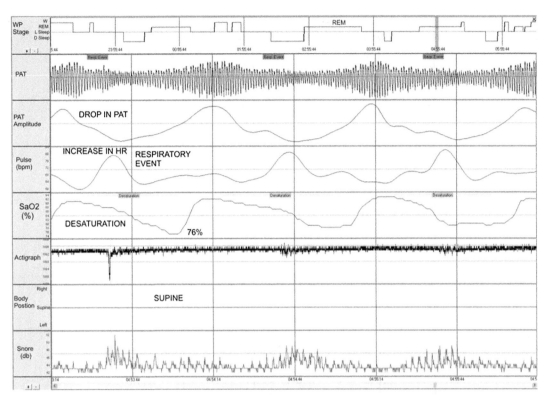

Fig. 3. Detection of a respiratory event using peripheral arterial tonometry (PAT). The PAT signal falls (increased sympathetic tone), associated with an increase then decrease in pulse (heart rate [HR]) and an arterial oxygen desaturation. (*From* Berry RB. Uses and limitations of portable monitoring for diagnosis and management of obstructive sleep apnea. Sleep Med Clin 2011;3:329; with permission.)

the preoperative clinic in identifying OSA, and patient-, clinician-, and device-related factors **(Box 1)**.[38] For example, is the goal of the preoperative clinic to conduct the portable monitoring itself, partner with sleep medicine provider(s) and sleep laboratories, or send a patient to a third-party sleep-testing company? Is the goal of the clinic to identify well in advance of surgery the presence of OSA to ensure adherence before surgery to minimize postoperative complications? Or is the goal of the clinic to identify the patients with the most severe forms of OSA in the case of urgent surgery to make sure such patients receive necessary monitoring postoperatively? These considerations and others will determine whether the clinic chooses to send patients for traditional in-laboratory sleep testing or to perform more or less complex forms of PM testing in the home.

Patient-related factors that should be considered in PM-device selection include the ease of setup of the device by the patient, the intrusiveness of the sensor used, the availability of technical support to assist the patient with device use, and whether return of equipment is planned to occur in person, via courier, or by certified

mail. Clinician-related factors include the simplicity of instructing patients how to use the PM device, the ease of use of the device and the ability to review the raw signals, to use automatic versus manual scoring, and to generate a report. There are also many important device-related factors that need to be considered. For example, the cost and maintenance of the device as well as the cost of replacement components and disposable sensors need to be considered. There are also considerations for the battery life and memory in PM devices, because some programs may attempt multi-night monitoring. Review of software requirements as well the cost of software upgrades is also important. The frequency with which a particular device can be redeployed could be a consideration in a high-volume clinic.

Another important factor in device selection is the accuracy and precision of sensors in diagnosing OSA. The AASM recently completed a technology assessment in 2011 examining the various sensors used to diagnose OSA.[21] **Table 6** summarizes the key questions asked and the conclusions of the task force. The report indicated that the use of thermal sensing devices alone were not

Table 5
SCOPER classification system

Sleep	Cardiovascular	Oximetry	Position	Effort	Respiratory
S1: Sleep by 3 EEG channels with EOG and chin EMG	C1: More than 1 ECG lead: events can be derived	O1: Oximetry (finger or ear) with recommended sampling at 3 s averaging and minimum of 10 Hz sampling	P1: Video or visual position measurement	E1: 2 respiratory inductive plethysmography (RIP) belts	R1: Nasal pressure and thermal sensing device
S2: Sleep by <3 EEG channels with or without EOG and chin EMG	C2: Peripheral arterial tonometry	O1x: Oximetry (finger or ear) without recommended sampling or not described	P2: Nonvisual position measurement	E2: 1 RIP belt	R2: Nasal pressure
S3: Sleep surrogate: eg, actigraphy	C3: Standard ECG measure (1 lead)	O2: Oximetry at alternative site (eg, forehead)		E3: Derived effort (eg, forehead pulsatile venous pressure)	R3: Thermal sensing device
S4: Other sleep measure	C4: Derived from pulse signal (e.g. oximetry)	O3: Other oximetry		E4: Other effort measure (including piezo belts)	R4: End-tidal CO_2 (EtCO$_2$)
	C5: Other cardiac measure				R5: Other respiratory measure

Data from Collop NA, Tracy SL, Kapur V, et al. Obstructive sleep apnea devices for out-of-center (OOC) testing: technology evaluation. J Clin Sleep Med 2011;7:531–48; and Collop NA, Anderson WM, Boehlecke B, et al. Clinical guidelines for the use of unattended portable monitors in the diagnosis of obstructive sleep apnea in adult patients. Portable Monitoring Task Force of the American Academy of Sleep Medicine. J Clin Sleep Med 2007;3(7):737–47; with permission.

acceptable; however, if performed in conjunction with the assessment of 2-channel respiratory effort, it was reasonably accurate. Nasal pressure monitoring was concluded to be adequate to diagnose OSA, although it was improved when 2 respiratory-effort channels were included. Insufficient data were available on the whether use of both nasal pressure and thermal sensing devices was better than either on its own. The task force also reviewed the ability of alternative devices that use nontraditional sensors for the diagnosis of OSA, such as the PAT device. Review of available studies indicated that a PAT-based PM device was adequate in the diagnosis of OSA. Other alternative devices assessed included those that use end-tidal CO_2 monitoring, acoustic signal as a substitute for airflow, and the use of cyclical variations in electrocardiography. In all situations it was deemed that there were insufficient data to determine whether these approaches were reasonably accurate in the diagnosis of OSA.

VALIDATION OF PM WITH PSG

The approach to validation of PM testing with PSG has taken several approaches.[39] First, devices

may be compared simultaneously on the same night, with the patient in the laboratory or in the home, to look at differences in the REI, AHI, and RDI. The overall advantage of the approach is that it allows comparison of the REI with an AHI or RDI without the concerns of night-to-night variability in measurements of sleep apnea severity. When performed in the laboratory setting, issues of sensor dislodgement are less likely than in the home. A disadvantage of this methodologic approach is that PM is not typically used in the laboratory, therefore generalizability to the home may be limited. Second, devices may be compared by conducting the PM in conjunction with PSG in the laboratory, then performing PM in the home and comparing sleep apnea severity between the 2 nights. Finally, studies have compared a PM-based strategy with an in-laboratory strategy, with comparison of outcomes over time (discussed later).

In 2011, the Agency for Healthcare Research and Quality (AHRQ) requested an update for a comparative effectiveness review to answer 7 key questions regarding the diagnosis and treatment of OSA.[40] One of the questions focused on the validity of PM devices as compared with in-laboratory PSG. As part of the study, 29 studies examining 18 different type III monitors and 70 studies examining 23 type IV monitors were reviewed. The quality of the studies was heterogeneous, but allowed for pooling of data for review. The investigators examined measures of agreement and the receiver-operating characteristics of the PM device types with PSG. Type III PM devices (-10 to $+24$ events/h) and type IV devices (-17 to $+12$ events/h) were found to have a wide range of mean biases (ie, the difference between the AHI by PM device and the AHI by PSG) and wide limits of agreement. The sensitivity and specificity of the type III device when defining OSA by an AHI of at least 5 events/h were 83% to 97% and 48% to 100%, respectively. The devices were less sensitive (64%–100%), but more specific (41%–100%) when OSA was defined by an AHI of at least 15 events/h. The sensitivity and specificity of the type IV devices substantially overlapped with those of type III devices. When defining OSA by an AHI of at least 5 events/h, the sensitivities ranged from 85% to 100% and specificities ranged from 50% to 100%, depending on the number of channels included in the type IV monitor assessed. At an AHI of at least 15 events/h, the devices were less sensitive (43%–100%) but had similar levels of specificity (43%–100%). The investigators looked at both positive and negative likelihood ratios in the ability of PM devices in predicting the sleep apnea severity category (ie, no OSA, mild OSA, moderate

Table 6
Summary of AASM technology evaluation

Key Question	Conclusion
1. Is a thermal sensing device without an effort measure adequate to diagnose OSA?	The literature was inadequate to state with confidence that thermal sensing devices alone are adequate in the diagnosis of OSA
2. Is a thermal sensing device with an effort measure adequate to diagnose OSA?	If using thermal sensor alone to measure respiration, 2 effort belts are required with either RIP or piezoelectric belts considered to be acceptable for the diagnosis of OSA
3. Is nasal pressure without an effort measure adequate to diagnose OSA?	Nasal pressure without an effort measure is adequate to diagnose OSA, although further studies would be ideal
4. Is nasal pressure with an effort measure adequate to diagnose OSA?	Nasal pressure with 2 RIP or piezoelectric belts is acceptable for the diagnosis of OSA
5. With an effort measure, is nasal pressure with thermal sensing significantly better than either a thermal sensor or nasal pressure alone?	There was insufficient evidence to state that both nasal pressure and thermal sensing devices are required for the diagnosis of OSA
6. What is the evidence for alternative sensors to diagnose OSA? (PAT, cardiac signal with oximetry, end-tidal CO_2, acoustic signals)	a. PAT signal: Adequate for the diagnosis of OSA, although scoring criteria variable in the validation studies reviewed b. Cardiac signals with oximetry: Shows promise, but inadequate data available c. End-tidal CO_2: Assessed only in the hospital setting, where it is adequate for OSA diagnosis d. Acoustic signal: Data are insufficient to determine whether the use of acoustic signals as a substitute for airflow is adequate in the diagnosis of OSA

Data from Collop NA, Tracy SL, Kapur V, et al. Obstructive sleep apnea devices for out-of-center (OOC) testing: technology evaluation. J Clin Sleep Med 2011;7:531–48.

OSA, and severe OSA). The investigators concluded that the strength of the evidence that both type III and type IV PM monitors were accurate in estimating OSA severity was moderate; however, there were insufficient data to compare specific monitors with one another. A significant limitation of the analysis was that more subtle respiratory events detected by PSG such as RERAs were not included in the definition of OSA severity by PSG, so it is possible that findings are even more disparate.

There are several reasons why the AHI by PM (AHI_{PM}) may vary relative to the AHI by PSG (AHI_{PSG}; **Box 2**). First, as discussed earlier, AHI_{PM} is based on recording time, in contrast to sleep time for most PM devices, which will most often result in an underestimation of OSA severity when compared with AHI_{PSG}. Second, because sleep-wake status is not assessed, disordered breathing events may be falsely scored while awake (eg, holding breath) and increase the AHI_{PM}. Third, disordered breathing events associated with arousals but insufficient oxyhemoglobin saturation will result in an underestimation of the OSA severity, unless the RDI is used. Fourth, night-to-night variability in OSA severity between the laboratory and the home may occur as a result of the relative amount of time spent supine or during rapid eye movement (REM) sleep. More supine time or REM sleep time may predispose to higher AHI values on those nights. Consumption of alcohol at home on the night of the PM or the use of sleeping medications could also elevate the AHI. Fifth, selection of sensors, particularly nontraditional sensors, may result in discordance in the AHI compared with traditional sensors. Thus, there are several sources of variability that can affect the OSA severity reported. This finding may argue for multi-night monitoring, rather than a single night of monitoring, to more accurately assess the variability in OSA severity and determination of an average AHI that may more accurately reflect the patient's clinical status. However, further research in this area is needed.

Box 2
Sources of variability in scoring sleep apnea severity between PM and PSG

1. Sleep time versus recording time
2. Scoring of disordered breathing events during time awake
3. Availability of arousal detection
4. Night-to-night variability
   a. Body position
   b. REM versus non-REM sleep time
   c. Alcohol consumption
   d. Use of hypnotics or opiates
   e. Fluid shifts
5. Differences in sensors used and scoring rules based on the sensors

Box 3
Advantages and limitations of PM relative to PSG testing

1. Advantages
   - Simple to self-administer
   - Sleep in more comfortable surroundings
   - Fewer sensors may improve sleep quality in the home
   - Less anxiety when at home
   - Lower cost
   - Greater frequency of monitoring possible (eg, oral appliance therapy)
   - Multi-night monitoring
2. Limitations
   - Validated only in the hands of sleep medicine specialists
   - Potential for false-negative results
   - Lack of sleep-time assessment
   - Inability to differentiate central versus OSA without effort measures
   - Inability to identify positional OSA, if no measure of body position
   - Increased likelihood of signal failure when unattended
   - Validity of automated scoring versus manual scoring

ADVANTAGES AND LIMITATIONS OF PM DEVICES

Based on the foregoing discussion, there are advantages and disadvantages to PM testing relative to PSG testing (**Box 3**). One advantage of PM testing is that it may allow the patient to sleep better in the home in familiar surroundings. Because of the lower number of sensors there may also be less intrusiveness for the patient, which may make it easier for him or her to sleep. In addition, some patients find video monitoring performed in the laboratory for determination of body position or parasomnia evaluation to be anxiety provoking, thus home testing without video monitoring may make such patients more comfortable. Another potential advantage of PM devices is that because of their lower cost and relative simplicity compared with a standard PSG study, the devices could be more widely implemented in a hospital setting for the monitoring of several patients. A technologist could help with the setup for such patients. PM devices could also allow more frequent monitoring of responses to therapies such as surgical interventions, oral appliances, or positional maneuvers. In addition, multi-night monitoring would be more viable with PM than with in-laboratory PSG. When access to a sleep laboratory is limited, PM monitoring is an alternative for the assessment of OSA in the appropriate patient.

There are, of course, limitations to the use of PM devices. The first is that almost all studies have looked at the use of PM devices in the hands of sleep medicine specialists, rather than primary care providers or other settings. Studies are needed to look at how implementation of PM devices may be similar or different in the hands of the non–sleep medicine provider. Second, there is a greater risk of false-negative results because the PM devices do not typically assess sleep. Owing to the higher false-negative rate, the PM device is not a good "screening" test because of its lower sensitivity. Third, the PM device generally does not determine sleep state and, thus, REM and non-REM sleep cannot be differentiated. Given the propensity for postsurgery REM sleep rebound that has been described, a patient's breathing during REM status may be important in preventing postoperative complications. Fourth, body position may not be assessed with some PM devices, which could lead to a false-negative finding if the patient sleeps nonsupine at home but sleeps supine postoperatively. Fifth, because PM devices are unattended, this can lead to increased failure rates in obtaining adequate data with which to make a diagnosis. In this situation, patients must be referred for in-laboratory PSG. Sixth, some PM devices may not assess respiratory effort, thus making assessment of OSA and central sleep apnea difficult. This situation can be problematic if the patient population being referred for PM testing has predisposing features for central sleep apnea such as congestive heart failure. Seventh, many systems have an automated scoring routine that is often a "black box." Understanding the limitations of PM devices will allow the clinician to provide appropriate care and referral for the chronic care of patients with SDB.

PATIENT SELECTION AND INDICATIONS FOR PM VERSUS PSG

Guidelines for patient selection were developed by the AASM in 2007 to guide the rational use of PM testing for OSA (**Box 4**).[41] These guidelines were developed based on the available evidence, whereby PM testing has been primarily tested in the hands of sleep medicine specialists. PM testing is best used for only the diagnosis of OSA because these devices primarily collect respiratory signals. Performing a comprehensive sleep evaluation in conjunction with PM testing ensures that a comprehensive diagnostic assessment is performed with accurate data collection and scoring, appropriate health care utilization, and effective patient management. PM testing is best used in patient populations with a high pretest probability of moderate to severe OSA (AHI $\geq$15 events/h). Furthermore, PM testing may have a role in monitoring response to non–continuous positive airway pressure (CPAP) therapies for OSA, and may be appropriate for patients in whom laboratory testing is not possible because of illness, safety, or immobility. PM testing is not recommended in patients with significant comorbid conditions such as moderate to severe pulmonary disease, neuromuscular disease, or congestive heart failure. With these conditions there is greater concern for nocturnal hypoventilation and/or central sleep apnea/Cheyne-Stokes respiration that may not be adequately detected by a PM device. In addition, PM testing should not be done when a patient is suspected of having another concomitant sleep disorder such as parasomnia, disorders of excessive sleepiness, sleep-related movement disorders, circadian rhythm disorders, or insomnia, whereby an in-laboratory sleep study would be more helpful. Furthermore, patients who may have difficulty in the self-application of sensors may find it difficult to use a PM device, in which case an in-laboratory sleep study may be more effective.

One approach to patient selection for a PM test is to use a Bayesian approach, as is commonly used with other medical disorders. With this approach a pretest probability is established for the likelihood of OSA. If the positive likelihood ratio (sensitivity/1 − specificity; LR+) is known for a given PM device, then a posttest probability can be determined for identifying moderate to severe OSA. Recent guidelines from the AASM suggest that the goal should be to have a posttest probability of 95%.[21] For example, if the pretest probability for moderate to severe OSA was 70%, a PM device should have an LR+ of at least 10 to have a posttest probability of 95% (**Fig. 4**).

Pretest probability can be determined based on the known prevalence of OSA in a patient population (eg, based on past experience), and can be improved by using questionnaires that have been developed to identify patients at high risk for moderate to severe OSA. Examples of questionnaires include the STOP, STOP-BANG,[15] ASA Checklist,[16] Berlin questionnaire,[16,42] Sleep Apnea Clinical Risk Score (SACS),[17] Multivariable Apnea Prediction (MAP),[18] and the OSA50.[13] The use of questionnaires for identifying patients at risk for OSA is reviewed elsewhere in this issue by Frances Chung and colleges in the article "A Screening tool of Obstructive Sleep Apnea: STOP-Bang Questionnaire", and can be referred to for further detail.

Box 4
Patient selection for PM studies

Patients in Whom PM Monitoring Can be Performed

1. In conjunction with a comprehensive sleep evaluation

2. To confirm the diagnosis of OSA in those with a high pretest probability

3. Monitor response to non-CPAP therapies (eg, oral appliance therapy)

4. Perform owing to issues of illness, safety, or immobility

Patients in Whom PM Monitoring Should Not be Performed

1. Moderate to severe pulmonary disease

2. Moderate to severe neuromuscular disease

3. Obesity hypoventilation syndrome

4. Concern for central sleep apnea or Cheyne-Stokes respiration (eg, congestive heart failure, brainstem stroke)

5. Concomitant sleep disorder (eg, parasomnia, narcolepsy, circadian rhythm disorder)

Data from Collop NA, Anderson WM, Boehlecke B, et al. Clinical guidelines for the use of unattended portable monitors in the diagnosis of obstructive sleep apnea in adult patients. Portable Monitoring Task Force of the American Academy of Sleep Medicine. J Clin Sleep Med 2007;3(7):737–47.

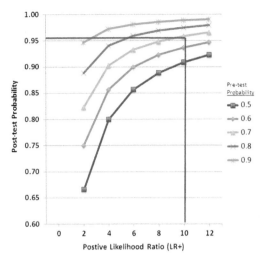

Fig. 4. Application of Bayes theorem to medical testing. The graph shows the posttest probability for a positive test, given a defined pretest probability and positive likelihood ratio (LR+). For example, for a pretest probability of 70%, if a portable monitor device has an LR+ of 10 for a diagnosis of OSA, the posttest probability of OSA will be approximately 96%. (*Data from* Collop NA, Tracy SL, Kapur V, et al. Obstructive sleep apnea devices for out-of-center (OOC) testing: technology evaluation. J Clin Sleep Med 2011;7:531–48.)

OUTCOMES BASED ON PM VERSUS IN-LABORATORY TESTING ALGORITHMS

The validation of PM in the diagnosis and management of OSA should not be limited to whether it correctly classifies the presence or absence of OSA. From a clinical standpoint, when PM is appropriately used, the question of comparison between outcomes from an ambulatory-based strategy and an in-laboratory–based strategy needs to be addressed. At least 7 studies have attempted to address this issue (**Table 7**), all of them suggesting that an ambulatory-based strategy can be noninferior to an in-laboratory–based strategy with respect to CPAP acceptance, improvement in sleep apnea severity, improvements in sleepiness, and improvements in quality of life.[43–49] In most of these studies, the ambulatory-based arm allowed for cross-over for an in-laboratory study when (1) the PM test was initially negative or there were technical difficulties in obtaining adequate data; or (2) initial therapy with autoCPAP was unsuccessful. Furthermore, all studies were conducted by centers skilled in the use of all sleep-testing diagnostic and therapeutic approaches, which may limit generalizability in other settings. Studies should be conducted whereby PM testing is performed in primary care settings and preoperative clinics, to understand whether there may be differences in outcomes when management is performed by a sleep center.

INTEGRATION OF OSA ASSESSMENT IN THE PREOPERATIVE CLINIC

Identification of OSA is only one of many goals within a busy preoperative clinic in maintaining patient safety in the perioperative and postoperative settings. With limited bed resources often available for postoperative monitoring, there is a need to effectively triage patients to the appropriate setting based on their risk profile. With both PSG and PM strategies for diagnostic testing available, development of an algorithm for OSA testing is desirable. **Fig. 5** demonstrates one possible algorithm that could be considered by integrating a concise questionnaire such as the Berlin or STOP-BANG to assess the risk of moderate to severe OSA. A review of comorbidities should be performed to identify conditions concerning for nocturnal hypoventilation. If any of these conditions exist or there are concerns for a concomitant sleep disorder, referral for a PSG study and evaluation by a sleep medicine clinician is most appropriate. If not, PM monitoring should be appropriate for OSA identification. Two attempts to obtain adequate data for PM could be made; if unsuccessful, the patient could be sent for PSG testing. Furthermore, if PM testing is negative but there is still suspicion for OSA, the patient should be considered for referral for PSG testing.

If testing is positive, patients can be referred for therapy, most likely with CPAP in the short term, with longer-term management considered after surgery. Programs may develop comfort with the use of in-laboratory CPAP titration or split-night sleep studies (a CPAP titration performed if significant OSA is identified in the first 1–2 hours of the night). Alternatively, in patients without the comorbidities discussed earlier, autoCPAP titration in the home for up to 1 week, followed by fixed CPAP or continued autoCPAP therapy, could be implemented. Patients who are compliant with CPAP may then be able to be managed postoperatively in the hospital setting without the need for monitoring in the intensive care unit or intermediate monitoring.

These strategies can be performed when surgery is elective; however, when surgery is more urgent or emergent, the luxury of time to perform the aforementioned approach is not available. In this situation, PM monitoring in patients at risk for moderate to severe OSA could be performed in the home or in the hospital the night before surgery, to determine the presence or absence of OSA and allow for triage of the patient to the appropriate setting postoperatively. Alternatively, strategies involving a 90-minute monitoring in the postanesthesia care unit for events concerning OSA have been implemented in some hospitals when OSA testing cannot be performed

Table 7
Review of studies examining in-laboratory PSG pathway versus PM pathway

Study,[Ref.] Year	Study Population	Arms	Screening Tool	Screened vs Enrolled	Prevalence of OSA	Repeat Testing	Inadequate Data	CPAP Adherence	Outcomes
Whitelaw et al,[49] 2005	Patients referred from family practice to a sleep clinic	Arm 1: PSG, followed by treatment with autoCPAP Arm 2: PM (Snoresat), followed by treatment with autoCPAP	None	Referred: 4767 Eligible: 2088 (44%) Enrolled: 307	AHI ≥10/h: PSG group: 68% PM group: 56%	None or not reported	None or not reported	PSG group: 3.8 h/night PM group: 3.3 h/night P = .4	Similar improvements in sleepiness (ESS) and sleep apnea related quality of life (SAQLI)
Mulgrew et al,[46] 2007	Patients referred to a hospital-based sleep center	Arm 1: PSG, CPAP titration, fixed CPAP therapy Arm 2: AutoCPAP × 1 wk, then fixed CPAP therapy	ESS ≥10, SACS ≥15, and overnight home oximetry (≥15/h)	Referred: 2216 Eligible: 79 (3.5%) Enrolled: 68	AHI ≥15/h: PSG group: 94%	None or not reported	None or not reported	PSG group: 5.4 h/night PM group: 6.0 h/night P = .02	Similar reductions in AHI observed between the 2 groups. Similar improvements in sleepiness (ESS) and SAQLI were observed
Berry et al,[44] 2008	Patients referred for a sleep study to a Veterans medical center	Arm 1: split night or PSG followed by CPAP titration, followed by fixed CPAP therapy Arm 2: PM (WatchPAT100), followed by autoCPAP therapy × 3 nights, then fixed CPAP therapy	None	Enrolled: 53	AHI ≥5/h: Overall: 93%	PM test: 4/53 (7.5%) AutoPAP: 7/50 (14%)	PM test: 2/53 (3.7%) AutoPAP: 45/53 (15%)	PSG group: 5.3 h/night 46% compliant PM group: 5.2 h/night 47% compliant P>.05	Similar improvements in sleepiness and sleep-related quality of life (FOSQ) and CPAP satisfaction
Antic, et al,[43] 2009	Patients referred to 3 academic sleep centers in Australia	Arm 1: Nurse model, autoCPAP × 4 nights followed by fixed CPAP therapy Arm 2: Physician model, full PSG, followed by CPAP titration, and fixed CPAP	ESS ≥8, snoring most or every night, ODI 2% >27/h)	Referred: 1427 Eligible: 195 Enrolled: 195	AHI in PSG group: Mean: 68 events/h	None or not reported	None or not reported	PM group: 4.1 h/night PSG group: 4.6 h/night P>.05	Similar improvements in sleepiness (ESS), quality of life, sleep-related quality of life, MWT, and executive function were observed

Skomro et al,[48] 2010	Tertiary-care sleep disorders clinic	Arm 1: Overnight PSG, 1 night PM (investigators and patients blinded to results), CPAP titration as split night (AHI ≥15) or separate night in those with AHI ≥5 Arm 2: PM (Embletta), 1 wk autoCPAP, 3 wk fixed CPAP therapy in those with RDI ≥5 (in-laboratory PSG and CPAP titration done; investigators and patients blinded to results)	ESS >10	Referred: 270 Eligible: 103 Enrolled: 102	AHI ≥5/h: Overall: 89/102 (87)%	None or not reported	None or not reported	PSG group: 5.6 h/night PM group: 5.4 h/night P = .49	Similar improvements in sleepiness (ESS), quality of life, sleep-related quality of life, and blood pressure were observed
VSATT Kuna et al,[45] 2011	Patients referred for to 2 Veterans medical centers sleep disorders clinic	Arm 1: In-laboratory pathway: PSG or split night with additional night for CPAP titration if needed, followed by fixed CPAP therapy Arm 2: Home testing pathway: PM (Embletta), AHI ≥15/h had autoCPAP × 5 d, followed by fixed CPAP therapy. Note: Patients with AHI <15/h or inadequate APAP titration had studies in the laboratory	None	Referred: ? Enrolled: 296	In-laboratory: 124/148 (84%) HST: 123/148 (83%) Overall: 247/296 (83%)	35/148 (24%) with repeat testing. 19% due to AHI <15/h on PM test 12/119 (10%) for autoCPAP	8/148 (6%) for PM testing 18/119 (15%) for autoCPAP	PSG group: 2.9 h/night PM group: 3.5 h/night P = .08	Similar improvements in sleepiness (ESS), quality of life, sleep-related quality of life, and depression scores were observed

(continued on next page)

Table 7
(continued)

Study,[Ref.] Year	Study Population	Arms	Screening Tool	Screened vs Enrolled	Prevalence of OSA	Repeat Testing	Inadequate Data	CPAP Adherence	Outcomes
HomePAP Rosen et al,[47] 2012	7 academic sleep disorders centers	Arm 1: PSG pathway: PSG or split night with additional night for CPAP titration if needed, followed by fixed CPAP therapy Arm 2: PM pathway: PM (Embletta X-30), AHI ≥15/h had autoCPAP × 7 d, followed by fixed CPAP therapy Note: Patients with AHI <15/h or inadequate APAP titration had studies in the laboratory	Modified SACS	Referred: ? Enrolled: 373	In-laboratory: 92/186 (49%) HST: 105/187 (56%) Overall: 197/373 (53%)	10/187(5%) with repeat testing. 19% due to AHI <15/h on PM test 10/105 (10%) for autoCPAP	Not reported for PM testing 7/105 (7%) for autoCPAP	PSG group: 2.9 h/ night PM group: 4.7 h/ night $P = .01$	Similar improvements in sleepiness (ESS), quality of life, sleep-related and sleep apnea quality of life were observed

Abbreviations: APAP, automatic positive airway pressure; ESS, Epworth Sleepiness Scale; FOSQ, Functional Outcomes of Sleep Questionnaire; HST, home sleep testing; MWT, maintenance wakefulness test; ODI, oxygen desaturation index; SACS, Sleep Apnea Clinical Risk Score.

From Collop NA, Anderson WM, Boehlecke B, et al. Clinical guidelines for the use of unattended portable monitors in the diagnosis of obstructive sleep apnea in adult patients. Portable Monitoring Task Force of the American Academy of Sleep Medicine. J Clin Sleep Med 2007;3(7):737–47; with permission.

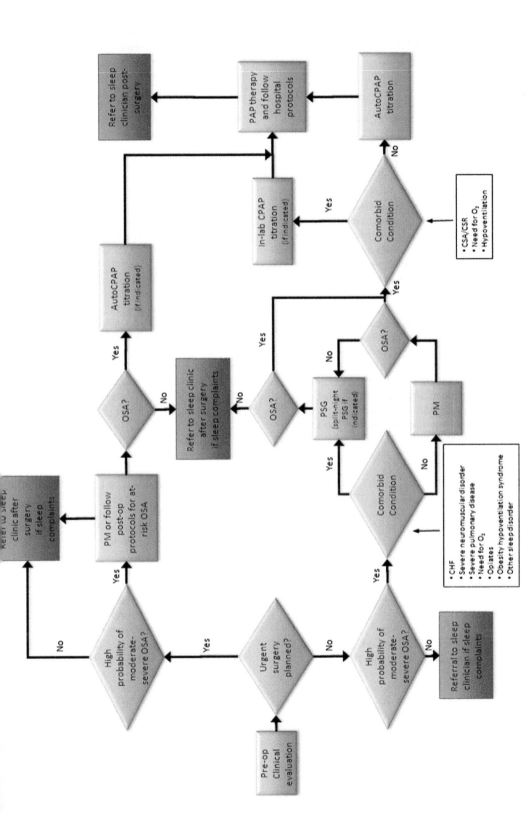

Fig. 5. Potential algorithm for diagnosis of obstructive sleep apnea (OSA) in a preoperative evaluation clinic incorporating portable monitoring (PM) and polysomnography (PSG) pathways. CHF, congestive heart failure; (C)PAP, (continuous) positive airway pressure; CSA, central sleep apnea; CSR, Cheyne-Stokes respiration.

before surgery.[50] Regardless of the strategy used, after surgery is completed, the patient should be referred for chronic care of OSA to a sleep medicine specialist or primary care provider.

SUMMARY

OSA is a highly prevalent condition; however, many patients remain undiagnosed or untreated, which could lead to postoperative complications in the surgical patient with unrecognized OSA. Timely identification of OSA and initiation of therapy before surgery can therefore represent an important target in improving postoperative outcomes. The use of PSG or PM can be used to identify these patients. PM is becoming more widely used to identify OSA; however, as with any diagnostic tool, clinicians using PM devices need to be familiar with which patients are most appropriate for PM, how to interpret PM data, and understanding the limitations of PM when using it for diagnosis. The PM device can be used only to confirm OSA, but does not rule out OSA when patients have OSA-related symptoms. PSG will continue to have a place in the management of OSA, particularly in more complicated patients. Clinicians in the preoperative clinic will need to develop pathways for OSA identification through partnership with local sleep centers and/or implementation of testing programs within the preoperative clinic.

REFERENCES

1. Young T, Palta M, Dempsey J, et al. The occurrence of sleep-disordered breathing among middle-aged adults. N Engl J Med 1993;328(17):1230–5.
2. Marin JM, Carrizo SJ, Vicente E, et al. Long-term cardiovascular outcomes in men with obstructive sleep apnoea-hypopnoea with or without treatment with continuous positive airway pressure: an observational study. Lancet 2005;365(9464):1046–53.
3. Mehra R, Benjamin EJ, Shahar E, et al. Association of nocturnal arrhythmias with sleep-disordered breathing: the Sleep Heart Health Study. Am J Respir Crit Care Med 2006;173(8):910–6.
4. Punjabi NM, Shahar E, Redline S, et al. Sleep-disordered breathing, glucose intolerance, and insulin resistance: the Sleep Heart Health Study. Am J Epidemiol 2004;160(6):521–30.
5. Barbe F, Pericas J, Munoz A, et al. Automobile accidents in patients with sleep apnea syndrome. An epidemiological and mechanistic study. Am J Respir Crit Care Med 1998;158(1):18–22.
6. Quan SF, Wright R, Baldwin CM, et al. Obstructive sleep apnea-hypopnea and neurocognitive functioning in the Sleep Heart Health Study. Sleep Med 2006;7(6):498–507.
7. Punjabi NM, Caffo BS, Goodwin JL, et al. Sleep-disordered breathing and mortality: a prospective cohort study. PLoS Med 2009;6(8):e1000132.
8. Young T, Finn L, Peppard PE, et al. Sleep disordered breathing and mortality: eighteen-year follow-up of the Wisconsin sleep cohort. Sleep 2008;31(8):1071–8.
9. Kaw R, Chung F, Pasupuleti V, et al. Meta-analysis of the association between obstructive sleep apnoea and postoperative outcome. Br J Anaesth 2012; 109(6):897–906.
10. Finkel KJ, Searleman AC, Tymkew H, et al. Prevalence of undiagnosed obstructive sleep apnea among adult surgical patients in an academic medical center. Sleep Med 2009;10(7):753–8.
11. Young T, Evans L, Finn L, et al. Estimation of the clinically diagnosed proportion of sleep apnea syndrome in middle-aged men and women. Sleep 1997;20(9): 705–6.
12. Kapur V, Strohl KP, Redline S, et al. Underdiagnosis of sleep apnea syndrome in U.S. communities. Sleep Breath 2002;6(2):49–54.
13. Chai-Coetzer CL, Antic NA, Rowland LS, et al. A simplified model of screening questionnaire and home monitoring for obstructive sleep apnoea in primary care. Thorax 2011;66(3):213–9.
14. Chung F, Ward B, Ho J, et al. Preoperative identification of sleep apnea risk in elective surgical patients, using the Berlin questionnaire. J Clin Anesth 2007; 19(2):130–4.
15. Chung F, Yegneswaran B, Liao P, et al. STOP questionnaire: a tool to screen patients for obstructive sleep apnea. Anesthesiology 2008;108(5):812–21.
16. Chung F, Yegneswaran B, Liao P, et al. Validation of the Berlin questionnaire and American Society of Anesthesiologists checklist as screening tools for obstructive sleep apnea in surgical patients. Anesthesiology 2008;108(5):822–30.
17. Flemons WW, Whitelaw WA, Brant R, et al. Likelihood ratios for a sleep apnea clinical prediction rule. Am J Respir Crit Care Med 1994;150(5 Pt 1):1279–85.
18. Maislin G, Pack AI, Kribbs NB, et al. A survey screen for prediction of apnea. Sleep 1995;18(3):158–66.
19. American Academy of Sleep Medicine. International classification of sleep disorders: diagnostic & coding manual. 2nd edition. Westchester (NY): American Academy of Sleep Medicine; 2005. p. 1–293.
20. Berry RB, Brooks R, Gamaldo CE, et al. The AASM manual for the scoring of sleep and associated events: rules, terminology and technical specifications, Version 2.0. Version 2.0. Darien (IL): American Academy of Sleep Medicine; 2012.
21. Collop NA, Tracy SL, Kapur V, et al. Obstructive sleep apnea devices for out-of-center (OOC) testing: technology evaluation. J Clin Sleep Med 2011;7(5):531–48.
22. Quan SF, Howard BV, Iber C, et al. The Sleep Heart Health Study: design, rationale, and methods. Sleep 1997;20(12):1077–85.

23. Berry RB. Uses and limitations of portable monitoring for diagnosis and management of obstructive sleep apnea. Sleep Med Clin 2011;6(3):309–33.

24. Collop NA. Portable monitoring for the diagnosis of obstructive sleep apnea. Curr Opin Pulm Med 2008;14(6):525–9.

25. Center for Medicare and Medicaid Services. Decision memo for sleep testing for obstructive sleep apnea (OSA) (CAG-00405N). 2009.

26. Ferber R, Millman R, Coppola M, et al. Portable recording in the assessment of obstructive sleep apnea. ASDA standards of practice. Sleep 1994; 17(4):378–92.

27. Pang KP, Gourin CG, Terris DJ. A comparison of polysomnography and the WatchPAT in the diagnosis of obstructive sleep apnea. Otolaryngol Head Neck Surg 2007;137(4):665–8.

28. Kim MJ, Lee GH, Kim CS, et al. Comparison of three actigraphic algorithms used to evaluate sleep in patients with obstructive sleep apnea. Sleep Breath 2012. http://dx.doi.org/10.1007/s11325-012-0689-z. [Epub ahead of print].

29. Hwang S, Chung G, Lee J, et al. Sleep/wake estimation using only anterior tibialis electromyography data. Biomed Eng Online 2012;11:26.

30. O'Driscoll DM, Turton AR, Copland JM, et al. Energy expenditure in obstructive sleep apnea: validation of a multiple physiological sensor for determination of sleep and wake. Sleep Breath 2012. http://dx.doi.org/10.1007/s11325-012-0662-x. [Epub ahead of print].

31. Senny F, Maury G, Cambron L, et al. The sleep/wake state scoring from mandible movement signal. Sleep Breath 2012;16(2):535–42.

32. Pitson DJ, Stradling JR. Value of beat-to-beat blood pressure changes, detected by pulse transit time, in the management of the obstructive sleep apnoea/hypopnoea syndrome. Eur Respir J 1998;12(3):685–92.

33. Pittman SD, Ayas NT, MacDonald MM, et al. Using a wrist-worn device based on peripheral arterial tonometry to diagnose obstructive sleep apnea: in-laboratory and ambulatory validation. Sleep 2004; 27(5):923–33.

34. Nakano H, Hayashi M, Ohshima E, et al. Validation of a new system of tracheal sound analysis for the diagnosis of sleep apnea-hypopnea syndrome. Sleep 2004;27(5):951–7.

35. Reichert JA, Bloch DA, Cundiff E, et al. Comparison of the NovaSom QSG, a new sleep apnea home-diagnostic system, and polysomnography. Sleep Med 2003;4(3):213–8.

36. Sanders MH, Kern NB, Costantino JP, et al. Accuracy of end-tidal and transcutaneous PCO_2 monitoring during sleep. Chest 1994;106(2):472–83.

37. Ayappa I, Norman RG, Seelall V, et al. Validation of a self-applied unattended monitor for sleep disordered breathing. J Clin Sleep Med 2008;4(1):26–37.

38. Hesselbacher S, Mattewal A, Hirshkowitz M, et al. Classification, technical specifications, and types of home sleep testing devices for sleep-disordered breathing. Sleep Med Clin 2011;6(3):261–82.

39. Kuna ST. Outcome measures for assessing portable monitor testing for sleep apnea. Sleep Med Clin 2011;6(3):293–307.

40. Balk EM, Moorthy D, Obadan NO, et al. Diagnosis and treatment of obstructive sleep apnea in adults. Rockville (MD): Agency for Healthcare Research and Quality (US); 2011.

41. Collop NA, Anderson WM, Boehlecke B, et al. Clinical guidelines for the use of unattended portable monitors in the diagnosis of obstructive sleep apnea in adult patients. Portable Monitoring Task Force of the American Academy of Sleep Medicine. J Clin Sleep Med 2007;3(7):737–47.

42. Netzer NC, Stoohs RA, Netzer CM, et al. Using the Berlin Questionnaire to identify patients at risk for the sleep apnea syndrome. Ann Intern Med 1999; 131(7):485–91.

43. Antic NA, Buchan C, Esterman A, et al. A randomized controlled trial of nurse-led care for symptomatic moderate-severe obstructive sleep apnea. Am J Respir Crit Care Med 2009;179(6):501–8.

44. Berry RB, Hill G, Thompson L, et al. Portable monitoring and autotitration versus polysomnography for the diagnosis and treatment of sleep apnea. Sleep 2008;31(10):1423–31.

45. Kuna ST, Gurubhagavatula I, Maislin G, et al. Noninferiority of functional outcome in ambulatory management of obstructive sleep apnea. Am J Respir Crit Care Med 2011;183(9):1238–44.

46. Mulgrew AT, Fox N, Ayas NT, et al. Diagnosis and initial management of obstructive sleep apnea without polysomnography: a randomized validation study. Ann Intern Med 2007;146(3):157–66.

47. Rosen CL, Auckley D, Benca R, et al. A multisite randomized trial of portable sleep studies and positive airway pressure autotitration versus laboratory-based polysomnography for the diagnosis and treatment of obstructive sleep apnea: the HomePAP study. Sleep 2012;35(6):757–67.

48. Skomro RP, Gjevre J, Reid J, et al. Outcomes of home-based diagnosis and treatment of obstructive sleep apnea. Chest 2010;138(2):257–63.

49. Whitelaw WA, Brant RF, Flemons WW. Clinical usefulness of home oximetry compared with polysomnography for assessment of sleep apnea. Am J Respir Crit Care Med 2005;171(2):188–93.

50. Gali B, Whalen FX, Schroeder DR, et al. Identification of patients at risk for postoperative respiratory complications using a preoperative obstructive sleep apnea screening tool and postanesthesia care assessment. Anesthesiology 2009;110(4): 869–77.

Obstructive Sleep Apnea and Perioperative Complications
From Mechanisms to Risk Modification

Satya Krishna Ramachandran, MD, FRCA

KEYWORDS

- Obstructive sleep apnea • Metabolic dysfunction • Sympathetic activation • Respiratory depression
- Risk modification

KEY POINTS

- Obstructive sleep apnea (OSA) is independently associated with significant postoperative morbidity and mortality.
- There are significant related metabolic, physiologic, and pathologic processes and conditions that potentially mediate these outcomes.
- The perioperative period signifies a high-risk period for these patients and risk-modification is traditionally attempted through multimodal approaches. There is need for comparative effectiveness research to identify best practice.

INTRODUCTION

Obstructive sleep apnea (OSA) is prevalent in a significant proportion of surgical patients, although most of these patients are undiagnosed. Patients with OSA pose unique challenges to perioperative care providers through identification, risk stratification, therapeutic safety, monitoring, and disposition. Interest into OSA as an independent risk factor for adverse perioperative outcomes is fairly recent. This reflects the growing trend of prospective research involving OSA and perioperative outcomes. Although the specific mechanisms of adverse outcomes are yet unclear, specialty bodies have recognized the challenges and provided expert guidance on the perioperative risk assessment and management of these complex patients.[1] This article reviews the key putative mechanisms for adverse outcomes and provides an overview of the effectiveness of risk modification strategies.

HEART RATE VARIABILITY, CONDUCTION ABNORMALITIES, AND OSA

The relationship between OSA and cardiovascular variability and conduction abnormalities has been studied extensively. Narkiewicz and colleagues[2] showed that the RR interval was significantly reduced in moderate to severe OSA, whereas RR interval variance was stunted across all disease severity in OSA. Although blood pressure was similar, systolic blood pressure variance was significantly heightened in moderate to severe OSA. These changes are consistent with a state of heightened sympathetic cardiovascular drive in sleep apnea.[3] Obstructive apneas are associated with significant negative intrathoracic pressures causing increased wall stress, diastolic dysfunction, and atrial remodeling.[4–7]

OSA also has significant effects on conduction abnormalities. QT prolongation, QT dispersion, and beat-to-beat variance in QT intervals have all been shown to correlate with OSA, and may serve to mark high risk of sudden cardiac death.[8–10] In addition, OSA is associated with prolongation of T-wave peak and end, a measure of increased ventricular arrhythmogenecity.[11] However, these dynamic conduction abnormalities occur more commonly than ventricular arrhythmias and may not be causal in arrhythmia genesis.[10] Sinus bradycardia, sinus arrest, and second-degree

Department of Anesthesiology, University of Michigan Medical School, 1500, East Medical Centre Drive, Ann Arbor, MI 48103, USA

E-mail address: rsatyak@med.umich.edu

Sleep Med Clin 8 (2013) 93–103

http://dx.doi.org/10.1016/j.jsmc.2012.12.004

(Mobitz type 1) heart block are not uncommon in young adults, whereas atrial arrhythmias and ventricular ectopics are commoner in older patients.[12–14] Severity of OSA is independently correlated to P-wave duration and prolonged electromechanical delay, signifying increased risk of atrial remodeling and arrhythmias.[15,16] It is unclear why these changes occur, but degree of hypoxemia, severity of OSA, obesity, severity of negative intrathoracic pressure, age, and gender are likely risk factors.[15,17]

The relationship between OSA and atrioventricular (AV) conduction delays is less clear. Some evidence exists to support the view that atrioventricular conduction is affected by OSA.[18–20] Nocturnal bradyarrhythmias were associated with obesity and severe OSA.[18] Interestingly, there is a 59% prevalence of OSA in patients with permanent pacemakers[21]; however, prolonged ventricular asystole during OSA is not due to fixed or anatomic disease of the sinus node or the AV conduction system.[22]

The perioperative implications of these data are evolving. There is heightened sympathetic nerve activity (SNA) because of the surgical insult and significant hypoxia that occurs postoperatively in patients with preoperative desaturation.[23] In addition, significant risks of postoperative airway obstruction and intrathoracic pressure changes exist because of the combined effects of analgesic medications, sleep disturbances, and changes in lung function. Postoperative atrial fibrillation occurs in 3% of noncardiac surgical patients and has significant impact on postoperative hospital costs, length of stay, and mortality.[24] Risk factors for OSA, including heart failure, hypertension, and obesity, are independently associated with risk of postoperative atrial fibrillation.

OSA AND SYMPATHETIC ACTIVATION

Significant episodic tachycardia and hypertension occur during sleep, closely following changes in SNA.[25] These can be explained by chemoreceptor responses to hypoxia and hypercapnia.[26–28] More severe hypoxemia during apneas results in greater frequency and amplitude of SNA, resulting in tachycardia and dynamic vasoconstriction that maintains muscle and splanchnic blood pressure during the low cardiac output state of obstructive apnea.[29,30] The vasoconstriction persists through resumption of breathing, when sudden increases in cardiac output occurs, causing large surges in blood pressure. Sleep stages have differing effects on the severity of nocturnal hypoxemia and SNA, with greatest effects seen in Stage 2 and rapid-eye movement (REM) sleep. This hypertonic SNA then

extends from being a primarily nocturnal phenomenon into heightened SNA during daytime hours, despite normal oxygen levels.[25] Thus, patients with untreated OSA have significantly elevated SNA, which is thought to contribute to development of hypertension, arrhythmias, and cardiac function abnormalities. The implications of these pathophysiological changes in the perioperative period are important. Sleep architecture changes are common after anesthesia and major surgery, either as a result of opioid medication effects or surgical insult. The end result is an abolition of REM sleep on the first night and a rebound of REM sleep on the third postoperative night. This period is also associated with significant nocturnal desaturation.[31] Both of these phenomena are likely to significantly enhance SNA and influence the risk of developing postoperative adverse cardiac outcomes.[32] Gogenur and colleagues[33] showed that 38% of postoperative episodes of ST segment changes were associated with a concurrent episode of desaturation, whereas tachycardia was seen in only 16% of ST segment abnormalities. The positive predictive value of desaturation or tachycardia on development of ST changes was poor at 4% and 1% respectively. Another study showed that presence of severe nocturnal hypoxemia adversely influenced outcomes following myocardial infarction. Simultaneous occurrence of episodic desaturation and arrhythmias was seen in 14% to 29% during the first 5 nights after myocardial infarction. Episodic desaturation occurred in conjunction with any electrocardiographic abnormalities in 53% to 72% of patients during the same time.[34] Previous studies have shown that nadir peripheral oxy-hemoglobin saturation ($SpO2$) less than 60% to 65% is associated with increase in the risk of ventricular arrhythmias.[35,36] In contrast, hypoxemia seen in patients with chronic obstructive pulmonary disease (COPD) does not increase risk of ventricular arrhythmias.[37] Hence, it can be summarized that the relationship among hypoxemia, SNA, and ischemic cardiac events is unlikely to be causal, but that SNA may significantly influence the outcomes of ischemic events because of its negative effect on the myocardial oxygen supply-demand balance, arrhythmogenicity, and other unmeasured effects.

Sudden unanticipated postoperative death in the early postoperative period follows patterns of sudden cardiac death seen in patients with OSA in the general population. Gami and colleagues[38] showed that patients with OSA were more likely to die during the hours from midnight to 6 AM and also showed a dose-dependent increase in this risk of sudden nocturnal death with increasing severity of OSA. This nocturnal pattern was is in striking contrast to the nadir of sudden death from cardiac causes during this time in persons without OSA and in the general population. In another study of postoperative patients with unanticipated life-threatening adverse respiratory events, a similar pattern was observed, with the greatest incidence of fatal events occurring during the nocturnal hours of midnight to 6 AM.[39] These findings either point to day-night variability in the quality of monitoring, nursing care, or pathophysiological phenomena that are common to these studies. What can these phenomena be? The higher incidence of sudden death in patients with OSA reflects the abnormal physiology of sleep, in which SNA is elevated (unlike the typical reduction in individuals who do not have OSA) and cardiac dysrhythmias are more likely to occur.

OSA AND INFLAMMATION

Several studies have demonstrated the significant association between OSA and inflammatory markers in a variety of disease states. The combination of repetitive hypoxemia and sleep deprivation in patients with OSA may be associated with increased levels of plasma cytokines, adhesion molecules,[40,41] serum amyloid,[42–44] and C-reactive protein (CRP).[41,45–47] There also is evidence for enhanced leukocyte activation in OSA.[48,49] The heightened inflammatory state may influence postoperative mortality and morbidity.

OSA AND METABOLIC DYSFUNCTION

OSA, both independent of and in conjunction with obesity, is associated with insulin resistance and leptin resistance.[50–53] Obesity, high SNA, and sleep deprivation are likely culprits in this association. The relationship between OSA and resting hyperglycemia or glucose intolerance may have significance in the setting of the heightened metabolic state and wound-healing processes after surgery. Systemic effects of insulin resistance may contribute to cardiovascular disease in OSA.[52] Ramachandran and colleagues[54] have previously shown that type 2 diabetes is an independent predictor of OSA diagnosis in surgical patients and that it is independently associated with early postoperative respiratory failure.[55]

OSA AND OXIDATIVE STRESS

Oxidative stress is a likely mechanism of adverse outcomes in patients with OSA, secondary to injury from cyclical deoxygenation-reoxygenation. Markers of oxidative stress injury are elevated in patients with OSA and include thiobarbituric acid–reactive substances, isoprostanes, nitrotyrosine, and oxidized low-density lipoprotein.[56–59]

OSA AND COEXISTING DISEASES

Perioperative outcomes research relevant to OSA suggests several important facts. First, OSA is independently associated with a twofold to sixfold increase in risk of adverse cardiopulmonary outcomes.[60] Second, high-risk features of OSA, namely morbid obesity (body mass index $\geq$40 kg.m^{-2}), diabetes, and hypertension are also independently associated with postoperative pulmonary outcomes.[55,61] Third, the first 3 days after surgery represents a high-risk period for unanticipated respiratory failure needing tracheal intubation. Ramachandran and colleagues[55] showed that half of all 30-day pulmonary outcomes occurred in the first 72 hours after surgery, affecting 0.8% to 0.9% of 222,094 patients. It is possible that severity of surgical insult and coexisting diseases explain most of the risk of postoperative pulmonary adverse outcomes, and the individual influence of preoperative hypoxemia and apneas is currently unknown. Postoperative desaturation has been linked to adverse outcomes in patients with OSA,[62] although the retrospective nature of this analysis and the lack of supportive data in ambulatory surgery patients with OSA suggests that severity of surgery may play an important confounding role in the association.[63] Surgical factors were the most prominent risk factors in predicting early postoperative respiratory failure in another study.[55]

OSA AND RESPIRATORY DEPRESSION

Respiratory depression (RD) is a plausible and an often-quoted mechanism of postoperative respiratory decline in patients with OSA. It is estimated that up to 20% of patients develop respiratory depression postoperatively.[64] Blake and colleagues[65] showed that patients with significant postoperative sleep-disordered breathing (SDB) received 3-times greater doses of morphine. The clinical significance and mechanisms of these findings are unknown, but the results signify the need explore the relationship between altered chemosensitivity and perioperative respiratory complications.

Several pathophysiological phenomena observed in patients with OSA make RD a plausible mechanism of perioperative adverse respiratory outcomes. Previous studies indicate that both static (wakeful state static measurements) and dynamic (sleep state measurements) aspects of the chemoreflex control are affected in OSA.

These studies indicate depressed chemosensitivity and an underdamped chemoreflex control as additional mechanisms that promote occurrence of periodic obstructive apneas.[66] Additionally, it appears that the changes in ventilatory sensitivity are correlated with the change in apnea-hypopnea index (AHI).[67] Several systemic conditions are associated with altered chemosensitivity in patients with OSA. Diabetic autonomic neuropathy may play an important role and alterations in peripheral and central chemosensitivity closely relate to the severity of neuropathy. A greater prevalence of OSA is observed in these patients.[68,69] Patients with COPD and OSA (overlap syndrome) experience more severe episodic nocturnal hypoxemia because of lower alveolar and blood oxygen stores, and longer apneas perhaps contributed to by depressed chemosensitivity.[70] Additionally, patients with overlap syndrome also have daytime hypercapnia and the severity of OSA may influence the degree of altered chemosensitivity seen in patients with COPD.[71] Peripheral chemosensitivity to hypoxia may mediate the association between OSA and hypertension.[72] A mutation in Phox2b causes congenital central hypoventilation syndrome in humans with lack of CO_2 chemosensitivity, fatal central apnea, and specific loss of parafacial neurons.[73] The dose-dependent relationship between opioids and RD is well known. Patients with OSA also show a dose-dependent worsening of central apnea and ataxic breathing during sleep, with increasing dosage of opioids for chronic pain.[74] Drugs may play an important role in modulating chemosensitivity in the perioperative period. Clonidine reversibly depresses both slope and threshold of CO_2 response, and selectively inhibits the response of hypoglossal nerve activity to CO_2.[75] Hypercapnic ventilatory response and peripheral chemosensitivity are enhanced by administration of the dopamine antagonist, domperidone, in patients with OSA.[76] Patients with mild-moderate OSA with higher awake central chemosensitivity had greater respiratory impairment during sleep with temazepam, suggesting that it might be possible to prospectively phenotype interindividual variability in risk of RD during wakefulness.[77] Thus, several mechanisms exist that make RD more likely to occur in patients with OSA. Obesity hypoventilation syndrome (OHS) or obesity-associated hypoventilation is defined as the triad of obesity, daytime hypoventilation, and SDB in the absence of an alternative cause for hypoventilation.[78] Patients with OHS are at greater risk of RD because of depressed hypercapnic ventilatory responses at rest. In addition, high inspired fraction during oxygen therapy is associated with increased risk of central apneas.[79]

Fair evidence exists to support the perioperative relationship between severe OSA and RD in pediatric literature. Brown and colleagues[80,81] have shown that children with OSA undergoing adenotonsillectomy are more likely to experience significant desaturation and require significantly lower doses of opioids postoperatively. In addition, the studies also showed that significant preoperative desaturation correlates with morphine requirements and the lower age group needs less morphine. Patients with severe preoperative desaturation required half morphine dose with equal analgesia and risk of side effect.[80] Unlike these data, the relationship between preoperative hypoxemia and postoperative opioid sensitivity is less clear in adults. Higher doses of opioids are associated with dose-dependent worsening of the apnea hypopnea index and frequency of respiratory dysrhythmia. Patients with OSA are predisposed to chronic pain states,[82] and are potentially more likely to be exposed to higher doses of opioid medications. Specific disease states may be indicative of higher risk of respiratory depression. Patients with OSA and pulmonary hypertension, OHS, and overlap syndrome may be associated with increased risk of adverse respiratory outcomes through RD. Ramachandran and colleagues[39] described 2 interesting findings in a retrospective study of patients who developed postoperative life-threatening adverse respiratory events. Patients who died received significantly lower doses of morphine equivalent daily dose, compared with patients who survived the events. Further, high-risk features of OSA were twice as frequent in patients with the adverse respiratory outcome compared with adult patients presenting to the same hospital for surgical care.

PERIOPERATIVE RISK MODIFICATION

The mainstay of perioperative RD risk modification remain patient selection, preoperative positive airway pressure (PAP) therapy, opioid reduction strategies, postoperative PAP therapy, and higher-quality monitoring. These form the key recommendations of the American Society of Anesthesiologists' practice guidelines.[1]

Patient Selection

The Society for Ambulatory Anesthesia[83] and the American Society of Anesthesiologists' practice guidelines[1] on management of patients with OSA provides a framework for patient selection. In general, patients with severe OSA (AHI >30/h), severe nocturnal desaturations (SpO_2 <60%), and untreated significant systemic conditions need to be identified, optimized, and managed in hospital settings. Severity of surgery plays an important role in determining the postoperative disposition and duration of monitoring after surgery. Several protocols have been described to manage patients at high risk of OSA,[84] with many using screening tools, such as the STOP-Bang[85] questionnaire, the sleep apnea clinical score,[84] and the American Society of Anesthesiologists screening tool.[86]

Preoperative CPAP Therapy

There is no randomized controlled trial–guided evidence of benefit with preoperative continuous positive airway pressure (CPAP) therapy and, more specifically, the duration of CPAP therapy needed for risk modification.

Despite this, there are several mechanisms for risk modification with preoperative CPAP therapy. Perhaps most importantly, CPAP therapy has a rapid effect on SNA, resulting in significant reduction of episodic hypertension and improving heart rate variability.[87] Cessation of CPAP therapy is associated with an instantaneous increase in SNA, pointing to the significance of compliance with PAP therapy in risk modification.[25] CPAP has been shown to improve hypoxemia, reduce arrhythmias,[14,19,88] reduce risk of postcardioversion atrial fibrillation,[89] and reduce the incidence of ventricular arrhythmias.[90] QT dispersion abnormalities are reversible with CPAP therapy.[9] CPAP also reverses the intrathoracic changes associated with atrial remodeling; however, it is unclear what the degree of risk modification is in a larger population. Although CPAP reduced resting heart rates, possibly because of reduced SNA,[91] it failed to improve risk of cardiovascular events[92] or arrhythmias.[91]

Direct evidence that preoperative CPAP therapy is associated with reduced RD in patients with OSA is lacking. Treatment with PAP therapy has complex and seemingly opposing effects on peripheral and central chemosensitivity. On the one hand, Spicuzza and colleagues[93] showed that reduced peripheral oxygen chemosensitivity may be a side effect of CPAP therapy. On the other hand, noninvasive ventilation (NIV) in patients with severe OHS has been shown to improve central apneas primarily through reduction in diurnal hypercapnia.[94] Although NIV treatment in mild OHS improves sleep and blood gas measurements, it does not change inflammatory, metabolic, and cardiovascular markers.[95] Similarly, CPAP therapy for 2 weeks caused significant increase in ventilatory responses to hypercapnia in patients with OSA.[96]

The effect of CPAP therapy on inflammation is variable, with some studies showing benefit and others showing no benefit. Appropriate CPAP therapy improved CRP values, suggesting its potentially beneficial role in reducing perioperative risk in patients with OSA.[97] This study showed that CRP decreased nonsignificantly in less than 3 months (Standard Mean Difference [SMD], 0.26, 95% confidence interval [CI] −0.08 to 0.60, $P = .138$), significantly decreased after 3 months (SMD, 0.68, 95% CI 0.34 to 1.02, $P = .000$), and further declined after 6 months (SMD, 0.74, 95% CI 0.43 to 1.05, $P = .000$) of CPAP treatment. Other studies describe a beneficial effect on pulmonary and nasal inflammatory markers but no effect on systemic markers.[59,98] Treatment with CPAP is associated with a reduction of the oxidative stress marker, nitrotyrosine.[59]

One of the bigger challenges with preoperative CPAP therapy is timely preoperative diagnosis and PAP titration. A recent study described a 40% adherence with treatment and median CPAP usage of just 2.5 hours among users.[99] Given that most patients with OSA are undiagnosed and most of known patients are untreated, significant challenges exist for risk modification using preoperative PAP therapy. Compared with continuing CPAP, 2 weeks of CPAP withdrawal was associated with a significant increase in morning blood pressures and heart rate. CPAP withdrawal is associated with an increase in urinary catecholamines but not markers of systemic inflammation, insulin resistance, or blood lipids.[100]

Postoperative CPAP Therapy

There is robust evidence for early treatment of postoperative hypoxemia using CPAP therapy. Squadrone and colleagues[101] performed a randomized control trial of CPAP versus face-mask oxygen therapy for treatment of hypoxemia after major elective abdominal surgery. CPAP treatment was associated with a 10-fold reduction in intubation rates and a 5-fold reduction in pneumonia rates. Direct evidence of benefit of postoperative CPAP therapy in patients with OSA is unclear. Utilization of perioperative OSA protocols and respiratory therapy teams is associated with improved outcomes.[102] An essential aspect of risk modification is developing protocols that address identification of the high-risk patient, use of appropriate monitoring, determination of thresholds for PAP initiation, and identification of parameters for escalation of care.[1]

Opioid Reduction Strategies

Increasing opioid doses increases clinically relevant side effects. The threshold dose for any clinically meaningful side effects was 30 mg for the day of surgery and postoperative day 1 following laparoscopic cholecystectomy. Additional 3-mg morphine equivalent increments increased the number of side effects in a stepwise manner. The threshold dose that produced sedation in that study was 8 mg. Opioid dose reduction is possible with several analgesic techniques and medications. Drug-specific and procedure-specific differences are important to recognize. Short-term pain control is improved by opioid dose reduction. Perioperative epidural analgesia was not protective against hypoxemia, and therapy with opioids did not seem to be of importance for the occurrence of late postoperative hypoxemia on nights 2 and 3 after coronary artery bypass grafting surgery.[103]

Opioid-induced respiratory depression may also be attributable to altered chemosensitivity in OSA. Despite the known relationship between opioid dose and postoperative respiratory disturbances, risk-reduction strategies aimed at reducing opioid dosage has not shown benefit in prospective studies. Brown and colleagues[80] did not find a relationship between prospective opioid dose prediction and reduced postoperative hypoxemia. Similarly, Blake and colleagues[65] showed no change in SDB with opioid sparing. These studies highlight a significant problem with using only opioid-sparing concepts in perioperative population risk reduction. The findings also signify the need to better phenotype patients at greatest risk of RD for targeted intervention.

Postoperative Monitoring and Surveillance

Expert societies and regulatory bodies have recently published guidelines to address the need for monitoring strategies to detect significant drug-induced respiratory depression in the postoperative period. Although this overall goal of better monitoring reflects the ideal end point, continuous postoperative monitoring is limited to hospitalized patients and current monitoring protocols often do not extend past 24 hours into the highest risk period for postoperative hypoxemia. Continuous pulse oximetry (CPOX) is superior to intermittent monitoring, but the clinical significance of episodic postoperative hypoxemia is still unclear, especially during opioid analgesic therapy. Previous studies did not demonstrate significant improvement in postoperative outcomes with CPOX.[104–107] Patient surveillance systems may provide a superior method of continuous monitoring by notifying desaturation and pulse rate abnormalities using threshold-based alert pages to nurses. Taenzer and colleagues[108] showed a reduction in rescue events and intensive

care unit transfers after institution of a threshold-based patient surveillance system. It must be noted that electronic patient monitoring systems have a greater chance of success when combined with robust protocols for escalation of care and clear expectations of responsibilities. The other concern with monitoring is technological intensification and the risk of alarm fatigue. The Emergency Care Research Institute continues to recognize alarm hazards as the top safety concern for health care. Specific aspects of concern include alarm overload, loss of communication of alarm data to paging interfaces, nuisance alarms, and lack of clarity on thresholds for escalation of care. The safety or risks of alarm thresholds are unknown largely. Thresholds of SpO_2 of less than 80% for longer than 30 seconds have been used to reduce alarm fatigue.[108] A recent study from the Johns Hopkins Hospital showed a reduction in nuisance alarms by 43% without loss of safety.[109,110] Data on the sensitivity and, therefore, the false-negative rates (ie, true desaturation events that do not trigger a paging alert) are unclear. The evidence for other modalities of continuous monitoring is sparse. In summary, the risks of technological intensification need to be balanced against the benefits of combined monitoring methods.

Postoperative Pulmonary Management

Lung volume maintenance is of crucial importance in reducing risk of obstructive apneas.[111] Postural change from supine to sitting reduces tendency to airway obstruction in patients with OSA.[112] Other factors that potentially augment lung volume include avoidance of 100% oxygen for longer than 15 minutes at emergence from anesthesia,[113] use of intraoperative lung recruitment,[114] and early use of CPAP therapy.[115,116]

Supplemental oxygen therapy is an important consideration in postoperative patients, especially in patients with OSA who may be at greater risk of developing RD. Pulse oximetry has value in assessment of hypoventilation in the absence of supplemental inspired oxygen. Arterial desaturation was fourfold higher in patients who breathed room air than in patients who breathed supplemental oxygen in the postanesthesia care unit.[117] Based on the alveolar gas equation, pulse oximetry would fail to detect an alveolar carbon dioxide value higher than 80 mm Hg with fairly modest increases in inspired oxygen fraction from 21% to 28%. This inspired oxygen fraction is easily achieved with 4-L to 6-L flow through a nasal cannula or face mask. Because oxygen therapy is usually the first response to postoperative desaturation, it may influence the safety of subsequent opioid therapy. Thus, there is need to develop better monitoring modalities in patients who need oxygen in the postoperative period. Perioperative caregivers need to be educated about the risk of routine oxygen therapy during opioid analgesic therapy.

SUMMARY

There are several putative mechanisms for the perioperative adverse events in patients with OSA. The mainstays of risk modification are patient selection, PAP therapy, opioid reduction strategies, and enhanced postoperative monitoring. Further research needs to be directed at phenotyping high-risk characteristics and evaluating specific interventions through the development of a high-quality sleep apnea perioperative outcomes registry.

REFERENCES

1. Gross JB, Bachenberg KL, Benumof JL, et al. Practice guidelines for the perioperative management of patients with obstructive sleep apnea: a report by the American Society of Anesthesiologists Task Force on Perioperative Management of patients with obstructive sleep apnea. Anesthesiology 2006;104:1081–93 [quiz: 1117–8].
2. Narkiewicz K, Montano N, Cogliati C, et al. Altered cardiovascular variability in obstructive sleep apnea. Circulation 1998;98:1071–7.
3. Narkiewicz K, Somers VK. Cardiovascular variability characteristics in obstructive sleep apnea. Auton Neurosci 2001;90:89–94.
4. Otto ME, Belohlavek M, Romero-Corral A, et al. Comparison of cardiac structural and functional changes in obese otherwise healthy adults with versus without obstructive sleep apnea. Am J Cardiol 2007;99:1298–302.
5. Romero-Corral A, Somers VK, Pellikka PA, et al. Decreased right and left ventricular myocardial performance in obstructive sleep apnea. Chest 2007;132:1863–70.
6. Buda AJ, Pinsky MR, Ingels NB Jr, et al. Effect of intrathoracic pressure on left ventricular performance. N Engl J Med 1979;301:453–9.
7. Somers VK, Dyken ME, Skinner JL. Autonomic and hemodynamic responses and interactions during the Mueller maneuver in humans. J Auton Nerv Syst 1993;44:253–9.
8. Voigt L, Haq SA, Mitre CA, et al. Effect of obstructive sleep apnea on QT dispersion: a potential mechanism of sudden cardiac death. Cardiology 2011;118:68–73.
9. Dursunoglu D, Dursunoglu N. Effect of CPAP on QT interval dispersion in obstructive sleep apnea patients without hypertension. Sleep Med 2007;8: 478–83.
10. Barta K, Szabo Z, Kun C, et al. The effect of sleep apnea on QT interval, QT dispersion, and arrhythmias. Clin Cardiol 2010;33:E35–9.
11. Kilicaslan F, Tokatli A, Ozdag F, et al. Tp-e interval, Tp-e/QT ratio, and Tp-e/QTc ratio are prolonged in patients with moderate and severe obstructive sleep apnea. Pacing Clin Electrophysiol 2012;35: 966–72.
12. Adlakha A, Shepard JW Jr. Cardiac arrhythmias during normal sleep and in obstructive sleep apnea syndrome. Sleep Med Rev 1998;2:45–60.
13. Ji KH, Kim DH, Yun CH. Severe obstructive sleep apnea syndrome with symptomatic daytime bradyarrhythmia. J Clin Sleep Med 2009;5:246–7.
14. Maeno K, Kasai A, Setsuda M, et al. Advanced atrioventricular block induced by obstructive sleep apnea before oxygen desaturation. Heart Vessels 2009;24:236–40.
15. Maeno KI, Kasai T, Kasagi S, et al. Relationship between atrial conduction delay and obstructive sleep apnea. Heart Vessels 2012 [Epub ahead of print]. Available at: http://link.springer.com/article/10.1007%2Fs00380-012-0288-8. Accessed December 18, 2012.
16. Cagirci G, Cay S, Gulsoy KG, et al. Tissue Doppler atrial conduction times and electrocardiogram interlead P-wave durations with varying severity of obstructive sleep apnea. J Electrocardiol 2011; 44:478–82.
17. Camen G, Clarenbach CF, Stowhas AC, et al. The effects of simulated obstructive apnea and hypopnea on arrhythmic potential in healthy subjects. Eur J Appl Physiol 2012 [Epub ahead of print]. Available at: http://link.springer.com/article/10.1007%2Fs00421-012-2457-y. Accessed December 18, 2012.
18. Becker HF, Koehler U, Stammnitz A, et al. Heart block in patients with sleep apnoea. Thorax 1998; 53(Suppl 3):S29–32.
19. Koehler U, Fus E, Grimm W, et al. Heart block in patients with obstructive sleep apnoea: pathogenetic factors and effects of treatment. Eur Respir J 1998;11:434–9.
20. Guilleminault C, Connolly SJ, Winkle RA. Cardiac arrhythmia and conduction disturbances during sleep in 400 patients with sleep apnea syndrome. Am J Cardiol 1983;52:490–4.
21. Garrigue S, Pepin JL, Defaye P, et al. High prevalence of sleep apnea syndrome in patients with long-term pacing: the European Multicenter Polysomnographic Study. Circulation 2007;115:1703–9.
22. Grimm W, Hoffmann J, Menz V, et al. Electrophysiologic evaluation of sinus node function and

atrioventricular conduction in patients with pro-longed ventricular asystole during obstructive sleep apnea. Am J Cardiol 1996;77:1310–4.

23. Isono S, Sha M, Suzukawa M, et al. Preoperative nocturnal desaturations as a risk factor for late postoperative nocturnal desaturations. Br J Anaesth 1998;80:602–5.

24. Bhave PD, Goldman LE, Vittinghoff E, et al. Incidence, predictors, and outcomes associated with postoperative atrial fibrillation after major noncardiac surgery. Am Heart J 2012;164:918–24.

25. Somers VK, Dyken ME, Clary MP, et al. Sympathetic neural mechanisms in obstructive sleep apnea. J Clin Invest 1995;96:1897–904.

26. Somers VK, Mark AL, Zavala DC, et al. Influence of ventilation and hypocapnia on sympathetic nerve responses to hypoxia in normal humans. J Appl Physiol 1989;67:2095–100.

27. Somers VK, Mark AL, Zavala DC, et al. Contrasting effects of hypoxia and hypercapnia on ventilation and sympathetic activity in humans. J Appl Physiol 1989;67:2101–6.

28. Somers VK, Mark AL, Abboud FM. Interaction of baroreceptor and chemoreceptor reflex control of sympathetic nerve activity in normal humans. J Clin Invest 1991;87:1953–7.

29. Guilleminault C, Motta J, Mihm F, et al. Obstructive sleep apnea and cardiac index. Chest 1986;89:331–4.

30. Katzenberg C, Olajos M, Morkin E, et al. Effects of changes in airway pressure on the left ventricle and left atrium of dogs. Cardiovasc Res 1986;20:853–62.

31. Rosenberg J, Ullstad T, Rasmussen J, et al. Time course of postoperative hypoxaemia. Eur J Surg 1994;160:137–43.

32. Rosenberg J, Rasmussen V, von Jessen F, et al. Late postoperative episodic and constant hypoxaemia and associated ECG abnormalities. Br J Anaesth 1990;65:684–91.

33. Gogenur I, Rosenberg-Adamsen S, Lie C, et al. Relationship between nocturnal hypoxaemia, tachycardia and myocardial ischaemia after major abdominal surgery. Br J Anaesth 2004;93:333–8.

34. Galatius-Jensen S, Hansen J, Rasmussen V, et al. Nocturnal hypoxaemia after myocardial infarction: association with nocturnal myocardial ischaemia and arrhythmias. Br Heart J 1994;72:23–30.

35. Shepard JW Jr, Garrison MW, Grither DA, et al. Relationship of ventricular ectopy to oxyhemoglobin desaturation in patients with obstructive sleep apnea. Chest 1985;88:335–40.

36. Valencia-Flores M, Orea A, Castano VA, et al. Prevalence of sleep apnea and electrocardiographic disturbances in morbidly obese patients. Obes Res 2000;8:262–9.

37. Shepard JW Jr, Garrison MW, Grither DA, et al. Relationship of ventricular ectopy to nocturnal oxygen desaturation in patients with chronic obstructive pulmonary disease. Am J Med 1985;78:28–34.

38. Gami AS, Howard DE, Olson EJ, et al. Day-night pattern of sudden death in obstructive sleep apnea. N Engl J Med 2005;352:1206–14.

39. Ramachandran SK, Haider N, Saran KA, et al. Life-threatening critical respiratory events: a retrospective study of postoperative patients found unresponsive during analgesic therapy. J Clin Anesth 2011;23:207–13.

40. Ohga E, Tomita T, Wada H, et al. Effects of obstructive sleep apnea on circulating ICAM-1, IL-8, and MCP-1. J Appl Physiol 2003;94:179–84.

41. Minoguchi K, Yokoe T, Tazaki T, et al. Silent brain infarction and platelet activation in obstructive sleep apnea. Am J Respir Crit Care Med 2007;175:612–7.

42. Kuramoto E, Kinami S, Ishida Y, et al. Continuous positive nasal airway pressure decreases levels of serum amyloid A and improves autonomic function in obstructive sleep apnea syndrome. Int J Cardiol 2009;135:338–45.

43. Poitou C, Coupaye M, Laaban JP, et al. Serum amyloid A and obstructive sleep apnea syndrome before and after surgically-induced weight loss in morbidly obese subjects. Obes Surg 2006;16:1475–81.

44. Svatikova A, Wolk R, Shamsuzzaman AS, et al. Serum amyloid a in obstructive sleep apnea. Circulation 2003;108:1451–4.

45. Shamsuzzaman AS, Winnicki M, Lanfranchi P, et al. Elevated C-reactive protein in patients with obstructive sleep apnea. Circulation 2002;105:2462–4.

46. Larkin EK, Rosen CL, Kirchner HL, et al. Variation of C-reactive protein levels in adolescents: association with sleep-disordered breathing and sleep duration. Circulation 2005;111:1978–84.

47. Punjabi NM, Beamer BA. C-reactive protein is associated with sleep disordered breathing independent of adiposity. Sleep 2007;30:29–34.

48. Dyugovskaya L, Lavie P, Lavie L. Increased adhesion molecules expression and production of reactive oxygen species in leukocytes of sleep apnea patients. Am J Respir Crit Care Med 2002;165:934–9.

49. Dyugovskaya L, Lavie P, Lavie L. Lymphocyte activation as a possible measure of atherosclerotic risk in patients with sleep apnea. Ann N Y Acad Sci 2005;1051:340–50.

50. Ip MS, Lam B, Ng MM, et al. Obstructive sleep apnea is independently associated with insulin resistance. Am J Respir Crit Care Med 2002;165:670–6.

51. Punjabi NM. Do sleep disorders and associated treatments impact glucose metabolism? Drugs 2009;69(Suppl 2):13–27.

52. Punjabi NM, Polotsky VY. Disorders of glucose metabolism in sleep apnea. J Appl Physiol 2005; 99:1998–2007.

53. Punjabi NM, Shahar E, Redline S, et al. Sleep-disordered breathing, glucose intolerance, and insulin resistance: the Sleep Heart Health Study. Am J Epidemiol 2004;160:521–30.

54. Ramachandran SK, Kheterpal S, Consens F, et al. Derivation and validation of a simple perioperative sleep apnea prediction score. Anesth Analg 2010; 110:1007–15.

55. Ramachandran SK, Nafiu OO, Ghaferi A, et al. Independent predictors and outcomes of unanticipated early postoperative tracheal intubation after nonemergent, noncardiac surgery. Anesthesiology 2011;115:44–53.

56. Schulz R, Mahmoudi S, Hattar K, et al. Enhanced release of superoxide from polymorphonuclear neutrophils in obstructive sleep apnea. Impact of continuous positive airway pressure therapy. Am J Respir Crit Care Med 2000;162:566–70.

57. Suzuki YJ, Jain V, Park AM, et al. Oxidative stress and oxidant signaling in obstructive sleep apnea and associated cardiovascular diseases. Free Radic Biol Med 2006;40:1683–92.

58. Lavie L. Obstructive sleep apnoea syndrome—an oxidative stress disorder. Sleep Med Rev 2003;7: 35–51.

59. Karamanli H, Ozol D, Ugur KS, et al. Influence of CPAP treatment on airway and systemic inflammation in OSAS patients. Sleep Breath 2012 [Epub ahead of print]. Available at: http://link.springer.com/article/10.1007/s11325-012-0761-8. Accessed December 18, 2012.

60. Memtsoudis S, Liu SS, Ma Y, et al. Perioperative pulmonary outcomes in patients with sleep apnea after noncardiac surgery. Anesth Analg 2011;112: 113–21.

61. Glance LG, Wissler R, Mukamel DB, et al. Perioperative outcomes among patients with the modified metabolic syndrome who are undergoing noncardiac surgery. Anesthesiology 2010;113: 859–72.

62. Liu SS, Chisholm MF, Ngeow J, et al. Postoperative hypoxemia in orthopedic patients with obstructive sleep apnea. HSS J 2011;7:2–8.

63. Liu SS, Chisholm MF, John RS, et al. Risk of postoperative hypoxemia in ambulatory orthopedic surgery patients with diagnosis of obstructive sleep apnea: a retrospective observational study. Patient Saf Surg 2010;4:9.

64. Cashman JN, Dolin SJ. Respiratory and haemodynamic effects of acute postoperative pain management: evidence from published data. Br J Anaesth 2004;93:212–23.

65. Blake DW, Yew CY, Donnan GB, et al. Postoperative analgesia and respiratory events in patients with symptoms of obstructive sleep apnoea. Anaesth Intensive Care 2009;37:720–5.

66. Asyali MH, Berry RB, Khoo MC. Assessment of closed-loop ventilatory stability in obstructive sleep apnea. IEEE Trans Biomed Eng 2002;49:206–16.

67. Beecroft JM, Duffin J, Pierratos A, et al. Decreased chemosensitivity and improvement of sleep apnea by nocturnal hemodialysis. Sleep Med 2009;10: 47–54.

68. Bottini P, Dottorini ML, Cristina Cordoni M, et al. Sleep-disordered breathing in nonobese diabetic subjects with autonomic neuropathy. Eur Respir J 2003;22:654–60.

69. Bottini P, Scionti L, Santeusanio F, et al. Impairment of the respiratory system in diabetic autonomic neuropathy. Diabetes Nutr Metab 2000;13: 165–72.

70. Fletcher EC. Chronic lung disease in the sleep apnea syndrome. Lung 1990;168(Suppl):751–61.

71. Franczuk M, Radwan L, Plywaczewski R, et al. Respiratory responses to CO2 stimulation in hypercapnic patients with obstructive sleep apnea syndrome. Pneumonol Alergol Pol 2006;74:383–90 [in Polish].

72. Garcia-Rio F, Racionero MA, Pino JM, et al. Sleep apnea and hypertension. Chest 2000;117: 1417–25.

73. Dubreuil V, Ramanantsoa N, Trochet D, et al. A human mutation in Phox2b causes lack of CO2 chemosensitivity, fatal central apnea, and specific loss of parafacial neurons. Proc Natl Acad Sci U S A 2008;105:1067–72.

74. Walker JM, Farney RJ, Rhondeau SM, et al. Chronic opioid use is a risk factor for the development of central sleep apnea and ataxic breathing. J Clin Sleep Med 2007;3:455–61.

75. Haxhiu MA, Dreshaj IA, Erokwu B, et al. Effect of I1-imidazoline receptor activation on responses of hypoglossal and phrenic nerve to chemical stimulation. Ann N Y Acad Sci 1995;763:445–62.

76. Osanai S, Akiba Y, Fujiuchi S, et al. Depression of peripheral chemosensitivity by a dopaminergic mechanism in patients with obstructive sleep apnoea syndrome. Eur Respir J 1999;13:418–23.

77. Wang D, Marshall NS, Duffin J, et al. Phenotyping interindividual variability in obstructive sleep apnoea response to temazepam using ventilatory chemoreflexes during wakefulness. J Sleep Res 2011;20:526–32.

78. Mokhlesi B. Obesity hypoventilation syndrome: a state-of-the-art review. Respir Care 2010;55: 1347–62 [discussion: 1363–5].

79. Wijesinghe M, Williams M, Perrin K, et al. The effect of supplemental oxygen on hypercapnia in subjects with obesity-associated hypoventilation: a randomized, crossover, clinical study. Chest 2011;139:1018–24.

80. Brown KA, Laferriere A, Lakheeram I, et al. Recurrent hypoxemia in children is associated with increased analgesic sensitivity to opiates. Anesthesiology 2006;105:665–9.

81. Brown KA, Laferriere A, Moss IR. Recurrent hypoxemia in young children with obstructive sleep apnea is associated with reduced opioid requirement for analgesia. Anesthesiology 2004;100:806–10 [discussion: 5A].

82. Khalid I, Roehrs TA, Hudgel DW, et al. Continuous positive airway pressure in severe obstructive sleep apnea reduces pain sensitivity. Sleep 2011;34:1687–91.

83. Joshi GP, Ankichetty SP, Gan TJ, et al. Special article: society for ambulatory anesthesia consensus statement on preoperative selection of adult patients with obstructive sleep apnea scheduled for ambulatory surgery. Anesth Analg 2012;115:1060–8.

84. Gali B, Whalen FX Jr, Gay PC, et al. Management plan to reduce risks in perioperative care of patients with presumed obstructive sleep apnea syndrome. J Clin Sleep Med 2007;3:582–8.

85. Chung F, Yegneswaran B, Liao P, et al. STOP questionnaire: a tool to screen patients for obstructive sleep apnea. Anesthesiology 2008;108:812–21.

86. Munish M, Sharma V, Yarussi KM, et al. The use of practice guidelines by the American Society of Anesthesiologists for the identification of surgical patients at high risk of sleep apnea. Chron Respir Dis 2012;9:221–30.

87. Belozeroff V, Berry RB, Sassoon CS, et al. Effects of CPAP therapy on cardiovascular variability in obstructive sleep apnea: a closed-loop analysis. Am J Physiol Heart Circ Physiol 2002;282:H110–21.

88. Abe H, Takahashi M, Yaegashi H, et al. Efficacy of continuous positive airway pressure on arrhythmias in obstructive sleep apnea patients. Heart Vessels 2010;25:63–9.

89. Kanagala R, Murali NS, Friedman PA, et al. Obstructive sleep apnea and the recurrence of atrial fibrillation. Circulation 2003;107:2589–94.

90. Ryan CM, Usui K, Floras JS, et al. Effect of continuous positive airway pressure on ventricular ectopy in heart failure patients with obstructive sleep apnoea. Thorax 2005;60:781–5.

91. Craig S, Pepperell JC, Kohler M, et al. Continuous positive airway pressure treatment for obstructive sleep apnoea reduces resting heart rate but does not affect dysrhythmias: a randomised controlled trial. J Sleep Res 2009;18:329–36.

92. Barbe F, Duran-Cantolla J, Sanchez-de-la-Torre M, et al. Effect of continuous positive airway pressure on the incidence of hypertension and cardiovascular events in nonsleepy patients with obstructive sleep apnea: a randomized controlled trial. JAMA 2012;307:2161–8.

93. Spicuzza L, Bernardi L, Balsamo R, et al. Effect of treatment with nasal continuous positive airway pressure on ventilatory response to hypoxia and hypercapnia in patients with sleep apnea syndrome. Chest 2006;130:774–9.

94. Redolfi S, Corda L, La Piana G, et al. Long-term non-invasive ventilation increases chemosensitivity and leptin in obesity-hypoventilation syndrome. Respir Med 2007;101:1191–5.

95. Borel JC, Tamisier R, Gonzalez-Bermejo J, et al. Noninvasive ventilation in mild obesity hypoventilation syndrome: a randomized controlled trial. Chest 2012;141:692–702.

96. Tun Y, Hida W, Okabe S, et al. Effects of nasal continuous positive airway pressure on awake ventilatory responses to hypoxia and hypercapnia in patients with obstructive sleep apnea. Tohoku J Exp Med 2000;190:157–68.

97. Guo Y, Pan L, Ren D, et al. Impact of continuous positive airway pressure on C-reactive protein in patients with obstructive sleep apnea: a meta-analysis. Sleep Breath 2012 [Epub ahead of print]. Available at: http://link.springer.com/article/10.1007/s11325-012-0722-2. Accessed December 18, 2012.

98. Gelardi M, Carbonara G, Maffezzoni E, et al. Regular CPAP utilization reduces nasal inflammation assessed by nasal cytology in obstructive sleep apnea syndrome. Sleep Med 2012;13:859–63.

99. Guralnick AS, Pant M, Minhaj M, et al. CPAP adherence in patients with newly diagnosed obstructive sleep apnea prior to elective surgery. J Clin Sleep Med 2012;8:501–6.

100. Kohler M, Stoewhas AC, Ayers L, et al. Effects of continuous positive airway pressure therapy withdrawal in patients with obstructive sleep apnea: a randomized controlled trial. Am J Respir Crit Care Med 2011;184:1192–9.

101. Squadrone V, Coha M, Cerutti E, et al. Continuous positive airway pressure for treatment of postoperative hypoxemia: a randomized controlled trial. JAMA 2005;293:589–95.

102. Ramachandran SK, Kheterpal S, Haas CF, et al. Automated notification of suspected obstructive sleep apnea patients to the perioperative respiratory therapist: a pilot study. Respir Care 2010;55:414–8.

103. Lundstrom LH, Nygard E, Hviid LB, et al. The effect of thoracic epidural analgesia on the occurrence of late postoperative hypoxemia in patients undergoing elective coronary bypass surgery: a randomized controlled trial. Chest 2005;128:1564–70.

104. Pedersen T, Moller AM, Hovhannisyan K. Pulse oximetry for perioperative monitoring. Cochrane Database Syst Rev 2009;(4):CD002013.

105. Moller JT. Anesthesia related hypoxemia. The effect of pulse oximetry monitoring on perioperative events and postoperative complications. Dan Med Bull 1994;41:489–500.

106. Moller JT, Svennild I, Johannessen NW, et al. Perioperative monitoring with pulse oximetry and late postoperative cognitive dysfunction. Br J Anaesth 1993;71:340–7.

107. Moller JT, Johannessen NW, Espersen K, et al. Randomized evaluation of pulse oximetry in 20,802 patients: II. Perioperative events and postoperative complications. Anesthesiology 1993;78:445–53.

108. Taenzer AH, Pyke JB, McGrath SP, et al. Impact of pulse oximetry surveillance on rescue events and intensive care unit transfers: a before-and-after concurrence study. Anesthesiology 2010;112:282–7.

109. Cvach M. Monitor alarm fatigue: an integrative review. Biomed Instrum Technol 2012;46:268–77.

110. Graham KC, Cvach M. Monitor alarm fatigue: standardizing use of physiological monitors and decreasing nuisance alarms. Am J Crit Care 2010;19:28–34 [quiz: 35].

111. Isono S. Obesity and obstructive sleep apnoea: mechanisms for increased collapsibility of the passive pharyngeal airway. Respirology 2012;17:32–42.

112. Tagaito Y, Isono S, Tanaka A, et al. Sitting posture decreases collapsibility of the passive pharynx in anesthetized paralyzed patients with obstructive sleep apnea. Anesthesiology 2010;113:812–8.

113. Benoit Z, Wicky S, Fischer JF, et al. The effect of increased FIO(2) before tracheal extubation on postoperative atelectasis. Anesth Analg 2002;95:1777–81 [table of contents].

114. Talab HF, Zabani IA, Abdelrahman HS, et al. Intraoperative ventilatory strategies for prevention of pulmonary atelectasis in obese patients undergoing laparoscopic bariatric surgery. Anesth Analg 2009;109:1511–6.

115. Boeken U, Schurr P, Kurt M, et al. Early reintubation after cardiac operations: impact of nasal continuous positive airway pressure (nCPAP) and noninvasive positive pressure ventilation (NPPV). Thorac Cardiovasc Surg 2010;58:398–402.

116. Neligan PJ, Malhotra G, Fraser M, et al. Continuous positive airway pressure via the Boussignac system immediately after extubation improves lung function in morbidly obese patients with obstructive sleep apnea undergoing laparoscopic bariatric surgery. Anesthesiology 2009;110:878–84.

117. Fu ES, Downs JB, Schweiger JW, et al. Supplemental oxygen impairs detection of hypoventilation by pulse oximetry. Chest 2004;126:1552–8.

Perioperative Clinical Pathways to Manage Sleep-Disordered Breathing

Edwin Seet, MBBS, MMed (Anesthesia)[a], Tee Lik Han, MBBS[a], Frances Chung, MBBS, FRCPC[b],*

KEYWORDS

- Obstructive sleep apnea • Perioperative clinical pathways • Screening • Perioperative management
- STOP-bang questionnaire

KEY POINTS

- Obstructive sleep apnea (OSA) is the most common type of sleep-disordered breathing.
- OSA is an independent risk factor for increased perioperative adverse events.
- Effective screening tools are available for the detection and risk stratification of OSA.
- The perioperative care of the OSA patient is challenging, and various strategies are available for risk mitigation.
- More research is required to formulate evidence-based clinical pathways for the perioperative management of OSA patients.

INTRODUCTION

The obstructive sleep apnea (OSA) syndrome is a disease characterized by recurrent episodic cessation of breathing lasting 10 or more seconds during sleep. In this condition, there is exaggerated depression of pharyngeal muscle tone during sleep and anesthesia, resulting in a cyclical pattern of partial or complete upper airway obstruction with impaired respiration.[1] Clinically this manifests as repeated nocturnal arousals and increased sympathetic output, daytime hypersomnolence, memory loss, and executive and psychomotor dysfunction.[2]

OSA is the most common type of sleep-disordered breathing.[3] There is a wide variation in the reported prevalence of this disorder because of the diversity between the different study populations, differing definitions for the disease, and the varying diagnostic methods. Its estimated prevalence is 1 in 4 males and 1 in 10 females for mild OSA,[4] and 1 in 9 males and 1 in 20 females for moderate OSA.[5,6] The economic cost of OSA is considerable.[7]

A significant number of patients with OSA are undiagnosed when they present for elective surgery.[8] In an observational study, approximately one-fourth (24%) of elective surgical patients were found to be at high risk based on screening, of whom 4 of 5 (81%) had not been previously diagnosed with OSA.[9] A similar trend is seen in the setting of ambulatory surgery.[10] More importantly, OSA has been linked with an increased incidence of postoperative complications. The perioperative management of OSA patients is challenging, and a sound understanding of the condition is required of anesthesiologists involved in the care of such patients.

This review article endeavors to summarize the principles in the perioperative management of OSA patients, including preoperative evaluation, perioperative risk mitigation, and postoperative

[a] Department of Anesthesia, Khoo Teck Puat Hospital, Alexandra Health Private Limited, 90 Yishun Central, Singapore 768828; [b] Department of Anesthesia, Toronto Western Hospital, University Health Network, University of Toronto, 399 Bathurst Street, McL 2-405, Toronto, Ontario M5T 2S8, Canada
* Corresponding author.
E-mail address: Frances.Chung@uhn.ca

Sleep Med Clin 8 (2013) 105–120
http://dx.doi.org/10.1016/j.jsmc.2012.11.005
1556-407X/13/$ – see front matter © 2013 Elsevier Inc. All rights reserved.

care. Functional algorithms are presented as a guide to managing such patients presenting for surgery. Where evidence in the form of published literature is lacking, certain recommendations have been made based on consensus or expert opinion. The clinical pathways suggested here serve as aids to the anesthesiologist. Clinical judgment should be exercised at all times; and exceptions made to accommodate for the various circumstantial and patient-related factors.

DIAGNOSTIC CRITERIA

Classically the gold standard for the definitive diagnosis of OSA requires an overnight polysomnography or sleep study. The Apnea-Hypopnea Index (AHI), defined as the average number of abnormal breathing events per hour of sleep, is used to determine the presence of and the severity of OSA. An apneic event refers to cessation of airflow for at least 10 seconds, and hypopnea occurs when there is reduced airflow with desaturation of 4% or more.[11] The American Academy of Sleep Medicine (AASM) diagnostic criteria for OSA require either an AHI of 15 or more, or AHI greater than or equal to 5, with symptoms such as excessive daytime sleepiness, unintentional sleep during wakefulness, unrefreshing sleep, loud snoring reported by partner, or observed obstruction during sleep.[12] The Canadian Thoracic Society guidelines for the diagnosis of OSA specify the presence of an AHI of at least 5 on polysomnography, and either of (1) daytime sleepiness not attributable to other factors or (2) at least 2 other symptoms of OSA (eg, choking or gasping during sleep, recurrent awakenings, unrefreshing sleep, daytime fatigue, or impaired concentration).[13] OSA severity is mild for AHI between 5 and 15, moderate for AHI 15 to 30, and severe for AHI greater than 30.[12]

COMORBIDITIES ASSOCIATED WITH OSA

OSA is associated with multiple comorbidities such as myocardial ischemia, heart failure, hypertension, arrhythmias, cerebrovascular disease, metabolic syndrome, insulin resistance, gastroesophageal reflux, and obesity. In one study, the prevalence of OSA was 41% in patients with a body mass index of greater than 28 kg/m^2, and 78% in morbidly obese patients planned for bariatric surgery.[14] Various pathophysiologic, demographic, and lifestyle factors also predispose to OSA. These factors include anatomic abnormalities that cause a mechanical reduction in airway-lumen diameter (eg, craniofacial deformities, macroglossia, retrognathia), endocrine diseases (eg, Cushing disease, hypothyroidism), connective tissue diseases (eg, Marfan syndrome), male gender, age older than 50 years, neck circumference greater than 40 cm, and lifestyle factors of smoking and alcohol consumption.[15]

POSTOPERATIVE COMPLICATIONS IN PATIENTS WITH OSA

Chronic untreated OSA leads to multisystemic adverse consequences and is an independent risk factor for increased all-cause mortality in the general population.[16,17] The anatomic inherent collapsibility of the airway and the systemic effects of the disease also place the surgical patient with OSA at increased risk of serious complications perioperatively.

In a retrospective study of patients who underwent hip or knee replacements conducted by Gupta and colleagues,[18] 24% of patients with known OSA developed serious complications after surgery, including unplanned admission to the intensive care unit (ICU), reintubation, and cardiac events, as opposed to 9% in the control group. Subsequent studies on similar outcomes conducted by Liao and colleagues[19] and Chung and colleagues[20] reported complication rates of 44% and 27.4%, respectively following elective surgery in patients with OSA versus 28% and 12.3%, respectively in those without OSA. Gali and colleagues[21] reported increased rates of pneumonia and the need for noninvasive ventilation in high-risk OSA patients. Kaw and colleagues[22] demonstrated an increased risk of postoperative hypoxemia, transfer to ICU, and longer duration of hospitalization in OSA patients following noncardiac surgery. Memtsoudis and colleagues[23] found a 2-fold higher risk of pulmonary complications in OSA patients after noncardiac surgery in comparison with matched controls with no OSA. In bariatric surgical patients, the presence of OSA was found to be an independent risk factor for adverse postoperative events.[24] A recent prospective observational study by Flink and colleagues[25] reported a 53% incidence of postoperative delirium in OSA patients compared with 20% in patients without OSA (odds ratio 4.3). A summary of the relevant studies and the complications reported is presented in **Table 1**.

More recently, a meta-analysis by Kaw and colleagues[26] showed that the presence of OSA increased the odds of postoperative cardiac events including myocardial infarction, cardiac arrest, and arrhythmias (odds ratio 2.1), respiratory failure (odds ratio 2.4), desaturation (odds ratio 2.3), transfers to ICU (odds ratio 2.8), and reintubations (odds ratio 2.1). Given the body of evidence associating a diagnosis of OSA with adverse perioperative outcomes, precautions should be taken perioperatively to reduce complications in this vulnerable group of patients.

CLINICAL PATHWAYS AND PRINCIPLES OF PERIOPERATIVE MANAGEMENT

In an attempt to improve the perioperative care for OSA patients, various investigators have constructed guidelines or clinical pathways.[27–32] Preoperatively, the use of sensitive clinical criteria to identify and risk-stratify potential OSA patients is advocated. The Sleep Apnea Clinical Score proposed by Flemons[27] used a combination of clinical variables, including neck circumference of at least 43 cm, snoring, disturbed breathing during sleep, daytime somnolence, obesity, and hypertension, to determine the likelihood of OSA. The American Society of Anesthesiologists 2006 guidelines on the perioperative management of OSA patients recommended screening patients using a 16-item checklist comprising clinical criteria categorized into physical characteristics, symptoms, and complaints. The patient's perioperative risk was then predicted by a scoring system based on OSA severity, invasiveness of procedure, and expected postoperative opioid requirement.[28] Recent review articles have supported the use of questionnaire-based screening tools to predict the probability and severity of OSA.[20,29,31] Patients who exhibit high-risk features on screening should undergo formal evaluation with confirmatory sleep studies. Positive airway pressure (PAP) therapy should be commenced preoperatively if polysomnographic evidence of moderate to severe OSA is present.[27–29]

Intraoperative measures have focused on the anticipation and management of difficult airways, mitigating the risk of aspiration of gastric acid, and the judicious use of pharmacologic agents to avoid problems of excessive sedation and respiratory depression in the immediate postoperative period.[28,29,31] Issues of monitoring and intervention are pertinent in the postoperative period. Based on expert opinion by the American Sleep Association (ASA) taskforce, if discharge to an unmonitored facility is planned, the observation period for OSA patients in the postanesthesia care unit (PACU) should be prolonged by a median of 3 hours more than for non-OSA patients, or 7 hours if respiratory events occur.[28] Another algorithm proposed by Adesanya and colleagues[29] recommended that patients with known OSA or at high risk on screening be observed for a minimum of 2 hours in the PACU, and be considered for continuous PAP in the event of oxygen desaturation. Subsequent inpatient care should include continuous monitoring of oxygen saturation in an appropriate environment. PAP therapy should be considered for patients already on PAP treatment or who have been noncompliant before surgery, as well as those at high risk of OSA.

This article provides an updated discussion on the preoperative evaluation of the diagnosed and suspected OSA patient, strategies for intraoperative risk mitigation, and postoperative patient disposition, with illustrations of published clinical algorithms.[30,33]

PREOPERATIVE EVALUATION OF THE PATIENT WITH DIAGNOSED OSA

A thorough history and physical examination are essential. Focused questions regarding OSA symptoms should be asked. Polysomnography results should be reviewed to confirm the diagnosis of OSA and evaluate the severity of the disease.

Patients with long-standing OSA may manifest a myriad of signs and symptoms suggesting the development of systemic complications, such as hypoxemia, hypercarbia, polycythemia, and cor pulmonale. The patient should also be assessed for significant comorbidities including morbid obesity, uncontrolled hypertension, arrhythmias, cerebrovascular disease, heart failure, and metabolic syndrome. Pulmonary arterial hypertension is a fairly common long-term complication of OSA, occurring in 15% to 20% of patients.[34] Its significance lies in the fact that certain physiologic derangements may raise pulmonary artery pressures further and should be avoided intraoperatively. The American College of Chest Physicians does not recommend routine evaluation for pulmonary arterial hypertension in patients with known OSA.[35] However, should there be anticipated intraoperative triggers for acute elevations in pulmonary arterial pressures (eg, high-risk surgical procedures of long duration), a preoperative transthoracic echocardiography may be considered.[29] Simple bedside investigations may be performed in the preoperative clinic to screen for OSA-related complications. In the absence of other attributable causes for hypoxemia, a baseline oximetry reading of 94% or less on room air suggests severe long-standing OSA, and may be a red flag signaling postoperative adverse outcome.[36]

Frequently OSA patients may be on PAP devices for treatment, for example, continuous positive airway pressure (CPAP), bilevel positive airway pressure (BiPAP), and automatically adjusting positive airway pressure (APAP) machines. Automatically adjusting PAP devices provides respiratory assistance based on airflow measurements,

Table 1
Adverse outcomes in OSA patients after surgery

	Gupta et al,[18] 2001	Liao et al,[19] 2009	Chung et al,[20] 2008	Kaw et al,[22] 2012	Gali et al,[21] 2009	Memtsoudis et al,[23] 2011	Flum et al,[24] 2009	Flink et al,[25] 2012
Study design	Retrospective case control study	Retrospective matched cohort study	Prospective cohort study	Retrospective cohort study	Prospective cohort study	Retrospective cohort study	Observational study	Prospective cohort study
Method of OSA diagnosis	Polysomnogram, nocturnal oximetry	Hospital discharge records	Polysomnogram	Polysomnogram	Sleep Apnea Clinical Score	Hospital discharge records	Patients' report of prior diagnosis	Polysomnogram
Nature of surgery	Orthopedic (hip and knee replacements)	Cardiothoracic Noncardiac[a] ENT[b]	Noncardiac[a] Ophthalmic Neurosurgery	Noncardiac[a] ENT[b]	Surgeries with postoperative stay ≥48 h	Noncardiac[a]	Bariatric surgery	Orthopedic (knee replacement), age >65 y
No. of Subjects								
OSA group	101	240	147	282	221	113960	2354[c]	15
Non-OSA group	101 (control)	240 (control)	64 (control)	189 (control)	472	5937742 (control)	2354[d]	91
Complication Rate								
OSA, n (%)	24 (24)	104 (43)	40 (27.4)	40 (14.2)	23 (10.4)	7828[e] (6.87)	112 (5.0)	8 (53%)
Non-OSA, n (%)	9 (9)	67 (28)	8 (12.3)	5 (2.6)	19 (4.02)	221651[e] (3.73)	77 (3.3)	19 (20%)
P value	0.004	<0.001	0.02	0.003	0.043	OR 1.95, 95% CI (1.91–1.98)	0.02 (unadjusted)	0.0123, OR 4.3

Complications

Complications						
Respiratory[f]	Yes	Yes	Yes	Yes	Yes	
Cardiac[g]	Yes	Yes	Yes	Yes	Yes	
Neurologic[h]	Yes	Yes	Yes			
Unplanned ICU admission	Yes	Yes	Yes	Yes		
Reintubation/ emergency intubation		Yes	Yes		Yes	
Lengthened hospital stay		Yes	Yes		Yes	
Other		NIV Pneumonia		Pneumonia ARDS PE	Death VTE Reintervention	Delirium

Abbreviations: ARDS, acute respiratory distress syndrome; CI, confidence interval; ENT, ear/nose/throat; ICU, intensive care unit; NIV, noninvasive ventilation; OR, odds ratio; PE, pulmonary embolism; VTE, venous thromboembolism.

[a] Noncardiac surgery: general surgery, urology, gynecology, orthopedic surgery, plastic surgery.
[b] ENT surgery not including upper airway surgery.
[c] Number of patients who reported a diagnosis of OSA preoperatively.
[d] Number of patients who did not report an established diagnosis of OSA preoperatively.
[e] Data for incidence of tracheal intubation only.
[f] Respiratory complications: desaturation, hypoxia, hypercapnia, respiratory failure, bronchospasm, laryngospasm, pulmonary edema.
[g] Cardiac complications: myocardial ischemia, myocardial infarction, arrhythmia.
[h] Neurologic complications: Confusion, agitation, stroke, transient ischemic attack, motor or sensory deficits.

fluctuations in pressure, or airway resistance.[37] The compliance of OSA patients to such treatment should be evaluated. The patient's updated PAP therapy settings should be obtained. Reassessment by a sleep medicine physician may be indicated in patients who have defaulted follow-up, have been noncompliant to treatment, have had recent exacerbation of symptoms, or have undergone upper airway surgery to relieve OSA symptoms. Patients who default PAP use should be advised to resume therapy.

To date there is insufficient evidence to prove conclusively the benefit of PAP therapy in the preoperative setting, and the duration of therapy required to effectively reduce perioperative risks has not been delineated. A retrospective matched cohort study by Liao and colleagues[19] suggested that preoperative PAP therapy may possibly be beneficial based on the observation that OSA patients who did not use home PAP devices before surgery but required PAP therapy after surgery had increased complication rates.

Current guidelines recommend that patients with moderate or severe OSA who are already on PAP therapy should continue to use PAP before surgery.[28] The anesthesia team should be informed early to allow for advanced planning of intraoperative management and risk mitigation. Mild OSA may not be a significant disease entity for patients undergoing surgery and anesthesia. According to the published results of the Busselton Health Cohort Study, mild OSA was not an independent risk factor for higher mortality in the general population.[17] Based on expert opinion and symptomatology of OSA patients, preoperative PAP use may not be indicated in patients with mild OSA. **Fig. 1** suggests an algorithm for the preoperative evaluation and management of the patient already diagnosed with OSA.[30,33]

METHODS FOR PERIOPERATIVE SCREENING FOR OSA

An overnight polysomnography is the gold-standard diagnostic test for OSA. However, routine screening with polysomnography is costly and resource intensive, because of equipment constraints and the requirement for special technical expertise. As a result, several tools have been developed to meet this need for simple, economical, and sensitive screening tests for the detection of patients with suspected OSA. These tools include questionnaire-based methods such as the Epworth Sleepiness Scale,[38] the Berlin Questionnaire,[39] the ASA checklist,[28] the Sleep Apnea Clinical Score,[27] the P-SAP score,[40] and the STOP-Bang questionnaire.[41] The STOP-Bang

questionnaire was originally developed in the surgical population but has been validated in various patient populations.[41,42] This concise scoring system consists of 8 easily administered questions framed with the acronym STOP-Bang (**Table 2**). Each question is scored based on the answer "Yes" or "No." Patients are deemed to be at risk of OSA if they have a STOP-Bang score of at least 3 and at high risk of OSA if the STOP-Bang score is 5 or more.[41,43]

The purpose of a screening test is to detect as many subjects with disease as possible with a low false-negative rate, that is, high sensitivity at the expense of lower specificity. The STOP-Bang questionnaire has high sensitivity and a high negative predictive value, especially for patients with moderate to severe OSA.[41] A STOP-Bang score of less than 3 is reassuring, as the patient is unlikely to have moderate to severe OSA. On the other hand, the false-positive rate may be high. For moderate OSA (AHI >15) and severe OSA (AHI >30), the sensitivity of STOP-Bang score is 93% and 100%, respectively, whereas the specificity is 43% and 37%, respectively.[41]

STOP-Bang scores of 5 and greater are even more predictive for moderate to severe OSA. For higher cutoff values of 5, 6, and 7, the specificity of STOP-Bang questionnaire for severe OSA (AHI >30) was 74%, 88%, and 95% respectively.[43] Based on these test characteristics, patients with STOP-Bang scores of 0 to 2 may be considered to be at low risk, 3 to 4 at intermediate risk, and 5 to 8 at high risk of having OSA. To avoid overzealous testing and unnecessary postoperative monitoring resulting from the high false-positive rates associated with lower cutoff values, it may be more cost-effective to use a STOP-Bang cutoff between 5 and 8. In addition, patients identified as high risk on STOP-Bang have been shown to have increased rates of postoperative complications.[20,44] The STOP-Bang questionnaire is useful in the preoperative setting to predict OSA severity, triage patients for further confirmatory testing, and exclude those without disease.[42]

PREOPERATIVE EVALUATION OF THE PATIENT WITH SUSPECTED OSA

In patients suspected of OSA, a thorough clinical examination should be performed with emphasis on pertinent symptoms and signs of OSA (see **Fig. 1**). The bed partner's presence at the interview would be useful in the assessment of snoring and observed apnea. The subsequent management is determined by the urgency of surgery. In emergency situations, the patient should proceed for surgery. Extensive testing for OSA will result in

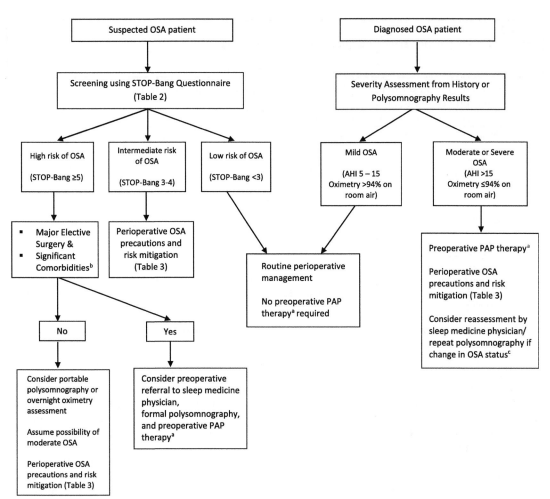

Fig. 1. Preoperative evaluation of a patient with known or suspected obstructive sleep apnea in the anesthesia clinic. [a] Positive airway pressure (PAP) therapy: includes continuous PAP, bilevel PAP, and automatically adjusting PAP. [b] Significant comorbidities: heart failure, arrhythmias, uncontrolled hypertension, pulmonary hypertension, cerebrovascular disease, metabolic syndrome, obesity (body mass index >35 kg/m²). [c] Change in OSA status: recent exacerbation of OSA symptoms, noncompliant to PAP therapy, recently underwent OSA-related surgery, lost to sleep medicine follow-up. AHI, Apnea-Hypopnea Index. (*Adapted from* Seet E, Chung F. Obstructive sleep apnea: preoperative assessment. Anesthesiol Clin 2010;28:199–215, with permission; and Seet E, Chung F. Management of sleep apnea in adults-functional algorithms for the perioperative period: continuing professional development. Can J Anaesth 2010;57:849–64. Copyright 2010 by Canadian Anesthesiologists' Society; with kind permission from Springer Science and Business Media.)

a delay of vital surgery. Perioperative precautions should be taken based on the clinical suspicion of OSA. A clinical algorithm is suggested regarding the elective setting (see **Fig. 1**).[30]

When nonurgent elective surgery is planned, the decision for further evaluation rests on (1) the risk of surgery and (2) the presence of other significant comorbidities suggestive of chronic OSA, such as uncontrolled hypertension, heart failure, arrhythmias, pulmonary hypertension, cerebrovascular disease, morbid obesity, and metabolic syndrome. For patients who are scored as high risk on STOP-Bang (score ≥5) who are planned for major elective surgery and have comorbid disease(s)

associated with long-standing OSA, a preoperative assessment by the sleep physician and a polysomnogram should be considered to confirm the diagnosis and establish the severity of disease. An early review by the sleep physician is recommended to allow for optimal PAP treatment and sufficient time for planning of the intraoperative and postoperative management.[28] Sometimes, major elective surgery may have to be deferred to allow adequate evaluation and optimization of suspected severe OSA. The eventual decision to evaluate a patient preoperatively should ultimately be made based on the clinical judgment of the attending physician, after taking into account

Table 2
Obstructive sleep apnea screening questionnaire: STOP-Bang

	STOP Questionnaire		
S	Snoring: Do you snore loudly (louder than talking or loud enough to be heard through closed doors)?	Yes	No
T	Tired: Do you often feel tired, fatigued, or sleepy during daytime?	Yes	No
O	Observed: Has anyone observed you stop breathing during your sleep?	Yes	No
P	Blood Pressure: Do you have or are you being treated for high blood pressure?	Yes	No
B	Body mass index: greater than 35 kg/m^2?	Yes	No
A	Age: Age over 50 y old?	Yes	No
N	Neck circumference: Neck circumference greater than 40 cm?	Yes	No
G	Gender: Male?	Yes	No

Low risk of OSA: Yes to fewer than 3 questions.
At risk of OSA: Yes to 3 or more questions.
High risk of OSA: Yes to 5 or more questions.
Modified from Chung F, Yegneswaran B, Liao P, et al. STOP questionnaire: a tool to screen patients for obstructive sleep apnea. Anesthesiology 2008;108:812–21; and Chung F, Subramanyam R, Liao P, et al. High STOP-Bang score indicates a high probability of obstructive sleep apnoea. Br J Anaesth 2012;108:768–75.

patient-related and logistic factors. The authors suggest that patients scored as high risk but without significant comorbidities be considered for further evaluation with portable monitoring devices, or to proceed with surgery with a presumed diagnosis of moderate OSA and undertaking perioperative OSA precautions.

Patients with an intermediate risk of OSA based on STOP-Bang may proceed for surgery without further testing with perioperative OSA precautions. This subset of patients may have previously undergone anesthesia uneventfully, and represent false positives on screening, or may have less severe OSA. Nonetheless, increased vigilance is prudent in managing these at-risk patients. If the subsequent intraoperative and postoperative course suggests a higher likelihood of OSA, for example, difficult airway,[45] or recurrent postoperative respiratory events such as desaturation, hypoventilation, or apnea,[21] a subsequent referral to the sleep physician and polysomnography may be indicated. OSA screening tests have a low false-negative rate. Patients deemed to be at low risk on screening with a score of less than 3 on STOP-Bang are unlikely to have OSA. These patients may proceed for surgery with routine perioperative care.

PORTABLE POLYSOMNOGRAPHY AND OVERNIGHT OXIMETRY

Home sleep testing may be a viable alternative to standard polysomnography for the diagnosis of OSA in certain subsets of patients.[46] Such monitoring equipment is classified into level 2 (full unattended polysomnography with $\geq$7 channels),

level 3 (devices limited to 4–7 channels), and level 4 (1–2 channels including nocturnal oximetry) devices. In particular, the level 2 portable polysomnograph has been shown to have a diagnostic accuracy similar to that of standard polysomnography,[47] while nocturnal oximetry is both sensitive and specific for detecting OSA in STOP-Bang–positive surgical patients.[48] The oxygen desaturation index derived from nocturnal oximetry correlates well with the AHI obtained from polysomnography.[48] Furthermore, a mean nocturnal oxygen saturation of 94.6% or less or mean oxygen desaturation index of greater than 9.2 are predictive of increased postoperative adverse events.[36]

The Portable Monitoring Task Force of the American Academy of Sleep Medicine (AASM) suggests that portable devices may be considered when there is high pretest likelihood for moderate to severe OSA without other substantial comorbidities.[49] Following the AASM 2007 guidelines, the Canadian Thoracic Society 2011 update on the diagnosis and treatment of sleep-disordered breathing recommended that portable monitoring devices of levels 2, 3, and 4, including nocturnal oximetry, may be used as confirmatory tests for the diagnosis of OSA, provided that proper standards for conducting the test and interpretation of results are met.[50] These portable devices are useful surrogates for the detection of OSA, especially if standard polysomnography is not available. The devices may also help with risk stratification of patients with suspected OSA, allowing preoperative PAP therapy and ample perioperative measures to be instituted for those identified to be at increased risk of complications.

INTRAOPERATIVE RISK-MITIGATION STRATEGIES FOR OSA PATIENTS

Various strategies may be used to mitigate the risks and avert adverse outcomes in OSA patients in the immediate perioperative and intraoperative periods, and these are listed in **Table 3**. Preoperatively, sedative premedication should be avoided.[51] Pain adjuvants such as the α2-agonists (dexmedetomidine) have an opioid-sparing effect and also reduce anesthetic requirement.[52]

Intraoperatively, the anesthesiologist may often be presented with a difficult airway. A history of OSA may be associated with difficult mask ventilation[53] as well as difficult intubation, with a difficult tracheal intubation occurring 8 times as often in OSA patients than in those without OSA.[54] Advanced planning of airway management is required. In addition, a backup action plan should be in place in anticipation of the possibility that the intended technique turns out to be unsuitable. Adequately skilled personnel and appropriate equipment, including a range of airway adjuncts, should be available before induction of anesthesia.[55] The entire anesthesia team should be familiar with a specific difficult airway algorithm,

Table 3
Perioperative precautions and risk mitigation for OSA patients

Anesthetic Concern	Principles of Management
Premedication	Avoid sedating premedication[51] Consider α2-adrenergic agonists (clonidine, dexmedetomidine)[52]
Potential difficult airway (difficult mask ventilation and tracheal intubation)[53,54]	Optimal positioning (Head Elevated Laryngoscopy Position) if patient obese Adequate preoxygenation Consider CPAP preoxygenation[57] Two-handed triple-airway maneuvers Anticipate difficult airway. Personnel familiar with a specific difficult-airway algorithm[56]
Gastroesophageal reflux disease[59]	Consider proton-pump inhibitors, antacids, rapid sequence induction with cricoid pressure
Opioid-related respiratory depression[51]	Minimize opioid use Use of short-acting agents (remifentanil) Multimodal approach to analgesia (NSAIDs, acetaminophen, tramadol, ketamine, gabapentin, pregabalin, dexmedetomidine, clonidine, dexamethasone, melatonin) Consider local and regional anesthesia where appropriate
Carry-over sedation effects from longer-acting intravenous and volatile anesthetic agents	Use of propofol/remifentanil for maintenance of anesthesia Use of insoluble potent anesthetic agents (desflurane) Use of regional blocks as a sole anesthetic technique
Excessive sedation in monitored anesthetic care	Use of intraoperative capnography for monitoring of ventilation[28]
Postextubation airway obstruction	Verify full reversal of neuromuscular blockade[28] Extubate only when fully conscious and cooperative[28] Nonsupine posture for extubation and recovery[28] Resume use of positive airway pressure device after surgery[28]

Abbreviations: CPAP, continuous positive airway pressure; NSAID, nonsteroidal anti-inflammatory drug.

Adapted from Seet E, Chung F. Management of sleep apnea in adults—functional algorithms for the perioperative period: continuing professional development. Can J Anaesth 2010;57:849–64. Copyright © 2010 by Canadian Anesthesiologists' Society; with kind permission from Springer Science and Business Media.

such as the ASA guidelines for the management of a difficult airway.[56] Preoxygenation using 100% oxygen with continuous PAP of 10 cm H_2O for 3 to 5 minutes with a 25° head-up tilt has been reported to achieve higher end-tidal concentrations of oxygen.[57,58] Triple-airway maneuvers and two-handed mask ventilation may be needed to attain adequate ventilation. Obese patients may have to be positioned on an incline to achieve optimal alignment to facilitate laryngoscopy—the Head Elevated Laryngoscopy Position or HELP. This action may be taken by simply stacking up multiple towels or blankets, or by using specially designed devices such as the Troop Elevation Pillow (Mercury Medical, Clearwater, FL, USA). Gastroesophageal reflux disease secondary to hypotonia of the lower esophageal sphincter is common among patients with OSA.[59] Measures to decrease the risk of aspiration of gastric acid should be considered, and include preoperative proton-pump inhibitors, antacids, and rapid sequence induction and cricoid pressure. Of note, use of cricoid pressure may further impede mask ventilation and tracheal intubation.[60]

Many of the anesthetic agents, for example, volatile agents, anxiolytics, and opioids, cause respiratory depression. OSA patients have a heightened sensitivity to the respiratory depressant effects of these drugs because of their increased susceptibility for airway collapse, chronic sleep deprivation, and blunted response to hypercarbia and hypoxia. Short-acting agents such as propofol, remifentanil, and desflurane are preferred, whereas long-acting agents should be avoided or their use minimized. Pulmonary hypertension is a known complication of chronic OSA. Intraoperative triggers for elevation of pulmonary artery pressures, namely hypercarbia, hypoxemia, hypothermia, and acidosis, should be avoided.

Intraoperative use of opioid-sparing agents such as nonsteroidal anti-inflammatories, cyclooxygenase-2 inhibitors, paracetamol, tramadol, and adjuvants such as the anticonvulsants pregabalin and gabapentin are helpful in reducing postoperative opioid requirements. Previous studies showed that desaturation was 12 to 14 times more common in patients with OSA who received opioids postoperatively than in those who were given nonopioid analgesic agents.[61] Other novel opioid-sparing adjuvants being investigated include corticosteroids such as dexamethasone, the N-methyl-D-aspartate receptor antagonist ketamine,[62] the α2-agonists clonidine and dexmedetomidine,[63] and melatonin.[64] A recent study investigating the beneficial effects of intraoperative intravenous doxapram found that postanesthetic recovery and outcomes of OSA patients

undergoing bariatric surgery were improved with the use of central respiratory stimulants.[65]

At the end of surgery, neuromuscular blockade should be fully reversed. An objective assessment of the neuromuscular junction using train-of-4 or other methods is ideal. It has been reported that even minute amounts of residual neuromuscular blockade can result in greater postoperative morbidity with increased risks of aspiration, airway obstruction, hypoventilation, hypoxia, and reintubation.[66] Patients should be extubated only when awake: fully conscious, obeying commands, and with airway patency confirmed. Purposeful movements must be distinguished from involuntary actions such as coughing and reflex reaching for the endotracheal tube. After extubation, patients should be nursed in a semi-upright or lateral position.[28]

Local and regional anesthesia techniques may be preferable to general anesthesia, as they avoid manipulation of the airway and reduce the postoperative requirement for sedating analgesic medication.[28] Wound infiltrations, peripheral nerve-block infusions, and epidural infusions of local anesthetic reduce opioid requirements postoperatively and may be of benefit. However, owing to the paucity of published literature in this field, there is currently no good-level evidence supporting one technique over the other. Patients receiving sedation for surgical procedures under monitored anesthetic care should be monitored for adequacy of ventilation by capnography. Patients previously on PAP therapy at home should continue the use of their PAP devices during procedures under mild to moderate sedation.[67] A secured airway is preferred to an unprotected one for procedures requiring deep sedation.[28]

POSTOPERATIVE DISPOSITION OF KNOWN AND SUSPECTED OSA PATIENTS AFTER GENERAL ANESTHESIA

The postoperative disposition of the OSA patient depends on 3 main components: the invasiveness of the surgery, the severity of OSA, and the requirement for postoperative opioids (**Fig. 2**). To illustrate, a patient with severe OSA who just had major surgery and is receiving high-dose opioids would be more likely to require continuous monitoring than another patient with suspected OSA undergoing minor surgery. The final decision regarding the level of monitoring is determined by the attending anesthesiologist, taking into account all patient-related, logistic, and circumstantial factors.

A practical algorithm (see **Fig. 2**) has been formulated based on the ASA 2006 guidelines on

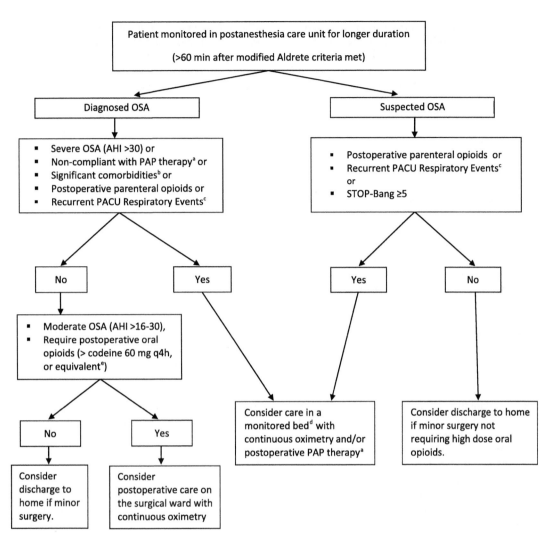

Fig. 2. Postoperative management of the patient with known or suspected obstructive sleep apnea after general anesthesia. [a] Positive airway pressure (PAP) therapy: includes continuous PAP, bilevel PAP, or automatically adjusting PAP. [b] Significant comorbidities: heart failure, arrhythmias, uncontrolled hypertension, cerebrovascular disease, metabolic syndrome, obesity (body mass index >35 kg/m²). [c] Recurrent postanesthesia care unit (PACU) respiratory event: repeated occurrence of oxygen saturation less than 90%, or bradypnea less than 8 breaths/min, or apnea 10 seconds and longer, or pain-sedation mismatch (high pain and sedation scores concurrently).[21] [d] Monitored bed: environment with continuous oximetry and the possibility of early medical intervention (eg, intensive care unit, step-down unit, or remote pulse oximetry with telemetry in surgical ward). [e] Equianalgesic doses of oral opioids: codeine 60 mg every 4 hours (q4h), Oxycodone 5 mg q4h, Hydromorphone 2 mg q4h. (*Adapted from* Seet E, Chung F. Obstructive sleep apnea: preoperative assessment. Anesthesiol Clin 2010;28:199–215, with permission; and Seet E, Chung F. Management of sleep apnea in adults-functional algorithms for the perioperative period: continuing professional development. Can J Anaesth 2010;57:849–64. Copyright 2010 by Canadian Anesthesiologists' Society; with kind permission from Springer Science and Business Media.)

the perioperative management of patients with OSA, and on evidence from recent research.[30,33] All patients with known or suspected OSA who have received general anesthesia should have extended monitoring in the PACU with continuous oximetry. There are currently no evidence-based guidelines addressing the optimal length of monitoring required in the PACU. The ASA guidelines, which were based on expert opinion, recommended prolonged observation for 7 hours in the PACU if respiratory events such as apnea or airway obstruction occur. Such recommendations are difficult to adhere to, especially in the context of community hospitals.[67] The algorithm recommended in this article proposes extended PACU observation for an additional 60 minutes in a quiet environment after the modified Aldrete criteria for discharge has been met.[30,33]

The occurrence of recurrent respiratory events in the PACU is another indication for continuous postoperative monitoring.[21] PACU respiratory events are: (1) episodes of apnea for 10 seconds or more, (2) bradypnea fewer than 8 breaths per minute, (3) pain-sedation mismatch, or (4) repeated oxygen desaturation to less than 90%. Any of these events occurring repeatedly in separate 30-minute intervals may be considered recurrent PACU respiratory events. Patients with suspected OSA (ie, scored as high risk on screening questionnaires) and who develop recurrent PACU respiratory events postoperatively are at increased risk of postoperative respiratory complications.[20,21,44] Continuous monitoring with oximetry in a unit with ready access to medical intervention is advocated. These locations would include ICUs, step-down units, or surgical ward equipped with remote telemetry and oximetry monitoring. These patients may also require postoperative PAP therapy.[67]

Advances incorporating smart technologies have been made in monitoring equipment. Multiple parameters including heart rate, blood pressure, temperature, capnography, and oxygen saturation can be tracked continuously, and the trends analyzed and interpreted according to preprogrammed algorithms. Such monitoring will potentially improve the sensitivity in detecting at-risk patients during their recovery while reducing false alarms, making the postoperative care of OSA patients safer than before.[68,69]

One should consider discharging a patient with known OSA to a monitored environment if the patient has severe OSA, has been noncompliant to PAP therapy, or has experienced recurrent PACU respiratory events (see **Fig. 2**). Furthermore, monitoring with continuous oximetry is recommended if parenteral opioids are administered, in view of possible drug-induced respiratory depression.[70] Patients with moderate OSA who require high-dose oral opioids should be managed in a surgical ward with continuous oximetry (see **Fig. 2**) regardless of the number of PACU respiratory events.

Known OSA patients already on PAP devices should continue PAP therapy postoperatively. Although there is insufficient high-level evidence demonstrating an improvement of outcomes with postoperative PAP therapy in OSA patients, a recent retrospective review of 797 patients scheduled for bariatric surgery suggested that timely recognition and management of OSA with perioperative continuous PAP may mitigate the risk of postoperative complications.[71]

When possible, a multimodal approach to analgesia should be used to minimize the use of opioids postoperatively. Apart from oral or systemic administration of opioid-sparing agents, other effective techniques include local anesthetic wound infiltration, peripheral nerve block catheters, and neuraxial infusions of local anesthetic agents. If postoperative parenteral opioids are necessary, consideration should be made for the use of patient-controlled analgesia with no basal infusion and a strict hourly dose limit, as this may help reduce the total amount of opioid used. OSA patients may have an upregulation of the central opioid receptors secondary to recurrent hypoxemia, and are therefore more susceptible to the respiratory depressant effects of opioids. As such, they may benefit from supplemental oxygen while on parenteral opioids.[72] The Anesthesia Patient Safety Foundation advises that ventilation should be monitored (eg, capnography) for the detection of hypoventilation when supplemental oxygen is delivered.[70]

An interesting phenomenon has been described in recent studies: the AHI increased significantly on postoperative day 3, particularly in male patients with moderate to severe OSA.[73] The occurrence of late complications in OSA patients may be attributed to delayed normalization of sleep architecture and AHI after the fifth postoperative night.[74] At present, deciding on the optimal level and duration of monitoring for OSA patients remains a daunting challenge. The vulnerable OSA patient is at risk of serious postoperative complications and even death. Granted, the incidence of postoperative OSA-related mortality is low; however, it only takes one unnecessary death or one case of hypoxic encephalopathy to be the impetus for closer postoperative monitoring.[75,76]

AMBULATORY SURGERY FOR OSA PATIENTS

The 2006 ASA guidelines on the perioperative management of OSA patients advised that superficial surgery, minor orthopedic surgery under local anesthesia or regional anesthesia, and lithotripsy may be performed as day cases.[28] Since the publication of the ASA guidelines in 2006, there has been increasing interest in ambulatory surgery for OSA patients. The newly published Society for Ambulatory Anesthesia (SAMBA) consensus statement has provided guidelines addressing the selection of suitable OSA patients for ambulatory surgery. The committee found, on systematic review of studies involving ambulatory surgery in OSA patients, that despite a higher incidence of desaturation and the need for supplemental oxygen among OSA patients, there was no significant difference in rates of serious adverse outcomes such as reintubation, mechanical ventilation, surgical airway, or death. The investigators recommend that known OSA patients with well-controlled comorbid diseases and who will comply with postoperative PAP therapy may be considered for ambulatory surgery. Patients are advised to use their PAP devices when sleeping even in daytime for several days postoperatively. Patients presumed to have OSA based on screening, who have optimized comorbid conditions and who will not require oral opioids postoperatively, may also be safely discharged after ambulatory surgery.[77] Emphasis was placed on advanced planning of the intraoperative and postoperative anesthetic and analgesic options, and timely education of patients and caregivers regarding their postdischarge care. The authors similarly recommend that diagnosed or suspected OSA patients without significant comorbidities, recurrent PACU respiratory events, or the need for high-dose oral opioids be considered for discharge home after minor surgery at the discretion of the attending physician (see **Fig. 2**).[30,78] Patients with severe OSA and uncontrolled comorbid diseases are not suitable for ambulatory surgery.[77,78] With regard to the type of procedures suitable for day surgery, the SAMBA guidelines recommend that painful operations for which postoperative nonopioid analgesia would be inadequate should not be performed on an outpatient basis. Based on current evidence, the committee suggests that laparoscopic upper abdominal procedures may be performed as day cases, in contrast to the ASA 2006 recommendations.[77]

All OSA patients should be escorted home by a reliable adult upon discharge. Caution should be exercised if diagnosed or suspected OSA patients develop repeated respiratory events in the early postoperative period, and there should be a lower threshold for unanticipated hospitalization. Ideally ambulatory surgical centers that manage OSA patients should have transfer agreements with better equipped inpatient facilities, and should also have the capacity to handle the postoperative problems associated with OSA.

From recent publications, it appears that the safe conduct of ambulatory surgery for OSA patients may be possible. Retrospective observational studies have reported low (<0.5%) postoperative complication rates with ambulatory or short-stay surgery for OSA patients undergoing bariatric surgery.[79–81] Such approaches are still deemed unconventional.[82] Discriminating criteria for patient selection, meticulous preoperative risk stratification, and optimization of OSA and related comorbidities, together with well-trained medical personnel, experienced high-volume facilities, and strict discharge criteria are all essential for the delivery of safe ambulatory surgery for this subset of patients.

SUMMARY

It is well known that OSA patients can suffer serious postoperative consequences, and this has led to the formulation of various screening methods for the detection and risk stratification of OSA patients. Although every patient deserves individualized care, practical algorithms to guide the perioperative management of such high-risk patients would be advantageous. The authors have formulated clinical algorithms to guide the care of diagnosed and suspected OSA patients in the preoperative, intraoperative, and postoperative periods. To date, many care pathways and recommendations are based on consensus or expert opinion rather than on high-level evidence. Future research in these areas and collaboration between the fields of anesthesiology and sleep medicine will be instrumental in shedding light on these lingering OSA-related perioperative care issues.[83]

REFERENCES

1. Isono S. Obstructive sleep apnea of obese adults: pathophysiology and perioperative airway management. Anesthesiology 2009;110:908–21.
2. Beebe DW, Gozal D. Obstructive sleep apnea and the prefrontal cortex: towards a comprehensive model linking nocturnal upper airway obstruction to daytime cognitive and behavioral deficits. J Sleep Res 2002;11:1–16.
3. Kryger MH. Diagnosis and management of sleep apnea syndrome. Clin Cornerstone 2000;2:39–47.
4. Young T, Palta M, Dempsey J, et al. The occurrence of sleep-disordered breathing among middle-aged adults. N Engl J Med 1993;328:1230–5.
5. Bixler EO, Vgontzas AN, Ten HT, et al. Effect of age on sleep apnea in men: I. Prevalence and severity. Am J Respir Crit Care Med 1998;157:144–8.
6. Bixler EO, Vgontzas AN, Lin HM, et al. Prevalence of sleep-disordered breathing in women. Am J Respir Crit Care Med 2001;163:608–13.
7. Hillman DR, Murphy AS, Antic R, et al. The economic cost of sleep disorders. Sleep 2006;29:299–305.
8. Chung F, Ward B, Ho J, et al. Preoperative identification of sleep apnea risk in elective surgical patients using the Berlin Questionnaire. J Clin Anesth 2007;19:130–4.
9. Finkel KJ, Searleman AC, Tymkew H, et al. Prevalence of undiagnosed obstructive sleep apnea among adult surgical patients in an academic medical center. Sleep Med 2009;10:753–8.
10. Stierer TL, Wright C, George A, et al. Risk assessment of obstructive sleep apnea in a population of patients undergoing ambulatory surgery. J Clin Sleep Med 2010;6:467–72.

11. Iber C, Ancoli-Israel S, Cheeson A, et al. The AASM manual for the scoring of sleep and associated events, rules, terminology and technical specifications. Westchester (IL): American Academy of Sleep Medicine; 2007.

12. Epstein LJ, Kristo D, Strollo PJ, et al. Clinical guideline for the evaluation, management and long-term care of obstructive sleep apnea in adults. J Clin Sleep Med 2009;5:263–76.

13. Fleetham J, Ayas N, Bradley D, et al, CTS Sleep Disordered Breathing Committee. Canadian Thoracic Society guidelines: diagnosis and treatment of sleep disordered breathing in adults. Can Respir J 2006;13: 387–92.

14. Lopez PP, Stefan B, Schulman CI, et al. Prevalence of sleep apnea in morbidly obese patients who presented for weight loss surgery evaluation: more evidence for routine screening for obstructive sleep apnea before weight loss surgery. Am Surg 2008;74: 834–8.

15. Chung F, Elsaid H. Screening for obstructive sleep apnea before surgery: why is it important? Curr Opin Anaesthesiol 2009;22:405–11.

16. Young T, Finn L, Peppard PE, et al. Sleep disordered breathing and mortality: eighteen-year follow-up of the Wisconsin sleep cohort. Sleep 2008;31:1071–8.

17. Marshall NS, Wong KK, Liu PY, et al. Sleep apnea as an independent risk factor for all-cause mortality: the Busselton Health Study. Sleep 2008;31:1079–85.

18. Gupta RM, Parvizi J, Hanssen AD, et al. Postoperative complications in patients with obstructive sleep apnea syndrome undergoing hip or knee replacement: a case-control study. Mayo Clin Proc 2001; 76:897–905.

19. Liao P, Yegneswaran B, Vairavanathan S, et al. Postoperative complications in patients with obstructive sleep apnea: a retrospective matched cohort study. Can J Anaesth 2009;56:819–28.

20. Chung F, Yegneswaran B, Liao P, et al. Validation of the Berlin questionnaire and American Society of Anesthesiologists checklist as screening tools for obstructive sleep apnea in surgical patients. Anesthesiology 2008;108:822–30.

21. Gali B, Whalen FX, Schroeder D, et al. Identification of patients at risk for postoperative respiratory complications using a preoperative obstructive sleep apnea screening tool and postanesthesia care assessment. Anesthesiology 2009;110:869–77.

22. Kaw R, Pasupuleti V, Walker E. Postoperative complications in patients with obstructive sleep apnea. Chest 2012;141:436–41.

23. Memtsoudis S, Liu SS, Ma Y, et al. Perioperative pulmonary outcomes in patients with sleep apnea after noncardiac surgery. Anesth Analg 2011;112: 113–21.

24. Longitudinal Assessment of Bariatric Surgery (LABS) Consortium, Flum DR, Bella SH, et al. Perioperative safety in the longitudinal assessment of bariatric surgery. N Engl J Med 2009;361:445–54.

25. Flink BJ, Rivelli SK, Cox EA, et al. Obstructive sleep apnea and incidence of postoperative delirium after elective knee replacement in the nondemented elderly. Anesthesiology 2012;116:788–96.

26. Kaw R, Chung F, Pasupuleti J, et al. Meta-analysis of the association between obstructive sleep apnoea and postoperative outcome. Br J Anaesth 2012; 109(6):897–906.

27. Flemons WW. Obstructive sleep apnea. N Engl J Med 2002;347:498–504.

28. Gross JB, Bachenberg KL, Benumof JL, et al. Practice guidelines for the perioperative management of patients with obstructive sleep apnea: a report by the American Society of Anesthesiologists Task Force on perioperative management of patients with obstructive sleep apnea. Anesthesiology 2006;104: 1081–93.

29. Adesanya AO, Lee W, Greilich NB, et al. Perioperative management of obstructive sleep apnea. Chest 2010;138:1489–98.

30. Seet E, Chung F. Management of sleep apnea in adults—functional algorithms for the perioperative period: continuing professional development. Can J Anaesth 2010;57:849–64.

31. Porhomayon J, El-Solh A, Chhangani S, et al. The management of surgical patients with obstructive sleep apnea. Lung 2011;189:359–67.

32. Meoli AL, Rosen CL, Kristo D, et al. Upper airway management of the adult patient with obstructive sleep apnea in the perioperative period—avoiding complications. Sleep 2003;26:1060–5.

33. Seet E, Chung F. Obstructive sleep apnea: preoperative assessment. Anesthesiol Clin 2010;28:199–215.

34. Bady E, Achkar A, Pascal S, et al. Pulmonary hypertension in patients with sleep apnoea syndrome. Thorax 2000;55:934–9.

35. Atwood CW, McCrory D, Garcia JG, et al. Pulmonary artery hypertension and sleep-disordered breathing: ACCP evidence-based clinical practice guidelines. Chest 2004;126:72S–7S.

36. Chung F, Zhou L, Liao P. Association of preoperative oximetry parameters with postoperative adverse events [abstract: 12-A-2312-ASAHQ]. Anesthesiology 2012.

37. Berry RB, Parish JM, Hartse KM. The use of autotitrating continuous positive airway pressure for treatment of adult obstructive sleep apnea. An American Academy of Sleep Medicine review. Sleep 2002;25:148–73.

38. Johns MW. A new method of measuring daytime sleepiness: the Epworth sleepiness scale. Sleep 1991;14:540–5.

39. Netzer NC, Hoegel JJ, Loube D, et al. Prevalence of symptoms and risk of sleep apnea in primary care. Chest 2003;124:1406–14.

40. Ramachandran SK, Kheterpal S, Consens F, et al. Derivation and validation of a simple perioperative sleep apnea prediction score. Anesth Analg 2010; 110:1007–15.

41. Chung F, Yegneswaran B, Liao P, et al. STOP questionnaire: a tool to screen patients for obstructive sleep apnea. Anesthesiology 2008;108:812–21.

42. Farney RJ, Walker BS, Farney RM, et al. The STOP-Bang equivalent model and prediction of severity of obstructive sleep apnea: relation to polysomnographic measurements of the apnea/hypopnea index. J Clin Sleep Med 2011;7:459–65.

43. Chung F, Subramanyam R, Liao P, et al. High STOP-Bang score indicates a high probability of obstructive sleep apnoea. Br J Anaesth 2012;108:768–75.

44. Vasu TS, Doghramji K, Cavallazzi R, et al. Obstructive sleep apnea syndrome and postoperative complications: clinical use of the STOP-Bang questionnaire. Arch Otolaryngol Head Neck Surg 2010; 136:1020–4.

45. Chung F, Yegneswaran B, Herrera F, et al. Patients with difficult intubation may need referral to sleep clinics. Anesth Analg 2008;107:915–20.

46. Collop NA. Home sleep testing: it is not about the test. Chest 2010;138:245–6.

47. Chung F, Liao P, Sun Y, et al. Perioperative practical experiences in using a level 2 portable polysomnography. Sleep Breath 2011;15:367–75.

48. Chung F, Liao P, Elsaid H, et al. Oxygen desaturation index from nocturnal oximetry: a sensitive and specific tool to detect sleep-disordered breathing in surgical patients. Anesth Analg 2012;114:993–1000.

49. Collop NA, Anderson WM, Boehlecke B, et al. Clinical guidelines for the use of unattended portable monitors in the diagnosis of obstructive sleep apnea in adult patients: portable Monitoring Task Force of the American Academy of Sleep Medicine. J Clin Sleep Med 2007;3:737–47.

50. Fleetham J, Ayas N, Bradley D, et al. Canadian Thoracic Society 2011 guideline update: diagnosis and treatment of sleep disordered breathing. Can Respir J 2011;18:25–47.

51. Chung S, Yuan H, Chung F. A systematic review of obstructive sleep apnea and its implications for anesthesiologists. Anesth Analg 2008;107:1543–63.

52. Bamgbade OA, Alfa JA. Dexmedetomidine anaesthesia for patients with obstructive sleep apnoea undergoing bariatric surgery. Eur J Anaesthesiol 2009;26:176–7.

53. Kheterpal S, Martin L, Shanks AM, et al. Prediction and outcomes of impossible mask ventilation: a review of 50,000 anesthetics. Anesthesiology 2009;110:891–7.

54. Siyam MA, Benhamou D. Difficult endotracheal intubation in patients with sleep apnea syndrome. Anesth Analg 2002;95:1098–102.

55. Cook TM, Woodall N, Harper J, et al, Fourth National Audit Project. Major complications of airway management in the UK: results of the fourth national audit project of the Royal College of Anaesthetists and the Difficult Airway Society. Part 2: intensive care and emergency departments. Br J Anaesth 2011;106:632–42.

56. American Society of Anesthesiologists Task Force on Management of Difficult Airway. Practice guidelines for management of the difficult airway: an updated report by the American Society of Anesthesiologists task force on management of the difficult airway. Anesthesiology 2003;98:1269–77.

57. Delay JM, Sebbane M, Jung B, et al. The effectiveness of noninvasive positive pressure ventilation to enhance preoxygenation in morbidly obese patients: a randomized controlled study. Anesth Analg 2008; 107:1707–13.

58. Dixon BJ, Dixon JB, Carden JR, et al. Preoxygenation is more effective in the 25 degrees head-up position than in the supine position in severely obese patients: a randomized controlled study. Anesthesiology 2005;102:1110–5.

59. Sabate JM, Jouet P, Merrouche M, et al. Gastroesophaegeal reflux in patients with morbid obesity: a role of obstructive sleep apnea syndrome? Obes Surg 2008;18:1479–84.

60. Ovassapian A, Salem MR. Sellick's maneuver: to do or not do. Anesth Analg 2009;109:1360–2.

61. Bolden N, Smith CE, Auckley D, et al. Perioperative complications during use of an obstructive sleep apnea protocol following surgery and anesthesia. Anesth Analg 2008;105:1869–70.

62. Eikermann M, Gross-Sundrup M, Zaremba S, et al. Ketamine activates breathing and abolishes the coupling between loss of consciousness and upper airway dilator muscle dysfunction. Anesthesiology 2012;116:35–46.

63. Ankichetty S, Wong J, Chung F. A systematic review of the effects of sedative and anesthetics in patients with obstructive sleep apnea. J Anaesthesiol Clin Pharmacol 2011;27:447–58.

64. Yousaf F, Seet E, Venkatraghavan L, et al. Efficacy and safety of melatonin as an anxiolytic and analgesic in the perioperative period: a qualitative systematic review of randomized trials. Anesthesiology 2010;113:968–76.

65. Bamgbade OA. Advantages of doxapram for postanaesthesia recovery and outcomes in bariatric surgery patients with obstructive sleep apnoea. Eur J Anaesthesiol 2011;28:387–91.

66. Murphy GS, Brull SJ. Residual neuromuscular block: lessons unlearned part 1: definitions, incidence, and adverse physiologic effects of residual neuromuscular block. Anesth Analg 2010;111:120–8.

67. Sundar E, Chang J, Smetana GW. Perioperative screening for and management of patients with

obstructive sleep apnea. J Clin Outcome Manag 2011;18:399–411.

68. Overdyk FJ, Carter R, Maddox RR, et al. Continuous oximetry/capnography monitoring reveals frequent desaturation and bradypnea during patient-controlled analgesia. Anesth Analg 2007;105:412–8.

69. Lynn LA, Curry JP. Patterns of unexpected in-hospital deaths: a root cause analysis. Patient Saf Surg 2011;5:3.

70. Weinger MB, Lee LA. "No patient shall be harmed by opioid-induced respiratory depression". In: proceedings of "Essential monitoring strategies to detect clinically significant drug-induced respiratory depression in the postoperative period" conference. APSF Newsletter 2011;26(2):21, 26–8.

71. Weingarten TN, Flores AS, McKenzie JA, et al. Obstructive sleep apnoea and perioperative complications in bariatric patients. Br J Anaesth 2011;106: 131–9.

72. Blake DW, Chia PH, Donnan G, et al. Preoperative assessment for obstructive sleep apnoea and the prediction of postoperative respiratory obstruction and hypoxaemia. Anaesth Intensive Care 2008;36: 379–84.

73. Chung F, Liao P, Fazel H, et al. What are the factors predicting the postoperative apnea-hypopnea index? Chest 2010;138:703A.

74. Chung F, Liao P, Fazel H, et al. Evolution of sleep pattern and sleep breathing disorders during first seven nights after surgery—a pilot study [abstract]. Sleep 2009;32:0667.

75. Gay PC. The value of assessing risk of obstructive sleep apnea in surgical patients: it only takes one. J Clin Sleep Med 2010;6:467–72.

76. Chung F, Liao P. Preoperative screening for obstructive sleep apnoea—one death is too many. Anaesth Intensive Care 2010;38:949–50.

77. Joshi GP, Ankichetty SP, Gan TJ, et al. Society for Ambulatory Anesthesia Consensus statement on peroperative selection of adult patients with obstructive sleep apnea scheduled for ambulatory surgery. Anesth Analg 2012;115(5):1060–8.

78. Ankichetty S, Chung F. Consideration for patients with obstructive sleep apnea undergoing ambulatory surgery. Curr Opin Anaesthesiol 2011;24:605–11.

79. Kurrek MM, Cobourn C, Wojtasik Z, et al. Morbidity in patients with or at high risk for obstructive sleep apnea after ambulatory laparoscopic gastric banding. Obes Surg 2011;21:1494–8.

80. Bergland A, Gaslason H, Raeder J. Fast-track surgery for bariatric laparoscopic gastric bypass with focus on anaesthesia and peri-operative care. Experience with 500 cases. Acta Anaesthesiol Scand 2008;52:1394–9.

81. Raeder J. Bariatric procedure as day/short stay surgery: is it possible and reasonable? Curr Opin Anaesthesiol 2007;20:508–12.

82. Schumann R. Anaesthesia for bariatric surgery. Best Pract Res Clin Anaesthesiol 2011;25:83–93.

83. Chung F, Hillman D, Lydic R. Sleep medicine and anesthesia—a new horizon for anesthesiologists. Anesthesiology 2011;114:1261–2.

Positive Airway Pressure Therapy for Perioperative Patients

Peter C. Gay, MD

KEYWORDS

- Positive airway pressure (PAP) therapy • Noninvasive ventilation (NIV) • Postoperative
- Perioperative • Obstructive sleep apnea (OSA) • Postoperative complications

KEY POINTS

- Positive airway pressure (PAP) therapy can be administered as a fixed pressure level (continuous PAP), a variable autotitrating pressure, or a bilevel setting, also referred to as noninvasive positive pressure ventilation.
- The best available evidence for use of PAP therapy in postoperative patients comes from patients with postextubation respiratory failure or from preemptive efforts to prevent reintubation.
- Patients with obstructive sleep apnea (OSA) or other forms of sleep-disordered breathing such as obesity hypoventilation are recognized as having additional risks for postoperative complications.
- Protocols are being proposed to manage postoperative patients with known or suspected OSA with PAP therapy.
- The role of preoperative diagnosis of OSA and preoperative PAP therapy treatment is also being explored.

INTRODUCTION

Positive airway pressure (PAP) therapy can be administered as a fixed pressure level or continuous PAP (CPAP), a variable autotitrating pressure (APAP), or bilevel setting (BPAP), also called noninvasive ventilation (NIV) and noninvasive positive pressure ventilation when delivered in the hospital setting. An APAP therapy intervention may occur preoperatively; most often in the case of untreated, recently diagnosed, or neglected patients with sleep-disordered breathing (SDB). Clinicians and investigators are also exploring preemptive PAP therapy in suspected or recently diagnosed obstructive sleep apnea (OSA), meaning that patients receive exposure to PAP therapy for some period before surgery in the hope of avoiding postoperative complications by allowing some time for early accommodation to the equipment. However, the most common scenario for PAP therapy in perioperative patients is postoperative intervention after a complication or impending event and it is best described in patients with respiratory failure issues receiving NIV, for whom the most randomized controlled trials (RCTs) exist. All 3 of these scenarios and the several forms of PAP therapy are discussed in this article.

HISTORICAL PERSPECTIVE

It is worthwhile reviewing the evolution of PAP therapy, because it provides insight into the function and usefulness of this therapy to facilitate oxygenation, ventilation, and relief of atelectasis or pneumonia. The earliest description of PAP therapy known to this author comes from a technique published in the Lancet in 1936 and labeled as a "pulmonary plus pressure machine."[1] This machine was fashioned from a vacuum cleaner

Pulmonary, Critical Care and Sleep Medicine, Mayo Clinic, 200 First Street SW, Rochester, MN 55905, USA
E-mail address: pgay@mayo.edu

Sleep Med Clin 8 (2013) 121–128
http://dx.doi.org/10.1016/j.jsmc.2012.12.002
1556-407X/13/$ – see front matter © 2013 Elsevier Inc. All rights reserved.

blower and used in patients with heart failure, pulmonary edema, and asthma to improve oxygenation.

The next innovation to be tried in PAP therapy was intermittent positive pressure ventilation (IPPV), which was used to improve ventilation in patients with Guillain-Barré syndrome, acute respiratory failure from pneumonia, pulmonary edema, and asthma.[2] Although IPPV became popular especially for postoperative patients to prevent hypoventilation and atelectasis, this procedure fell into disfavor when later randomized studies showed lack of benefit in patients with chronic obstructive pulmonary disease (COPD).[3] Patients were randomly assigned to treatment and closely followed by monthly home and quarterly clinic visits for an average of 33 months. The trial was hampered by disappointing compliance, with only half of the patients using their devices as prescribed; this is a challenge in many of the clinical trials described later: patient acceptance of the interventions is often not accepted. There was no statistically significant difference between the treatment groups in mortality, rate and duration of hospitalizations, or change in lung function or life quality with time, overall or for clinically relevant subgroups.

The investigator credited with the discovery of CPAP was Dr Colin Sullivan from Australia, who had pursued his interest in patients observed to obstruct their upper airway while asleep; he conceived the idea of applying PAP therapy in 1981. This idea resulted in a miraculous resolution of the disorder now known as OSA without requiring tracheostomy, which was the only previously known therapy.[4] Sullivan stated, "Continuous positive airway pressure completely prevented the upper airway occlusion in each of the five patients. The upper airway occlusion could be turned off and on simply by increasing or reducing the level of positive airway pressure," and thus CPAP was born.

It was later realized that a subgroup of patients with SDB are not completely responsive to CPAP and might require a differential between the levels of expiratory PAP (EPAP) and inspiratory PAP (IPAP) to eliminate SDB events. Sanders and colleagues[5] proposed that BPAP could have unique efficacy and introduced the first BPAP device for patients with OSA, which was called BiPAP (Philips Healthcare Respironics, Murrysville, PA). Studies showed that simple CPAP could not resolve continued hypopneas and flow limitation, as shown by squaring off of the flow signal before the arousal in a patient with SDB and severe obesity. When the IPAP level was increased to allow a greater differential or pressure support,

the flow limitation and arousals were resolved. In a group of 13 patients with OSA comparing CPAP and BPAP, both modes effectively reduced the mean number of apneas from 56 to 2/h and increased the minimum oxygen saturation from 47% to 87%. The mean PAP of 14 cm H_2O for CPAP could be reduced to near 9 cm H_2O EPAP with the BPAP therapy, leading to the presumption that BPAP would have comfort advantages in patients requiring high pressures to control OSA or perhaps what was likely a component of obesity hypoventilation.

Rideau and colleagues[6] were first to use a mask attached to a ventilator in patients with Duchenne muscular dystrophy to make clinicians realize that a high level of ventilation could result from NIV with improvement in chronic hypoventilation. Patients with hypercapnia could be supported and chronic hypoventilation disorders could potentially be reversed. This technology was later applied to patients with hypercapnic respiratory failure caused by acute COPD exacerbation, and NIV soon found a permanent place in the hospital environment for treatment of medical and surgical patients.[7]

PREOPERATIVE PAP PROTOCOLS

Patients with previously known OSA who are non-compliant with their PAP therapy are a challenge in the perioperative period; during a recent consecutive poll in our preoperative evaluation clinic, an average of 6 a week patients with OSA of all severities were not using their CPAP when evaluated (unpublished quality control data from Mayo Clinic, Rochester, MN). We normally urge reinitiation of PAP or repeat sleep consultation before surgery, but this is often not acceptable to the patient, and there are few outcome data to substantiate this approach. We encourage patients with OSA who have been using PAP to continue this preoperatively and to bring their equipment with them to the hospital on the day of surgery, as recommended by the Anesthesiologists Task Force on perioperative management of patients with OSA.[8] Many patients with OSA still forget to bring their equipment and subsequently cannot recall the pressure for their PAP treatment, so in the cooperative patient we use an APAP device, usually set with a floating pressure window between 5 and 15 cm H_2O while they are in the hospital. In January, 2012 alone, our respiratory therapists had 373 first-time visits to hospital patients' rooms for either a BPAP or CPAP setup, indicating the large volume of patients using PAP therapy monthly (unpublished quality control data from Mayo Clinic, Rochester, MN).

A recent study was presented in abstract form at the 2011 Society of Anesthesia and Sleep Medicine Annual Meeting by a team of investigators from Toronto.[9] Patients at high risk for OSA based on the STOP-Bang questionnaire underwent a home sleep study (Embeltta, ResMed, Poway, CA) and those patients with an apnea-hypopnea index (AHI) >15 events/h were subsequently randomized into APAP (64 patients with mean AHI = 28.6/h) or a control group (67 patients with mean AHI = 25/h). Patients in the APAP group received APAP for 3 nights preoperatively and then 5 nights postoperatively. Although APAP reduced the mean AHI to 3.2 events/h, less than half of the patients (N = 27) were still using APAP on the third postoperative night, indicating the difficulty with compliance in these recently diagnosed patients with OSA who were early users of APAP.

Another retrospective observational study in general surgery patients sought to objectively quantify CPAP adherence in a cohort of presurgical patients diagnosed with OSA during their preoperative workup, again using the STOP-Bang screening questionnaire.[10] The patients were seen in their anesthesia perioperative medicine clinic and underwent a laboratory-based split-night diagnostic and therapeutic titration polysomnogram (PSG) before surgery. Patients newly diagnosed with moderate to severe OSA (AHI of ≥15) were offered APAP to take home before surgery and asked to bring the device with them for the postoperative period. Of 431 referred patients, 211 returned and completed a PSG, and 65% of these patients required PAP therapy and started APAP an average of 4 days before surgery. In 75% of patients, the objective CPAP adherence was available from the first 30 days at 6 to 8 weeks with a sleep specialist-guided follow-up. The median adherence was very low, at 2.5 hours per night, with only 25% of patients using their CPAP devices for 4.5 hours or more per night. Independent predictors of reduced CPAP adherence included African American race, male gender, and depressive mood, but patients were not initially seen by a sleep physician before the PSG and home

APAP titration. Regardless, the protocol as designed did not provide strong encouragement to continue this method of preoperative introduction of PAP therapy in first-time users (**Table 1**).

POSTOPERATIVE PAP PROTOCOLS
General Protocol for Surgical and Medical Patients

We use a systematic approach in both surgical and medical hospitalized patients with suspected SDB OSA, called the obstructive apnea systematic intervention strategy (OASIS), guided by our sleep specialists, who now spend half a day in the hospital seeing these patients.[11] Patients with more hypercapnia and hypersomnolence or overt respiratory failure are transferred to the intensive care unit (ICU) for initiation of BPAP therapy. If patients are suspected to have OSA, as is common on the cardiology and surgical services, they are asked to undergo overnight oximetry. Depending on the severity of the findings, the patients may continue with supplemental oxygen and be offered an outpatient sleep laboratory follow-up or trial empiric APAP therapy in hospital or undergo portable cardiorespiratory studies without PSG to obtain an AHI to allow prescription of home-going PAP therapy. Although this method is only approved for uncomplicated OSA, we are not reimbursed for any hospital study in the Medicare population regardless, and in-hospital PSG studies are of notoriously poor quality. Those who are offered outpatient evaluations in the sleep laboratory return only about half the time for follow-up. We are continuing to pursue modifications of the OASIS protocol to optimize treatment plans for all our hospitalized patients with known or suspected OSA, but the process is far from finalized and verifiable outcome data are needed to guide us further. Protocols and data for postoperative care in more specific subsets of patients are discussed later.

General Surgery

Despite a paucity of data, interest remains high in improving outcomes in those with known or

Table 1			
Selected preoperative protocols			
Reference	**Patient Type**	**Intervention RCTs**	**Major Findings**
Liao et al,[9] 2011	General surgery	3 d preoperative PSG-APAP vs standard care	APAP resolves OSA but >50% do not use
Guralnick et al,[10] 2012	General surgery	4 d preoperative PSG-APAP vs standard care	Median APAP use at 30 d = 2.5 h/night

suspected SDB through protocol-directed PAP therapy. By reviewing several cases, Bolden and colleagues[12] identified issues in patients with OSA that occurred before and after implementation of a standardized OSA protocol. When continuous CPAP was becoming increasingly available in the early 1990s, 1 hospital mandated a treatment protocol for all postoperative patients with OSA with CPAP. This protocol came in response to a postoperative death in a patient with OSA in which CPAP was withheld, followed shortly thereafter by rescue of another postoperative patient from serious complications after treating with CPAP.[13] Of the subsequent 14 patients in whom CPAP was given preoperatively and for 24 to 48 hours after extubation with all subsequent sleep, none developed major respiratory complications. Although the data were limited, the investigators advocated for increased awareness of patients with OSA and argued for CPAP before and after surgery.

Abdominal Surgery

Squadrone and colleagues[14] performed a prospective, multicenter, RCT in patients with hypoxemia (ratio of arterial oxygen tension to inspiratory oxygen fraction [Pao_2/Fio_2] $\leq$ 300) after elective laparotomy and randomized patients (total n = 209) to receive either 50% oxygen for 6 hours by Venturi mask or added use of CPAP set at 7.5 cm H_2O. These investigators showed that CPAP and oxygen use can reduce the frequency of intubation (1% vs 10%, $P = .005$) and also reduce severe complications, including pneumonia, infections, and sepsis. There was no difference in mortality or hospital length of stay and no attempt was made to discern whether any of the patients had OSA or were at higher risk to have undiagnosed OSA. This trial used the helmet mask for CPAP delivery and may be a reason for the very high (96%) tolerance rate of CPAP in their patients, but this mask is not available in the United States or Canada.

A systematic review and meta-analysis of CPAP treatment in patients after abdominal surgery also concluded that there was a significant reduction in the rate of atelectasis and pneumonia, but the duration of use varied widely in these studies.[15] Whether or not patients had coexisting OSA was not specifically investigated in these trials, so the role that this treatment might have played for OSA is unknown.

Orthopedic Patients

Attempts have been made to provide just-in-time hospital introduction of APAP use in undiagnosed patients who prove to be at high risk for OSA based on a previously verified Sleep Apnea Clinical Score questionnaire.[16] These investigators applied APAP to patients at high risk for OSA in the postoperative period after elective total knee or hip arthroplasty and hypothesized that this would reduce postoperative complications and shorten hospital stays. The high-risk patients were randomized to receive standard care plus postoperative APAP or standard care alone, whereas low-risk patients received standard care alone. There were 115 patients of the total 138 (52 low-risk with median AHI = 12.7/h and 86 high-risk group with median AHI near 25 in both the APAP and control groups) enrolled, who also underwent a predismissal (median 3 days postoperatively) cardiorespiratory sleep study. In 38 of the 43 patients who received APAP with adherence data, the median time on PAP while in hospital was 184 minutes/d, although first-night use was higher, at 373 minutes. There were no significant differences in complication rates or length of stay ($P = .65$) for the high-risk randomized groups, but patients with an AHI of 15 or more randomized to APAP had a 1-day median longer postoperative stay ($P = .02$), possibly because of more sleep deprivation or reduced mobility. Although probably underpowered for the end points and no patients trialed CPAP before hospitalization, this study still could not show any benefit to empiric postoperative use of APAP in first-time users at high risk for OSA (**Table 2**).

Cardiac Surgery

Patients with known OSA undergoing cardiac surgery were suspected to be at higher risk of postoperative complications in a small matched cohort study (37 patients) compared with patients without known OSA, but there was no difference and no attempt to evaluate the effect of CPAP on the outcome.[17] Other investigators prospectively randomized 500 patients scheduled for elective cardiac surgery to receive nasal CPAP at 10 cm H_2O immediately after extubation in a control fashion for 10 minutes every 4 hours versus at least 6 h/d.[18] These investigators found that more prolonged aggressive use of CPAP (aCPAP) significantly improved the Pao_2/Fio_2 ratio and reduced pulmonary complications, including hypoxemia, pneumonia, and reintubation rate in the aCPAP patients compared with controls (12 of 232 aCPAP patients vs 25 of 236 control patients, $P<.03$) without altering heart rate and blood pressure. Readmission rates to higher-level care were also significantly lower in the aCPAP-treated group (7/232 aCPAP vs 14/236 controls, respectively; $P<.03$). The investigators

Table 2
Selected postoperative protocols

Reference	Patient Type	Intervention	Major Findings
Squadrone et al,[14] 2005	Abdominal surgery OSA unknown	RCT 6 h CPAP: O_2 vs O_2 alone	Reduced intubation and complications
Ferreyra et al,[15] 2008	Abdominal surgery OSA unknown	Meta-analysis CPAP treatment	Reduced atelectasis and pneumonia
O'Gorman et al,[16] 2012	General surgery High-risk OSA	RCT: APAP vs standard care	High-risk OSA more complications but CPAP no effect
Zarbock et al,[18] 2009	Cardiac surgery	RCT: 6 h vs 10 min CPAP; OSA status unknown	Patient oxygenation improved; reduced complications
Flum et al,[19] 2009	Gastric bypass	Observational only: known OSA	OSA increased risk
Jensen et al,[20] 2008	Gastric bypass	Observational: no OSA vs OSA CPAP compliant vs noncompliant	No significant difference in complications in all 3 groups
Huerta et al,[21] 2002	Gastric bypass	Observational: OSA CPAP compliant vs noncompliant	No increased risk of surgical wound dehiscence
Ebeo et al,[22] 2002	Gastric bypass	RCT: BPAP vs standard care	BPAP improved pulmonary function but complications and length of stay same

concluded that the administration of prophylactic aCPAP after cardiac surgery had a notable beneficial effect and does reduce pulmonary complications, even if the patients are not asked about or investigated for OSA.

Patients Undergoing Gastric Bypass Surgery

Patients undergoing bariatric surgery have a very high incidence of OSA, so the use of PAP therapy to reduce postoperative complications in this group may be most insightful in evaluating the efficacy of this treatment in patients expected to have SDB. Aside from SDB, respiratory complications also extend to atelectasis, abnormal gas exchange, and impaired clearance of secretions. A multicentered observational study[19] prospectively evaluated major adverse outcomes at 30 days in patients undergoing bariatric surgery at 10 sites within the United States. Diagnosis of OSA, impaired functional status, and history of deep vein thrombosis or pulmonary embolus were factors independently associated with an increased risk of the composite end points.

Although CPAP and BPAP effectively treat these problems, postgastric bypass PAP therapy has not been universally adopted out of concern that PAP therapy may lead to anastomotic dehiscence. Opponents of PAP therapy in the postoperative

setting report no differences in adverse outcomes when comparing known patients with OSA who were using preoperative PAP therapy or not, or with the patients who had no known OSA.[20] Most patients in that review (811) were without known OSA, followed by 144 PAP-dependent and 140 non-PAP-dependent patients with known OSA. In the absence of any reported anastomotic leaks or deaths, minimal pulmonary complications were noted in the PAP-dependent OSA, non-PAP OSA, and no known OSA groups.

Most clinicians would presumably have difficulty withholding postoperative PAP therapy from those who clearly need it for SDB on the theoretic basis of a decreased risk of pressurized air causing its own serious complications. To assess the safety and efficacy of postoperative PAP after Roux-en-Y gastric bypass, 1 study prospectively evaluated the risk of subsequent anastomotic leaks and pulmonary complications.[21] Of the 1067 patients included, 420 had known OSA, only 159 of whom were using CPAP. Although no episodes of pneumonia were diagnosed in any of the patients, only 2 of the 15 major anastomotic leaks occurred in patients treated with CPAP, and no correlation was found between the 2 ($P = .6$).

There is some evidence that BPAP therapy improves pulmonary function after open Roux-en-Y gastric bypass, based on a small single-center

Table 3
Selected NIV protocols

Reference	Patient Type	Intervention	Major Findings
Auriant et al,[24] 2001	Thoracic surgery	RCT: NIV vs standard care	Intubation rate and mortality reduced; no change in LOS; OSA status unknown
Liao et al,[25] 2010	Thoracic surgery	RCT: prophylactic BPAP vs standard care	Pulmonary complications unaffected but CT scan lung expansion better; OSA status unknown

prospective study.[22] Baseline pulmonary function tests were performed on 27 patients, who were randomized to then receive either conventional postoperative care or BPAP. Preoperative expiratory flow reduction found in both groups was not statistically significant between the groups. In the group receiving BPAP therapy, the forced vital capacity [FVC], forced expiratory volume in 1 second [FEV$_1$], and oxygen saturation were significantly higher compared with the control group. Despite these findings, BPAP did not translate into shorter length of stay or improved complication rates.

NIV

The use of NIV for both treatment and prevention of respiratory failure gained acceptance after several randomized trials were performed attesting to the efficacy of this therapy in surgical patients, as summarized by Conti and colleagues,[23] but no study specifically identified a subset of those known to have OSA. The use of NIV in specific categories of postoperative patients is reviewed in **Table 3**.

Cardiothoracic Surgery

A randomized prospective trial was performed in 48 patients who developed acute respiratory failure after lung resection.[24] This study compared NIV versus standard treatment, including oxygen supplementation, bronchodilators, analgesia, and aggressive chest physiotherapy. The respiratory and heart rate, in addition to the Pa_{O_2}/Fi_{O_2} ratio, were significantly better (all $P<.05$) for the NIV patients. The intubation rate (20.8% vs 50%) and ICU mortality (37.5% vs 12.5%) were also significantly better for the NIV group, despite the fact that there were no significant differences in ICU and hospital length of stay. The major reasons for reintubation were tachypnea and encephalopathy.

The prophylactic use of NIV in postthoracic surgery patients was also investigated in another

randomized prospective controlled study of 50 patients receiving either conventional postoperative care or NIV.[25] The NIV therapy was applied with BPAP for a mean ventilation time of 13.5 ± 4.9 hours using an average IPAP of 13 ± 3.2 cm H_2O and all were set to a minimum EPAP set of 4 cm H_2O. Although no significant adverse effects of NIV treatment were observed and an improvement in lung expansion judged by CT scanning was noted (3/23 vs 13/27, $P = .008$), there were no significant differences in pulmonary function parameters or other pulmonary complications postoperatively between the 2 groups ($P>.05$). In those who had pulmonary complications, multilogistic regression analysis showed that COPD was a risk factor, and perhaps prophylactic use in selected patients, such as those with COPD or OSA, might show a beneficial outcome.

SUMMARY

The role of just-in-time or preoperative PAP therapy intervention and effect on outcomes in patients with OSA has yet to be determined. Emphasis has been placed on preoperative screening for suspect OSA and minimizing risk for known and suspect patients with OSA perioperatively. Our institution and others have implemented in-hospital sleep-consultative services in combination with OASIS, with close follow-up through a protocol to aid workup and initial management of perioperative inpatients with suspected OSA, but outcomes-based research is sorely needed. Results in this population vary by institution, so perioperative outcomes in patients with OSA will likely be a future element for judging best practice performance.

In the absence of robust prospective outcomes data to guide us in the monitoring and postoperative management of patients with OSA undergoing surgery, we must continue to develop best practices to avoid situations that we do not realize are dangerous until a catastrophe occurs[26] and then we must face the consequences of what has become known as the prototypical SDB malpractice case. How do we know that the prototypical case relates to severe OSA, or could morbid obesity, the presence of an abdominal incision, type of narcotics, extubation without CPAP, an unmonitored setting, or some other factor(s) be the major culprit? Unexpected sudden death registries such as that kept in the American Society of Anesthesiologists Closed Claims Project, may help prevent future disasters. The purpose of the project is to identify major areas of life loss in anesthesia, patterns of injury, and strategies for prevention. It is to be hoped that by combining preoperative screening, identifying pertinent recurrent events in the postanesthesia care unit, and optimizing perioperative care, useful protocols will be constructed. Although disastrous postoperative consequences in patients with SDB are rare, 1 death is always too many.[27]

REFERENCES

1. Poulton EP, Oxon DM. Left-sided heart failure with pulmonary oedema: its treatment with the "pulmonary plus" pressure machine. Lancet 1936;228: 981–3.

2. Cournand A, Motley HL. Physiological studies of the effects of intermittent positive pressure breathing on cardiac output in man. Am J Physiol 1948;152:162–74.

3. Intermittent positive pressure breathing therapy of chronic obstructive pulmonary disease. A clinical trial. Ann Intern Med 1983;99(5):612–20.

4. Sullivan CE, Berthon-Jones M, Issa FG, et al. Reversal of obstructive sleep apnoea by continuous positive airway pressure applied through the nares. Lancet 1981;1:862–5.

5. Sanders MH, Kern N. Obstructive sleep apnea treated by independently adjusted inspiratory and expiratory positive airway pressures via nasal mask. Physiologic and clinical implications. Chest 1990;98(2):317–24.

6. Rideau Y, Gatin G, Bach J, et al. Prolongation of life in Duchenne's muscular dystrophy. Acta Neurol (Napoli) 1983;5:118–24.

7. Caples SM, Gay PC. Noninvasive positive pressure ventilation in the intensive care unit: a concise review. Crit Care Med 2005;33(11):2651–8.

8. Gross JB, Bachenberg KL, Benumof JL, et al. Practice guidelines for the perioperative management of patients with obstructive sleep apnea: a report by the American Society of Anesthesiologists Task Force on Perioperative Management of patients with obstructive sleep apnea. Anesthesiology 2006;104:1081–93.

9. Liao P, Chung F, Luo Q, et al. Randomized controlled trial (RCT) of perioperative auto-CPAP treatment in OSA patient: a preliminary report [abstract]. SASM 2011.

10. Guralnick AS, Pant M, Minhaj M, et al. CPAP adherence in patients with newly diagnosed obstructive sleep apnea prior to elective surgery. 2012; Oct 15;8(5):501–6.

11. Gay PC. Sleep and sleep-disordered breathing in the hospitalized patient. Respir Care 2010;55: 1240–54.

12. Bolden N, Smith CE, Auckley D. Avoiding adverse outcomes in patients with obstructive sleep apnea (OSA): development and implementation of a perioperative OSA protocol. J Clin Anesth 2009;21(4): 286–93.

13. Rennotte MT, Baele P, Aubert G, et al. Nasal continuous positive airway pressure in the perioperative management of patients with obstructive sleep apnea submitted to surgery. Chest 1995;107(2): 367–74.

14. Squadrone V, Coha M, Cerutti E, et al. Continuous positive airway pressure for treatment of postoperative hypoxemia: a randomized controlled trial. JAMA 2005;293:589–95.

15. Ferreyra GP, Baussano I, Squadrone V, et al. Continuous positive airway pressure for treatment of respiratory complications after abdominal surgery: a systematic review and meta-analysis. Ann Surg 2008;247:617–26.

16. O'Gorman SM, Gay PC, Morgenthaler TI. Does auto-titrating positive airway pressure therapy improve postoperative outcome in patients at risk for obstructive sleep apnea syndrome? A randomized controlled clinical trial. Chest, in press.

17. Kaw R, Golish J, Ghamande S, et al. Incremental risk of obstructive sleep apnea on cardiac surgical outcomes. J Cardiovasc Surg 2006;47(6):683–9.

18. Zarbock A, Mueller E, Netzer S, et al. Prophylactic nasal continuous positive airway pressure following cardiac surgery protects from postoperative pulmonary complications–a prospective, randomized, controlled trial in 500 patients. Chest 2009;135: 1252–9.

19. Flum DR, Belle SH, King WC, et al, The Longitudinal Assessment of Bariatric Surgery (LABS) Consortium. Perioperative safety in the longitudinal assessment of bariatric surgery. N Engl J Med 2009;361(5): 445–54.

20. Jensen C, Tejirian T, Lewis C, et al. Postoperative CPAP and BiPAP use can be safely omitted after laparoscopic Roux-en-Y gastric bypass. Surg Obes Relat Dis 2008;4(4):512–4.

21. Huerta S, DeShields S, Shpiner R, et al. Safety and efficacy of postoperative CPAP to prevent pulmonary complications after Roux en-Y gastric bypass. J Gastrointest Surg 2002;6(3):354–8.

22. Ebeo C, Benotti P, Byrd R, et al. The effect of BiPAP on postoperative pulmonary function following gastric surgery for obesity. Respir Med 2002;96(9):672–6.

23. Conti G, Costa R, Spinazzola G. Non-invasive ventilation (NIV) in surgical patients with post-operative acute respiratory failure. Curr Anaesth Crit Care 2006;17:329–32.

24. Auriant I, Jallot A, Hervé O, et al. Non-invasive ventilation reduces mortality in acute respiratory failure following lung resection. Am J Respir Crit Care Med 2001;164:1231–5.

25. Liao G, Chen R, He J. Prophylactic use of noninvasive positive pressure ventilation in post-thoracic surgery patients: a prospective randomized control study. J Thorac Dis 2010;2:205–9.

26. Ostermeier AM, Roizen MF, Hautkappe M, et al. Three sudden postoperative respiratory arrests associated with epidural opioids in patients with sleep apnea. Anesth Analg 1997;85:452–60.

27. Gay PC. The value of assessing risk of obstructive sleep apnea in surgical patients: it only takes one. J Clin Sleep Med 2010;6:473–4.

Perioperative Complications in Patients with Obstructive Sleep Apnea

Roop Kaw, MD

KEYWORDS

- Obstructive sleep apnea • Upper airway surgery • Anesthesia • Pain medications

KEY POINTS

- Factors to consider when evaluating how patients with suspected obstructive sleep apnea (OSA) should be monitored postoperatively include the preclinical suspicion of the severity of OSA; type of surgery; the anticipated need for pain medications, especially intravenous (IV) patient-controlled anesthesia in the postoperative period; and the availability of emergency airway and respiratory equipment and so forth.
- In general, all patients with OSA undergoing upper airway surgery should be strongly considered for inpatient surgery, even when the surgery can be performed on an outpatient basis in similar patients without OSA.
- Minor surgeries requiring local or regional anesthesia only, like arthroscopy and lithotripsy, can be safely performed on an outpatient basis in patients with OSA.
- Minor surgeries and procedures that are usually performed on an outpatient basis but require IV sedation or IV analgesia can also be safely performed on an outpatient basis in patients with OSA, but recent guidelines by American Society of Anesthesiologists (ASA) require continual observation of qualitative clinical signs and monitoring for the presence of exhaled carbon dioxide during moderate or deep sedation unless this is precluded or invalidated by the nature of the patient, procedure, or equipment.

The prevalence of obstructive sleep apnea (OSA) is increasing in the general population and is higher among patients undergoing surgery. It is estimated that between 1990 and 1998 there was a 12-fold increase in the diagnosis of OSA in surgical outpatients.[1] Recent studies report a prevalence of greater than 30% in neurosurgical patients[2] and up to 91% in patients undergoing bariatric surgery.[3] In another series of 305 patients undergoing elective surgery and screened for OSA by the Berlin questionnaire, about 24% of patients were noted to be at risk of having OSA.[4] Similar estimates using the Snoring, Tiredness, Observed Apneas and High Blood Pressure (STOP) questionnaire revealed a prevalence of 27.5%.[5] More recently, using the National Surgical Inpatient data (the largest all-payer inpatient discharge database sponsored by the Agency for Healthcare Research and Quality), Memtsoudis and colleagues[6] reported a prevalence of sleep apnea (billed diagnosis) of 2.7% among 1,710,000 general surgical patients and 5.5% among 1,513,137 orthopedic patients (**Fig. 1**). OSA can pose a significant challenge to anesthesiologists in the perioperative period because of possible difficult intubation,[7] increased sensitivity to narcotics, and postoperative upper airway obstruction. Among the many diverse reasons predisposing patients with OSA to postoperative complications is the worsening of sleep apnea in the supine position.[8] In addition, a smaller amount of upper airway collapse is required to cause obstruction in patients predisposed to postintubation edema, hematoma, nasal packing, or tubes and so forth.

Departments of Hospital Medicine and Outcomes Research, Anesthesiology, Cleveland Clinic, 9500 Euclid Avenue, Cleveland, OH 44195, USA
E-mail address: kawr@ccf.org

Sleep Med Clin 8 (2013) 129–134
http://dx.doi.org/10.1016/j.jsmc.2012.12.001
1556-407X/13/$ – see front matter © 2013 Elsevier Inc. All rights reserved.

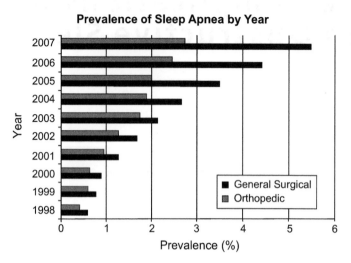

Prevalence of Sleep Apnea by Year

(Y-axis: Year; 2007, 2006, 2005, 2004, 2003, 2002, 2001, 2000, 1999, 1998)
(X-axis: Prevalence (%); 0 1 2 3 4 5 6)

■ General Surgical
▨ Orthopedic

Fig. 1. Prevalence of a diagnosis code for sleep apnea among patients undergoing orthopedic and general surgical procedures from 1998 to 2007. (*From* Memtsoudis S, Liu SS, Ma Y, et al. Perioperative pulmonary outcomes in patients with sleep apnea after non-cardiac surgery. Anesth Analg 2011;112(1):117; with permission.)

Sleep deprivation during the perioperative period has been associated with worsening of OSA, especially because of the emergence of rapid eye movement (REM) rebound, although this is controversial.[9] A recent study by Liao and colleagues[10] reported a higher apnea-hypopnea index (AHI) and oxygen desaturation index among patients with OSA on the third postoperative night compared with AHI preoperatively or on the first postoperative night. Several other possible mechanisms exist, such as fat distribution and the physiologic interaction of cross-sectional area, lung volume, and driving pressure changes.

An intriguing question has been whether severity of OSA relates to postoperative complications. The literature is divided, with some studies pointing to severe OSA associated with a greater complication rate[11–15] and others not confirming this association.[16–18] Respiratory failure is intuitively the main concern among postoperative complications in patients with OSA. These cases were first described by Esclamado and colleagues[11] in a retrospective review of 135 patients surgically treated for OSA from 1982 to 1987, with about 77% patients having airway problems and 1 patient who died. The earliest cases of postoperative respiratory failure among patients with OSA undergoing surgery unrelated to the treatment of OSA were reported by Rennotte and colleagues[19] in 1995, who suggested that nasal continuous positive airway pressure (CPAP) used before surgery and resumed immediately after extubation helped reduce postoperative complications in patients with OSA. In 1997, Ostermeier and colleagues[20] reported 3 cases of sudden postoperative respiratory arrest associated with epidural opioids in patients with sleep apnea. All three patients died. Depending on the definition used in the studies reported in the literature, as well as their

respective sample sizes, respiratory failure has not been consistently reported among patients with OSA. Moreover, some of the subsequent studies were initiated as quality improvement projects and hence, by design, report fewer postoperative respiratory complications than are reported in the overall surgical population.[15,21–23] Among other reasons for variations in reporting of postoperative complications between different studies are whether OSA was diagnosed clinically, by screening, or by a gold standard test; and, especially among case control studies, whether the comparison was against a group of true controls (OSA excluded by formal polysomnography). A large study of approximately 50,000 patients with OSA undergoing general surgery and 65,000 undergoing orthopedic surgery recently reported a 5-fold increase in intubation and mechanical ventilation after surgery (**Fig. 2**).[6] More recently, a meta-analysis of 3942 patients with OSA reported postoperative respiratory failure rates of 1.96% versus 0.70% (odds ratio [OR] 2.43, 95% confidence interval [CI] 1.34–4.39, $P = .003$) and a postoperative cardiac event rate of 3.76% versus 1.69% (OR 2.07, 95% CI 1.23–3.50, $P = .007$) (**Figs. 3** and **4**).[24] Early reports also show that the incidence of respiratory failure may be particularly high among patients with obesity hypoventilation syndrome, which is more likely to be unrecognized before elective noncardiac surgery.[25] Patients with OSA on chronic opiates have been shown to fail CPAP therapy more often than those who are not chronically on opioids for pain control.[26] This has been attributed to the detection of central sleep apnea during CPAP, a condition known as complex sleep apnea. Although postoperative desaturation in patients with OSA has attracted negative attention in the literature, these events can be an important clue to possible further worsening of

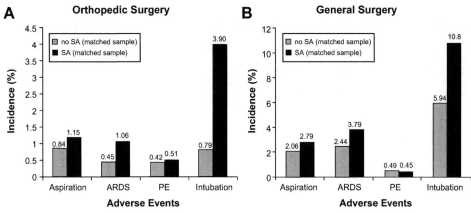

Fig. 2. Incidence of respiratory complications for patients with and without sleep apnea (SA) undergoing orthopedic (*A*) and general surgical (*B*) procedures for patients using the full and matched sample. AE, adverse event; ARDS, adult respiratory distress syndrome; PE, pulmonary embolism. (*From* Memtsoudis S, Liu SS, Ma Y, et al. Perioperative pulmonary outcomes in patients with sleep apnea after non-cardiac surgery. Anesth Analg 2011; 112(1):117; with permission.)

respiratory complications, particularly in patients whose OSA is unrecognized at the time of surgery.

Among the most common and consistently reported postoperative outcomes in patients with OSA is unanticipated transfer to the intensive care unit (ICU).[14,23,27] Liao and colleagues[16] reported the largest number of ICU transfers to date, but according to the investigators most of these transfers were planned. A wide range of isolated cardiac complications have also been reported after surgery in patients with OSA.[5,14,18,22,23] These complications include postoperative atrial fibrillation and other arrhythmias, myocardial ischemia and infarction, and major intraoperative fluctuations in systolic and diastolic blood pressure requiring pharmacologic agents.[28] In a small prospective study evaluating the incidence of arrhythmia in patients with OSA after coronary artery bypass surgery, those with an oxygen desaturation index (≥4% per hour) of at least 5 had

a relative risk of 2.8 for the development of atrial fibrillation postoperatively.[29] The two groups were not controlled for body mass index and the risk of postoperative atrial fibrillation was statistically insignificant among patients with AHI greater than or equal to 5.

Anecdotal reports and case series of sudden cardiac arrhythmias and sudden cardiac death associated with severe OSA and hypoxemia have been reported during overnight polysomnographic recordings in sleep laboratories.[30] The slow advent of inpatient polysomnography has supported to such claims. A study examining the prevalence of OSA in the medical ICU reported apneic periods of 30 to 90 seconds followed by prolonged periods of flat/absent electroencephalogram activity among 2 patients, 1 of whom arrested and died.[31] Gami and colleagues[32] reviewed 112 reports of sudden death and found that almost half of the patients with polysomnographically confirmed OSA died

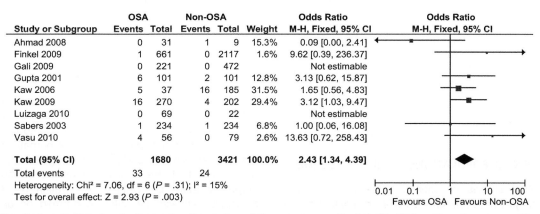

Fig. 3. Forest plots for Postoperative Respiratory failure among patients with OSA undergoing non-cardiac surgery.

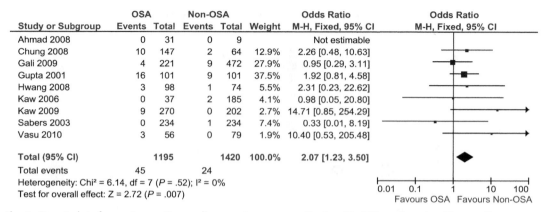

Fig. 4. Forest plots for postoperative cardiac events among patients with OSA undergoing Non-cardiac surgery.

during sleep hours (12:00 midnight to 6:00 AM) compared with 21% of those without OSA (relative risk 2.57). The risk of sudden death was related to disease severity of OSA. More recently, recurrent episodes of cardiopulmonary arrest were reported in a hospitalized patient with undiagnosed severe OSA during REM sleep, with oxygen desaturation to 30% documented on polysomnography. No subsequent near-arrest events were noted with the use of CPAP.[33] Sudden cardiac death (or near death) has been attributed to depressed or failed arousal followed by life-threatening hypoxemia in patients with severe OSA, which may be true among some obese patients who may average 50 or more severe cyclic desaturations per hour of sleep every night and may be at particular risk for acquired arousal failure.[34] Others have attributed the depressed arousal mechanism to sleep deprivation and fragmentation among hospitalized patients.[35] Narcotics, especially patient-controlled analgesia, spinal anesthesia, and sedatives, can further increase or delay the arousal threshold and thereby compromise airway patency and survival among such patients. Further studies are needed to reveal the mechanisms of apnea termination and arousal response, particularly among acutely ill hospitalized patients, postoperative patients, and patients receiving sedatives and narcotics. Although no studies to date have reported any postoperative deaths directly attributable to OSA, it has been reported that most unexpected and unexplained postoperative deaths occur at night within 7 days of surgery.[36]

SPECIAL POPULATIONS: BARIATRIC SURGERY

Most studies of patients undergoing bariatric surgery have not reported OSA as a risk factor for postoperative complications.[37–39] In a recent study of 4776 patients undergoing bariatric surgery, self-

reported OSA did not predict 30-day major composite outcome including death, thromboembolic event, surgical reintervention, or increased length of stay.[40] These findings may not apply to patients with unrecognized OSA at the time of undergoing surgery. In the bariatric surgery population, given the high prevalence of OSA, most patients are tested for OSA preoperatively, prescribed CPAP or biphasic positive airway pressure, and resumed at admission to post-anesthesia care unit. Most patients are closely monitored for at least the first 24 hours. Earlier reports have suggested treatment with CPAP as a predictor for anastomotic leaks postoperatively,[41,42] but larger series of patients having bariatric surgery did not confirm this.[17,43–45]

AMBULATORY VERSUS INPATIENT SURGERY

Factors to consider when evaluating how patients with suspected OSA should be monitored postoperatively include the preclinical suspicion of the severity of OSA, type of surgery, the anticipated need for pain medications (especially IV patient-controlled anesthesia in the postoperative period), and the availability of emergency airway and respiratory equipment and so forth. In general, all patients with OSA undergoing upper airway surgery should be strongly considered for inpatient surgery, even when the surgery can be performed on an outpatient basis in similar patients without OSA.[39] Minor procedures requiring local or regional anesthesia only, like arthroscopy and lithotripsy, can be safely performed on an outpatient basis in patients with OSA.[39] Minor surgeries and procedures that are usually performed on an outpatient basis but require IV sedation or IV analgesia can also be safely performed on an outpatient basis in patients with OSA, but recent guidelines by ASA require continual observation of qualitative clinical signs and monitoring for the presence of exhaled carbon dioxide during moderate or deep sedation unless this is precluded or invalidated by the nature of the patient, procedure, or equipment.[46]

REFERENCES

1. Namen AM, Dunagan DP, Fleischer A, et al. Increased physician-reported sleep apnea: the National Ambulatory Medical Care Survey. Chest 2002;121:1741–7.

2. Pollak L, Shpirer I, Rabey JM, et al. Polysomnography in patients with intracranial tumors before and after operation. Acta Neurol Scand 2004;109:56–60.

3. Hallowell PT, Stellato TA, Schuster M, et al. Potentially life threatening sleep apnea is unrecognized without aggressive evaluation. Am J Surg 2007; 193(3):364–7.

4. Chung F, Ward B, Ho J, et al. Preoperative identification of sleep apnea risk in elective surgical patients using the Berlin questionnaire. J Clin Anesth 2007; 19:130–4.

5. Chung F, Yegneswaran B, Liao P, et al. STOP questionnaire: a tool to screen patients for obstructive sleep apnea. Anesthesiology 2008;108:812–21.

6. Memtsoudis S, Liu SS, Ma Y, et al. Perioperative pulmonary outcomes in patients with sleep apnea after non-cardiac surgery. Anesth Analg 2011; 112(1):113–21.

7. Siyam MA, Benhamou D. Difficult endotracheal intubation in patients with sleep apnea syndrome. Anesth Analg 2002;95:1098–102.

8. Morganthaler TI, Kapen S, Lee-Chiong T, et al. Practice parameters for the medical therapy of obstructive sleep apnea. Sleep 2006;29:1031–5.

9. Rosenberg J, Rasmussen GI, Wejdemann KR, et al. Ventilatory pattern and associated episodic hypoxemia in the late postoperative period in the general surgical ward. Anaesthesia 1999;544:323–8.

10. Liao P, Sun F, Amirshahi B, et al. A significant exacerbation of sleep breathing disorders in OSA patients undergoing surgery with general anesthesia. Sleep 2009;A223, 0684.

11. Esclamado RM, Glenn MG, McCulloch TM, et al. Perioperative complications and risk factors in the surgical treatment of obstructive sleep apnea syndrome. Laryngoscope 1989;99:1125.

12. Riley RW, Powell NB, Guillenminault C, et al. Obstructive sleep apnea surgery: risk management and complications. Otolaryngol Head Neck Surg 1997;117:648.

13. Meoli AL, Rosen CL, Kristo D, et al. Upper airway management of the adult patient with obstructive sleep apnea in the perioperative period–avoiding complications. Sleep 2003;26:1060.

14. Gupta RM, Parvizi J, Hanssen AD, et al. Postoperative complications in patients with obstructive sleep apnea syndrome undergoing hip or knee replacement: a case- control study. Mayo Clin Proc 2001; 76:897–905.

15. Hwang D, Shakir N, Limann B, et al. Association of sleep-disordered breathing with postoperative complications. Chest 2008;133(5):1128–34.

16. Liao P, Yeneswaran B, Vairavanathan S, et al. Postoperative complications in patients with obstructive sleep apnea: a retrospective matched cohort study. Can J Anaesth 2009;56(11):819–28.

17. Weingarten TN, Flores AS, McKenzie JA, et al. Obstructive sleep apnoea and perioperative complications in bariatric patients. Br J Anaesth 2011; 106(1):131–9.

18. Kaw R, Pasupuleti V, Walker E, et al. Postoperative complications in patients with obstructive sleep apnea. Chest 2012;141(2):436–41.

19. Rennotte MT, Baele P, Aubert G, et al. Nasal continuous positive airway pressure in the perioperative management of patients with obstructive sleep apnea submitted to surgery. Chest 1995;107(2): 367–74.

20. Ostermeier AM, Roizen MF, Hautkappe M, et al. Three sudden postoperative respiratory arrests associated with epidural opioids in patients with sleep apnea. Anesth Analg 1997;85(2):452–60.

21. Gali B, Whalen FX, Gay PC, et al. Management plan to reduce risks in perioperative care of patients with presumed obstructive sleep apnea syndrome. J Clin Sleep Med 2007;3:582–8.

22. Finkel KJ, Searleman AC, Tymkew H. Prevalence of undiagnosed obstructive sleep apnea among adult surgical patients in an academic medical center. Sleep Med 2009;10:753–8.

23. Gali B, Whalen FX, Schroeder DR, et al. Identification of patients at risk for postoperative respiratory complications using a preoperative obstructive sleep apnea screening tool and post-obstructive anesthesia care assessment. Anesthesiology 2009; 110:869–77.

24. Kaw R, Chung F, Pasupuleti V, et al. Meta-analysis of the association between obstructive sleep apnoea and postoperative outcome. Br J Anaesth 2012; 109(6):897–906.

25. Kaw R, Pasupuleti V, Walker E, et al. Obesity hypoventilation syndrome: an emerging and unrecognized risk factor among surgical patients. Am J Respir Crit Care Med 2011;183:A3147.

26. Guillenminault C, Cao M, Yue HJ, et al. Obstructive sleep apnea and chronic opioid use. Lung 2010; 188:459–68.

27. Kaw R, Golish J, Ghamande S, et al. Incremental risk of obstructive sleep apnea in cardiac surgical outcomes. J Cardiovasc Surg (Torino) 2006;47: 683–9.

28. Stierer TL, Wright C, George A, et al. Risk assessment of obstructive sleep apnea in a population of patients undergoing ambulatory surgery. J Clin Sleep Med 2010;6(5):467–72.

29. Mooe T, Gullsby S, Rabben T, et al. Sleep-disordered breathing: a novel predictor of atrial fibrillation after coronary artery bypass surgery. Coron Artery Dis 1996;7:475–8.

30. Chokroverty S, Sahota P. Preface V. Acute and emergent events in sleep disorders. New York: Oxford University Press; 2011.

31. Dyken ME, Yamada T, Glenn CL, et al. Obstructive sleep apnea associated with cerebral hypoxemia and death. Neurology 2004;62(3):491–3.

32. Gami AS, Howard DE, Olson EJ, et al. Day-night pattern of sudden death in obstructive sleep apnea. N Engl J Med 2005;352(21):1206–14.

33. Khoo SM, Mukherjee JJ, Phua J, et al. Obstructive sleep apnea presenting as recurrent cardiopulmonary arrest. Sleep Breath 2009;13:89–92.

34. Peppard PE, Ward NR, Morrell MJ. The impact of obesity on oxygen desaturation during sleep-disordered breathing. Am J Respir Crit Care Med 2009;180(8):788–93.

35. Guillenminault C, Rosekind M. The arousal threshold: sleep deprivation, sleep fragmentation obstructive sleep apnea syndrome. Bull Eur Physiopathol Respir 1981;17:341–9.

36. Rosenberg J, Pedersen MH, Ramsingh T, et al. Circadian variation in unexpected postoperative death. Br J Surg 1992;79(12):1300–2.

37. Ahmad S, Nagle A, McCarthy RJ, et al. Postoperative hypoxemia in morbidly obese patients with and without obstructive sleep apnea undergoing laparoscopic bariatric surgery. Anesth Analg 2008;107(1):138–43.

38. Ballantyne GH, Svahn J, Capella RF, et al. Predictors of prolonged hospital stay following open and laparoscopic gastric bypass for morbid obesity: body mass index, length of surgery, sleep apnea, asthma and metabolic syndrome. Obes Surg 2004; 14:1042–50.

39. Gross JB, Bachenberg KL, Benumof JL, et al. Practice guidelines for the perioperative management of patients with obstructive sleep apnea: a report by the American Society of Anesthesiologists Task Force on Perioperative Management of patients with obstructive sleep apnea. Anesthesiology 2006;104(5):1081.

40. Flum DR, Belle SH, King WC, et al. Perioperative safety in the longitudinal assessment of bariatric surgery. N Engl J Med 2009;36(5):445–54.

41. Fernandez AZ Jr, DeMaria EJ, Tichansky DS, et al. Experience with over 3000 open and laparoscopic bariatric procedures: multivariate analysis of factors related to leak and resultant mortality. Surg Endosc 2004;18(2):193–7.

42. Vasquez TL, Hoddinott K. A potential complication of bi-level positive airway pressure after gastric bypass surgery. Obes Surg 2004;14(2):282.

43. Huerta S, DeShields S, Shpiner R, et al. Safety and efficacy of postoperative continuous positive airway pressure to prevent pulmonary complications after Roux-en-Y gastric bypass. J Gastrointest Surg 2002;6:354–8.

44. Livingston EH, Huerta S, Arthur D, et al. Male gender is a predictor of morbidity and age a predictor of mortality for patients undergoing gastric bypass surgery. Ann Surg 2002;236:576–82.

45. Podnos YD, Jimenez JC, Wilson SE, et al. Complications after laparoscopic gastric bypass: a review of 3464 cases. Arch Surg 2003;138:957–61.

46. Weaver J. The latest ASA mandate: CO_2 monitoring for moderate and deep sedation. Anesth Prog 2011; 58(3):111–2.

Obesity Hypoventilation Syndrome and Anesthesia

Edmond H.L. Chau, MD[a], Babak Mokhlesi, MD, MSc[b],
Frances Chung, MBBS, FRCPC[a],*

KEYWORDS

- Obesity hypoventilation syndrome • Perioperative management • Positive airway pressure

KEY POINTS

- Obesity hypoventilation syndrome (OHS) is an important disease entity that requires the anesthesiologist's thorough understanding.
- Patients with OHS present with severe upper airway obstruction, restrictive pulmonary physiology, blunted central respiratory drive, and pulmonary hypertension. The primary therapy for OHS is positive airway pressure (PAP) therapy.
- Screening questionnaires such as the validated STOP-Bang questionnaire can identify patients at high risk of obstructive sleep apnea.
- Before major elective surgery, these patients should be referred to sleep medicine for polysomnography and PAP titration.
- Future research should focus on the perioperative strategies of screening, monitoring, and treatment of OHS and associated complications.

INTRODUCTION

Obesity is a global health concern. One of the complications associated with morbid obesity is obesity hypoventilation syndrome (OHS). OHS is defined by the triad of obesity (body mass index [BMI] $\geq$30 kg/m^2), daytime hypoventilation with hypercapnia (partial pressure of arterial carbon dioxide [Paco$_2$] $\geq$45 mm Hg at sea level), and hypoxemia (partial pressure of arterial oxygen [Pao$_2$] less than 70 mm Hg at sea level), and sleep-disordered breathing.[1] OHS is diagnosed after excluding other known causes of hypoventilation, such as severe obstructive or restrictive parenchymal lung disease, kyphoscoliosis, severe hypothyroidism, neuromuscular disease, and congenital central hypoventilation syndrome. In 90% of cases of OHS, the sleep-disordered breathing present is obstructive sleep apnea (OSA).[2] The prevalence of OHS in the general adult population is estimated to be 0.15% to 0.3%.[2] In patients undergoing bariatric surgery, approximately 8% present with OHS.[3]

Patients with OHS have a higher burden of comorbidities and increased risk for perioperative morbidity and mortality.[4–6] Therefore, a thorough plan of evaluation and management is essential for patients with OHS who undergo surgery. Currently, information on the perioperative management of OHS is extremely limited in the literature. As the prevalence of OHS is likely to increase as a result of the current global obesity epidemic, it is crucial for physicians to recognize and manage patients with this syndrome. This review examines the current data on OHS and discusses its optimal perioperative management.

[a] Department of Anesthesiology, Toronto Western Hospital, University Health Network, University of Toronto, Bathurst Street, Toronto, Ontario M5T2S8, Canada; [b] Section of Pulmonary and Critical Care Medicine, Department of Medicine, Sleep Disorders Center, University of Chicago Pritzker School of Medicine, Maryland Avenues, Chicago, IL 60637, USA
* Corresponding author. Department of Anesthesia, Room 405, 2McL, 399 Bathurst Street, Toronto, Ontario, Canada M5T 2S8.
E-mail address: frances.chung@uhn.on.ca

Sleep Med Clin 8 (2013) 135–147
http://dx.doi.org/10.1016/j.jsmc.2012.11.006
1556-407X/13/$ – see front matter © 2013 Elsevier Inc. All rights reserved.

PATHOPHYSIOLOGY

Daytime hypercapnia is a distinguishing feature in OHS and is entirely due to hypoventilation; a short course of noninvasive positive airway pressure (PAP) therapy (<2 weeks) improves hypercapnia without any significant changes in body weight, carbon dioxide (CO_2) production, or dead space volume.[7] There are currently 3 main hypotheses regarding the development of OHS: obesity-induced impairment in respiratory mechanics, leptin resistance, and impaired compensation for acute hypercapnia in OSA.[2,8]

Obesity-Induced Impairment in Respiratory Mechanics

Obesity induces hypoventilation by increasing the mechanical load on the respiratory system, resulting in fatigue and weakness of the respiratory muscles.[9–11] In several studies, patients with OHS were shown to have higher BMI than eucapnic obese individuals.[12–15] However, because less than one third of morbidly obese individuals develop hypercapnia, other mechanisms may contribute to hypoventilation.[14–16]

Leptin Resistance

Leptin is a protein secreted specifically by adipocytes to regulate appetite and energy expenditure.[17–19] Leptin crosses the blood-brain barrier and exerts its effect by binding to leptin receptors in various areas of the brain.[18] In obese individuals, a higher level of leptin is found to be associated with an increase in ventilation to compensate for the increased CO_2 production by excess body mass.[17,20,21] Patients with OHS have an even higher serum leptin level than eucapnic individuals matched for BMI.[22,23] Although the precise relationship between leptin and OHS remains to be determined, it is speculated that leptin resistance may lead to central hypoventilation in OHS.

Impaired Compensation of Acute Hypercapnia in OSA

Hypoventilation during sleep secondary to obstructive apneas and hypopneas results in transient episodes of acute hypercapnia and serum bicarbonate (HCO_3^-) retention. Eucapnic patients with OSA present several compensatory mechanisms to maintain acid-base homeostasis. During sleep, they hyperventilate between periods of apnea.[24] In addition, during wakefulness in daytime, acute hypercapnia is corrected and the excess HCO_3^- is excreted. On the other hand, patients with OHS have a reduced duration of ventilation between periods of apnea while sleeping.[25] The resulting acute hypercapnia persists during wakefulness and HCO_3^- retention occurs, causing gradual adaptation by chemoreceptors and further blunting of ventilatory CO_2 responsiveness. In a computer model, when both CO_2 response and the rate of renal HCO_3^- excretion was abnormally low, an increase in awake Pa_{CO_2} and HCO_3^- developed over multiple days.[26]

DISTINGUISHING CLINICAL FEATURES

Compared with eucapnic obese individuals with and without OSA, patients with OHS demonstrate more severe upper airway obstruction, restrictive pulmonary physiology, blunted central respiratory drive, and increased incidence of pulmonary hypertension. Patients with OHS display increased upper airway resistance in both the sitting and supine position in comparison with obese individuals with eucapnia.[27] In perioperative settings, patients with OHS are at increased risk of life-threatening apneic events because sedatives and narcotics increase the collapsibility of the upper airway and attenuate respiratory drive.[28,29]

Spirometric values from morbidly obese patients typically reveal a restrictive pattern with a reduction in forced expiratory volume in the first second (FEV_1) and forced vital capacity (FVC) but normal FEV_1/FVC ratio. This restrictive pulmonary physiology is further impaired in OHS.[3] Chest wall compliance is reduced and respiratory resistance is increased, likely secondary to the reduction in functional residual capacity and expiratory reserve volume. As a result, the work of breathing in OHS patients is twice that of obese eucapnic individuals[30,31] and increases further when these patients are positioned supine from sitting as a result of the cephaled shift of abdominal contents.[30,32]

In contrast to obese eucapnic individuals who possess a substantially increased central respiratory drive,[32] patients with OHS have a blunted central respiratory drive to both hypercapnia and hypoxia. They do not hyperventilate to the same extent as obese eucapnic individuals when forced to rebreathe CO_2[33–35] or breathe a hypoxic gas mixture.[35]

The prevalence of pulmonary hypertension in patients with OHS is high, ranging from 30% to 88%.[4,36–38] Seventy-seven percent of patients with OHS with respiratory failure in the intensive care unit have moderate to severe pulmonary hypertension (pulmonary systolic pressure >45 mm Hg).[37] The cause of pulmonary hypertension is likely secondary to chronic alveolar hypoxia and hypercapnia. In morbidly obese patients, left-heart failure is not uncommon and may increase pulmonary arterial pressure.[39]

MORBIDITY AND MORTALITY

Obesity and OSA are associated with a spectrum of comorbidities such as coronary artery disease, heart failure, stroke, and metabolic syndrome, which result in increased morbidity and mortality.[40–44] Furthermore, patients with OSA are at increased risk of developing postoperative complications including arrhythmias and hypoxemia.[45–47] An increased risk of transfer to the intensive care unit and increased length of hospital stay were also observed among patients with OSA who underwent noncardiac surgery.[46]

Several studies have shown that patients with OHS may experience higher morbidity and mortality than patients who are similarly obese and have OSA. Compared with obese individuals with eucapnia, patients with OHS were more likely to develop heart failure (odds ratio [OR] 9, 95% confidence interval [CI] 2.3–35), angina pectoris (OR 9, 95% CI 1.4–57.1), and cor pulmonale (OR 9, 95% CI 1.4–57.1).[4] They also received higher rates of long-term care at discharge (19% vs 2%, $P = .01$), and invasive mechanical ventilation (6% vs 0%, $P = .01$).[48]

Hospitalized patients with untreated OHS had a high mortality rate of 46% during a 50-month follow-up period after discharge.[49] In addition, their mortality rate is higher compared with obese eucapnic patients after hospital discharge at 18 months (23% vs 9%).[48] In patients undergoing open bariatric surgery, those with either OHS or OSA suffered a surgical mortality rate of 4%, significantly higher than those without the disease (0.2%, $P<.01$).[50] In patients with OHS with additional risk factors (previous history of venous thromboembolism, BMI $\geq$50 kg/m^2, male sex, hypertension and age $\geq$45 years) undergoing bariatric surgery, mortality ranges between 2% and 8%.[5,6,51]

In summary, patients with OHS experience higher morbidity and mortality than those with eucapnia who are obese. Previous history of venous thromboembolism, morbid obesity, male sex, hypertension, increasing age, and noncompliance with PAP treatment may further increase mortality risk. The surgical mortality rate in high-risk patients with OHS undergoing bariatric surgery is between 2% and 8%.

TREATMENT

Therapeutic interventions for OHS include 4 main components: PAP therapy, supplemental oxygen, bariatric surgery, and pharmacologic respiratory stimulants.

PAP Therapy

The 2 main forms of PAP therapy currently being used are continuous positive airway pressure (CPAP) and bilevel PAP. The overall short-term and long-term benefits were summarized in a recent systematic review.[3]

Short-term benefits of PAP include an improvement in gas exchange and sleep-disordered breathing. A short course ($\leq$3 weeks) of PAP results in a significant decrease in $Paco_2$ and an increase in Pao_2.[49,52–54] Furthermore, sleep study parameters, including the apnea-hypopnea index (AHI) and oxygen saturation during sleep, were reported to be significantly improved.[53–56]

Long-term benefits of PAP include an improvement in pulmonary function and central respiratory drive to CO_2. A course of PAP therapy for 24 to 48 weeks significantly increased FEV_1 and FVC.[57–59] The effect of PAP on central respiratory drive, measured as the change in minute ventilation per unit change in end-tidal CO_2, was reported in several studies to be favorable.[52,58,60]

PAP may also reduce mortality in OHS. Two retrospective studies have reported a mortality rate of 13% to 19% in patients with OHS on PAP throughout a mean period of 4 years.[57,61] Through indirect comparison, this mortality rate is lower than the 23% mortality rate reported in patients with untreated OHS at 18 months of follow-up.[48]

CPAP failure, defined by a residual AHI of 5 or more or a mean nocturnal pulse oximeter oxygen saturation (Spo_2) less than 90%, has been reported.[62] A recent prospective randomized study compared the long-term efficacy of bilevel PAP versus CPAP.[63] Two groups of 18 patients with OHS who underwent successful CPAP titration were randomized to either bilevel PAP or CPAP for 3 months. Both groups experienced a similar degree of improvement in $Paco_2$ and daytime sleepiness. Overall, bilevel PAP was not considerably superior to CPAP if CPAP titration was successful. However, if CPAP titration is unsuccessful, bilevel PAP should be strongly considered and treatment should be individualized to each patient.[2] Bilevel PAP should be instituted if the patient is intolerant of higher CPAP pressure (>15 cm H_2O) or if hypoxemia persists despite adequate resolution of obstructive respiratory events.[64] A therapeutic algorithm for CPAP titration in OHS patients is shown in **Fig. 1**.

A new treatment modality in patients with OHS is average volume-assured pressure-support (AVAPS) ventilation. This mode of PAP therapy

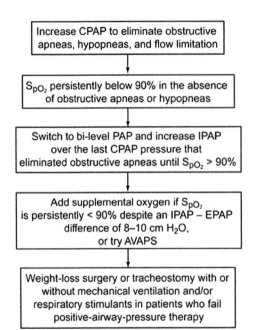

Fig. 1. Algorithm for continuous PAP titration in patients with OHS. AVAPS, average volume-assured pressure-support ventilation; CPAP, continuous positive airway pressure; EPAP, expiratory positive airway pressure; IPAP, inspiratory positive airway pressure.

ensures the delivery of a preset tidal volume during bilevel PAP mode. The expiratory tidal volume and leak are estimated based on pneumotacographic inspiratory and expiratory flows. Target tidal volume is typically set at 8 to 10 mL/kg of ideal body weight. The expiratory PAP is set to resolve upper airway obstruction and the inspiratory PAP is automatically adjusted to achieve the targeted tidal volume. This mode of PAP also provides a backup rate to alleviate central apneas that may emerge during PAP therapy.[65] In 1 clinical trial, AVAPS was more effective in improving nocturnal hypoventilation compared with CPAP and bilevel PAP in ST mode (activated backup rate). However, the degree of improvement in daytime $Paco_2$ did not reach statistical significance.[66] In a recent randomized controlled trial of patients with OHS, there was no significant difference between AVAPS and bilevel PAP ST mode in the degree of improvement in daytime and nocturnal gas exchange.[67] However, in this study, those randomized to bilevel PAP ST mode underwent aggressive bilevel PAP titration focusing on achieving adequate tidal volumes (mean inspiratory PAP of 23 cm H_2O and mean expiratory PAP of 10 cm H_2O), as recommended by the American Academy of Sleep Medicine guidelines on noninvasive ventilation.[68]

In summary, PAP therapy improves gas exchange, sleep-disordered breathing, lung function, and central respiratory drive to CO_2. Long-term PAP therapy also lowers the mortality rate in patients with OHS. Because of its noninvasiveness and effectiveness, PAP is the first-line therapy for OHS. CPAP is usually the initials modality of choice because of its relative simplicity and low cost. However, if CPAP titration fails, bilevel PAP or AVAPS should be applied. A need for a backup rate should be strongly considered because central apneas occur commonly in patients with OHS undergoing PAP therapy.

Supplemental Oxygen

Approximately 20% to 30% of patients with OHS continue to desaturate to Spo_2 less than 90% during sleep while on adequate CPAP or bilevel PAP settings, thereby requiring supplemental oxygen.[55] Administration of high-concentration supplemental oxygen without PAP therapy may induce hypoventilation and worsen hyercapnia.[69,70] In a recent study, a significant decrease in minute ventilation, resulting in an increase in transcutaneous CO_2 tension by 5 mm Hg, was found in patients with OHS while breathing 100% oxygen compared with those breathing room air.[71] Therefore, clinicians should administer the lowest concentration of oxygen to patients with OHS to avoid worsening of hypercapnia while maintaining optimized oxygenation, particularly in patients with OHS experiencing an exacerbation or recovering from sedatives/narcotics or general anesthesia.[72]

Bariatric Surgery

Bariatric surgery is a mainstay treatment of obesity, especially for morbidly obese patients in whom more conservative approaches have failed or who have developed comorbidities. Bariatric surgery improves gas exchange and lung function in OHS. At 1 year after surgery, Pao_2, $Paco_2$, FEV_1, and FVC all improved significantly.[50,73] To better understand the effect of surgical weight loss on OSA, Greenburg and colleagues[74] performed a meta-analysis of 12 studies including a total of 342 patients in whom polysomnography before and after maximum weight loss were available. They found that bariatric surgery led to significant weight loss with a mean reduction in BMI from 55.3 kg/m^2 to 37.7 kg/m^2. This robust weight loss was accompanied by a reduction in the AHI from baseline values of 55 events/h (95% CI 49–60) to 16 events/h (95% CI 13–19). However, many of these patients (62%) had persistent OSA of moderate severity (AHI $\geq$15 events/h). Thus, although improvements should be anticipated, OSA does not resolve in all patients after surgically achieved weight loss. CPAP therapy could still benefit patients with residual OSA after maximum weight loss. Similarly, 14% of patients with OHS still require PAP therapy after weight loss.[73] Therefore, patients with OHS should undergo reevaluation after bariatric surgery before discontinuing PAP therapy. As patients age and/or regain some weight over the years, the severity of OSA can increase.

Bariatric surgery is associated with significant risk. The overall perioperative mortality ranges between 0.5% and 1.5%.[75,76] The presence of OSA and extreme preoperative weight are independent risk factors associated with perioperative death and adverse events including venous thromboembolism, surgical reintervention, and prolonged hospital stay.[76,77] Ideally, PAP should be initiated in all patients with OHS and bariatric surgery should be considered as a second-line intervention.

Pharmacotherapy

Medications that increase respiratory drive have been investigated for the treatment of OHS. Limited evidence is available for 2 respiratory stimulants: medroxyprogesterone acetate and acetazolamide.

Medroxyprogesterone acetate stimulates respiration at the hypothalamic level.[78] Its role in OHS is uncertain. An early study reported an increase in Pao_2 and a decrease in $Paco_2$ in patients with OHS treated with medroxyprogesterone acetate.[79] However, a later study did not demonstrate the same benefits.[7] Because medroxyprogesterone acetate increases the risk of venous thromboembolism,[80] administration to patients with OHS whose mobility is limited may be unsafe.

Acetazolamide is a carbonic anhydrase inhibitor that increases minute ventilation by inducing metabolic acidosis through increased excretion of bicarbonate by the kidneys. Acetazolamide has been shown to improve AHI, increase Pao_2, and reduce $Paco_2$ in patients with OSA.[81,82] More recently, in mechanically ventilated patients with OHS, acetazolamide reduced plasma HCO_3^- and increased hypercapnic drive response.[83] Given the limited data on pharmacotherapy and because it is not widely used, the authors do not recommend it as a mainstay therapy but rather an adjunctive therapy in patients with OHS who remain hypercapnic despite adequate adherence to optimally titrated PAP therapy. Specifically, OHS patients requiring high doses of loop diuretics, which can lead to further HCO_3^- retention, may be ideal candidates for acetazolamide. Caution should be exercised in prescribing a respiratory stimulant in patients with ventilatory limitation because it can lead to exacerbation of acidosis and worsening of dyspnea. Acetazolamide should not be prescribed as a respiratory stimulant if a patient cannot normalize or near normalize their $Paco_2$ (or end-tidal CO_2) levels with 1 to 2 minutes of voluntary hyperventilation.

PREOPERATIVE ASSESSMENT OF PATIENTS WITH OHS

The 3 main challenges in OHS are OSA, obesity, and hypoventilation (hypercapnia and hypoxemia). For a patient with suspected OHS presenting for elective surgery, the preoperative assessment should begin with the history and physical examination directed to identify comorbidities in OHS, including coronary artery disease, congestive heart failure, pulmonary hypertension, and diabetes mellitus. A detailed examination of the airway and sites for venous access should also be performed. Further laboratory and imaging investigations should be focused on screening for sleep-disordered breathing and stratification of surgical risk. An algorithm for the perioperative evaluation and management of OHS is given in **Fig. 2**.

Preoperative Screening for OHS

OHS is often undiagnosed and may increase perioperative risk. Appropriate screening facilitates the identification of patients at risk for OHS, referral to sleep medicine for PAP therapy, and modifications in the surgical approach, anesthetic technique, and postoperative monitoring.

The definitive test for alveolar hypoventilation is an arterial blood gas performed on room air during wakefulness. As this is a relatively invasive procedure, several screening tools have been proposed. Mokhlesi and colleagues[15] suggested 3 clinical predictors of OHS: serum HCO_3^-, AHI, and lowest oxygen saturation during sleep. Increased serum HCO_3^- level caused by metabolic compensation of chronic respiratory acidosis is common in patients with OHS. In a cohort of obese patients with OSA referred to the sleep laboratory for suspicion of OSA, a serum HCO_3^- threshold of 27 mEq/L demonstrated a 92% sensitivity in predicting hypercapnia on arterial blood gas.[15] To complement the highly sensitive serum HCO_3^-, a highly specific (95%) AHI threshold of 100 was identified. A 2-step screening process was proposed, with serum HCO_3^- as the initial test to exclude patients without OHS and then AHI as

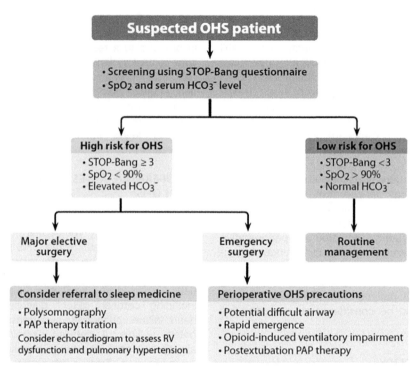

Fig. 2. Perioperative management of the patient suspected to have OHS. HCO_3^-, serum bicarbonate; RV, right ventricular. (*Adapted from* Mokhlesi B. Obesity hypoventilation syndrome: a state-of-the-art review. Respir Care 2010;55:1347–62; with permission.)

the second test to improve specificity. In addition, hypoxemia (Spo_2 <90%, corresponding to Pao_2 <60 mm Hg)[84] during wakefulness should lead clinicians to suspect OHS in patients with OSA. In a recent meta-analysis, patients with OSA and higher BMI, higher AHI, and more restrictive chest wall mechanics were more likely to develop OHS.[85] In these patients with OHS, the mean BMI, AHI, percent predicted FEV_1, and percent predicted FVC were 39 kg/m², 64 events/h, 71%, and 85%, respectively.

In summary, patients presenting with a high BMI and AHI should alert the physician to screen for OHS. The serum HCO_3^- is an easy initial screening test. If it is increased or hypoxemia by room air Spo_2 during wakefulness is present, a measurement of arterial blood gases, or end-tidal CO_2, is recommended. Once hypercapnia is confirmed, referral to sleep medicine and further testing, such as pulmonary function testing, chest imaging, measurement of thyroid-stimulating hormone level, and clinical assessment of neuromuscular strength, should be considered to rule out other important causes of hypoventilation.

Preoperative Screening for OSA

OSA screening in patients suspected to have OHS provides valuable information that may modify perioperative management. Approximately 90% of patients with OHS present with OSA, therefore a positive screen increases the index of suspicion for OHS. Multiple screening tools have been developed to evaluate patients at risk for OSA. The STOP-Bang questionnaire was used in preoperative patients.[86,87] It is a scoring model combining the STOP (snoring, tiredness, observed apneas, and increased blood pressure) questionnaire and Bang (BMI ≥35 kg/m², age >50 years, neck circumference >40 cm, and male gender). A systematic review has suggested using the STOP-Bang questionnaire in the surgical population due to its high methodological quality and easy-to-use features.[88] A positive screen (≥3 questions answered yes) is highly sensitive for moderate to severe OSA and is useful to exclude patients with the disease. On the other hand, patients with an STOP-Bang score of 5 to 8 have been shown to be at higher risk for moderate to severe OSA.[89] If these patients present with concurrent morbid obesity, they are at high risk for OHS and should be referred to sleep medicine for further evaluation.

In summary, the STOP-Bang questionnaire is a validated and easy tool to screen for OSA as part of the preoperative evaluation for patients with suspected OHS. A high STOP-Bang score with coexisting morbid obesity indicates an increased risk for OHS.

Preoperative Risk Stratification and Cardiopulmonary Testing

The Lee revised cardiac risk index represents a valuable tool to predict cardiac risk for elective major noncardiac surgery in the general population.[90] However, other risk factors specifically related to OHS, such as pulmonary hypertension and a history of venous thromboembolism, should be considered when evaluating perioperative risk. The Obesity Surgery Mortality Risk Score was developed for patients undergoing gastric bypass, and includes 5 risk factors: hypertension, BMI of 50 kg/m^2 or greater, male sex, age 45 years or more, and known risk factors for pulmonary embolism (OHS, previous thromboembolism, preoperative vena cava filter, pulmonary hypertension).[5,6,51] This risk score stratifies mortality risk into low (0 or 1 comorbidity), intermediate (2 to 3 comorbidities) and high (4 to 5 comorbidities). Mortality rates were 0.2%, 1.2%, and 2.4% for low-risk, intermediate-risk, and high-risk classes, respectively.[6] The most common causes of death were pulmonary embolism (30%), cardiac causes (27%), and gastrointestinal leak (21%).

A 12-lead electrocardiogram and chest radiograph should be obtained in patients suspected to have OHS to evaluate for coronary artery disease, congestive heart failure, and pulmonary hypertension. Indications for further cardiovascular testing should be based on the patient's cardiovascular risk factors and the invasiveness of surgery according to current American Heart Association guidelines.[90,91] The assessment of functional capacity is of particular importance in obese individuals because cardiorespiratory fitness levels and the postoperative complication rate are inversely related to BMI.[92,93] If these patients are undergoing major surgery and present with multiple cardiac risk factors, stress testing and transthoracic echocardiogram may be considered if management may be changed.[91]

Studies evaluating postoperative pulmonary complications have generally found no increased risk attributable to obesity.[94] However, patients with OSA were found to have a higher risk of pulmonary complications than patients without OSA in a recent retrospective study.[95] Routine pulmonary function tests may not translate into an effective risk prediction for postoperative pulmonary complications in noncardiothoracic surgery.[96] However, if coexisting chronic obstructive pulmonary disease is suspected in the patient with OHS, spirometry may be considered for diagnosis and subsequent optimization.

INTRAOPERATIVE MANAGEMENT OF OHS

Key considerations specific to the intraoperative management of OHS include airway management and emergence from anesthesia.

Airway Management

OSA is a risk factor for both difficult mask ventilation and tracheal intubation.[97] In addition, patients with severe OSA (AHI $\geq$40 events/h) showed a significantly higher prevalence of difficult intubation than patients with lower AHI.[98]

Obesity results in a threefold increase in difficulty with mask ventilation.[99] Whether obesity increases the difficulty of tracheal intubation is more controversial. A retrospective study of 18,500 surgical patients reported that obesity is a risk factor for difficult intubation.[100] However, other studies have not found an association between BMI and intubation difficulties.[101,102] More recently, Kheterpal and colleagues[103] identified 5 risk factors (limited mandibular protrusion, thick/obese neck anatomy, OSA, snoring, and BMI more than 30 kg/m^2) as independent predictors of difficult mask ventilation and intubation during anesthesia induction, which suggests that patients with OHS with limited mandibular protrusion are in the highest risk group for airway complications.

During induction of anesthesia, patients with OHS should be placed in the ramp position with tilting of the torso and head by 25°. This position has been shown to improve the glottic view during intubation and reduce atelectasis.[104] Preoxygenation for more than 3 minutes with a tightly fitted mask can increase apnea tolerance time. A variety of airway adjuncts and skilled anesthesiology assistance should be made available in advance. Awake fiber optic intubation should be considered in patients with OHS with markers for difficult mask ventilation and intubation. In situations during which a patient with OHS is hypoxemic, concomitant use of PAP during fiber optic intubation prevents further deterioration of oxygen saturation.[105,106] In addition, PAP splints the airway open and thus facilitates the visualization of anatomic landmarks.[107]

Emergence from Anesthesia

Patients with OHS are sensitive to the respiratory depressant effects of anesthetic agents due to the propensity for airway collapse, sleep deprivation, and blunting of physiologic response to hypercapnia and hypoxemia. A semi-upright or lateral position is recommended at the end of surgery for better oxygenation and airway maintenance.[108] Rapid emergence from anesthesia is preferred because tracheal extubation should be performed only after the patient is fully conscious. A systematic analysis of the literature comparing postoperative recovery after propofol, isoflurane, desflurane, and sevoflurane-based anesthesia in adults demonstrated that early recovery was faster in the desflurane and sevoflurane groups.[109] Another strategy to accelerate emergence is to decrease volatile anesthetic requirement and minimize washout time from fat/muscle by using other short-acting anesthetic adjuvants, such as remifentanil, or a combined general regional anesthetic.[29]

POSTOPERATIVE MANAGEMENT OF OHS

Key considerations specific to the postoperative management of OHS include monitoring for opioid-induced ventilatory impairment (OIVI) and prompt use of PAP therapy. The dual roles of postoperative PAP therapy are to prevent and treat respiratory failure secondary to sleep-disordered breathing.

OIVI

OIVI induces central respiratory depression, decreased level of consciousness, and upper airway obstruction, ultimately resulting in alveolar ventilation. The incidence of OIVI after major surgery varies with the different routes of opioid administration. The incidence of decreased respiratory rate was 0.8%, 1.2%, and 1.1% for intramuscular, intravenous patient-controlled analgesia, and epidural analgesia, respectively.[110] The incidence of oxygen desaturation was 37%, 11.5%, and 15.1% for intramuscular, intravenous patient-controlled analgesia, and epidural analgesia, respectively.[110] Patients with OHS could be at significant risk for OIVI because of their susceptibility to upper airway obstruction, depressed central respiratory drive, and impaired pulmonary mechanics. An opioid-sparing analgesic regimen, including local anesthetic–infused nerve block catheters and nonopioid adjuncts (acetaminophen, nonsteroidal antiinflammatory drugs), should be considered in these patients.

Improved postoperative monitoring is key in reducing the risk of OIVI. Patient-specific, anesthetic, and surgical factors determine the requirements for postoperative monitoring. Patients with OHS undergoing major surgery who require high doses of postoperative opioid should be monitored with continuous oximetry. Recurrent respiratory events in the postanesthesia care unit, including apnea for 10 seconds or more, bradypnea of less than 8 breaths/min, pain-sedation mismatch, or desaturations to less than 90%, can be used to identify patients at high risk of postoperative respiratory complications.[111] Recently, Macintyre and colleagues[112] proposed that sedation level is a more reliable sign of OIVI than respiratory rate because multiple reports suggest that OIVI is not always accompanied by a decrease in respiratory rate.[112–114] Thus, sedation scoring systems should be used postoperatively to recognize OIVI so that appropriate interventions are triggered. In patients with OHS requiring high doses of postoperative opioids, sedation monitoring should be considered every 1 to 2 hours for the first 24 hours.[115]

Postoperative PAP Therapy: Prevention of Respiratory Failure

There is limited evidence demonstrating a reduction in postoperative complications with PAP in patients with OHS. However, a case series of 14 patients with OSA suggested that the use of CPAP continuously for 24 to 48 hours after extubation may reduce the risk of postoperative complications.[116] In addition, PAP was found to decrease respiratory failure after extubation in severely obese patients admitted to the intensive care unit (absolute risk reduction of 16%).[117] Subgroup analysis of patients with hypercapnia showed reduced hospital mortality in the PAP group compared with the control group. Other potential benefits of postoperative PAP include reduced hemodynamic fluctuations and arrhythmia related to hypoxemia.

In summary, patients with OHS who were previously on PAP should resume therapy as soon as possible postoperatively. In patients suspected to have OHS experiencing postoperative ventilatory impairment, PAP should be considered. Based on the available literature, patients with OHS typically require an inspiratory PAP and the expiratory PAP of 16 to 22 cm H_2O and 9 to 10 cm H_2O, respectively, to achieve adequate resolution of upper airway obstruction and to improve ventilation. Bilevel PAP can be empirically set at these pressures in patients suspected of having OHS.

Postoperative PAP Therapy: Treatment of Respiratory Failure

Although the incidence of postoperative respiratory failure in patients with OHS is unknown, these patients are particularly susceptible to cardiopulmonary complications secondary to increased respiratory load, blunted central drive, pulmonary hypertension, and impaired ventricular function. In the postoperative period, these patients may decompensate acutely due to multiple factors, including sedation, sleep deprivation, and deconditioning.[118] Of concern, misdiagnosis is common if the physician is not aware of the potential for sleep-disordered breathing causing acute cardiopulmonary failure.[37,118] It was reported that 77% of patients with OHS admitted to the intensive care unit for hypercapnic respiratory failure were erroneously diagnosed and treated for chronic obstructive pulmonary disease/asthma.[37]

Four presentations of acute cardiopulmonary failure may be encountered postoperatively: hypercapnic respiratory failure, acute congestive heart failure, acute cor pulmonale, and sudden death, an extreme manifestation. The mechanisms leading to the development of such complications were described by Carr and colleagues[118] in detail. A high index of suspicion and early initiation of PAP therapy are key in managing patients with suspected OHS who develop respiratory failure postoperatively. Adjunctive interventions include judicious sedation/analgesia, minimal sleep disruption at night, and close follow-up with a sleep specialist.

SUMMARY

OHS is an important disease entity that requires the anesthesiologist's thorough understanding. The prevalence of OHS is estimated to be 0.15% to 0.3% in the general population and 8% in patients undergoing bariatric surgery.[2,3] Patients with OHS present with severe upper airway obstruction, restrictive pulmonary physiology, blunted central respiratory drive, and pulmonary hypertension. The primary therapy for OHS is PAP.

Perioperative management begins with a high index of suspicion for OHS in the morbidly obese patient. Screening questionnaires such as the validated STOP-Bang questionnaire can identify patients at high risk of OSA. This screening tool can be further complemented by the presence of low Spo_2, increased end-tidal CO_2 or $Paco_2$, and serum HCO_3^- level to identify patients at high risk of OHS. Before major elective surgery, these patients should be referred to sleep medicine for polysomnography and PAP titration. An echocardiogram should be considered to assess right ventricular function and pulmonary hypertension. Perioperative precautions for OHS include prudent airway management, rapid emergence, monitoring for ventilatory impairment, and early resumption of PAP therapy. Future research should focus on the perioperative strategies of screening, monitoring, and treatment of OHS and associated complications.

REFERENCES

1. Olson A, Zwillich C. The obesity hypoventilation syndrome. Am J Med 2005;118:948–56.
2. Mokhlesi B. Obesity hypoventilation syndrome: a state-of-the-art review. Respir Care 2010;55: 1347–62.
3. Chau E, Lam D, Wong J, et al. Obesity hypoventilation syndrome: a review of epidemiology, pathophysiology, and perioperative considerations. Anesthesiology 2012;117:188–205.
4. Berg G, Delaive K, Manfreda J, et al. The use of health-care resources in obesity-hypoventilation syndrome. Chest 2001;120:377–83.
5. DeMaria E, Portenier D, Wolfe L. Obesity surgery mortality risk score: proposal for a clinically useful score to predict mortality risk in patients undergoing gastric bypass. Surg Obes Relat Dis 2007; 3:134–40.
6. DeMaria E, Murr M, Byrne TK, et al. Validation of the obesity surgery mortality risk score in a multi-center study proves it stratifies mortality risk in patients undergoing gastric bypass for morbid obesity. Ann Surg 2007;246:578–82.
7. Rapoport DM, Garay SM, Epstein H, et al. Hypercapnia in the obstructive sleep apnea syndrome. A reevaluation of the "Pickwickian syndrome". Chest 1986;89:627–35.
8. Piper AJ, Grunstein RR. Obesity hypoventilation syndrome: mechanisms and management. Am J Respir Crit Care Med 2011;183:292–8.
9. Aldrich T, Arora NS, Rochester DF. The influence of airway obstruction and respiratory muscle strength on maximal voluntary ventilation. Am Rev Respir Dis 1982;126:195–9.
10. Ladosky W, Botelho MA, Albuquerque JP Jr. Chest mechanics in morbidly obese non-hypoventilated patients. Respir Med 2001;95:281–6.
11. Lavietes M, Clifford E, Silverstein D, et al. Relationship of static respiratory muscle pressure and maximum ventilatory ventilation. Respiration 1979; 38:121–6.
12. Akashiba T, Akahoshi T, Kawahara S, et al. Clinical characteristics of obesity-hypoventilation syndrome in Japan: a multi-center study. Intern Med 2006;45: 1121–5.
13. Kawata N, Tatsumi K, Terada J, et al. Daytime hypercapnia in obstructive sleep apnea syndrome. Chest 2007;132:1832–8.
14. Laaban J, Chailleux E. Daytime hypercapnia in adult patients with obstructive sleep apnea syndrome in France, before initiating nocturnal

nasal continuous positive airway pressure therapy. Chest 2005;127:710–5.

15. Mokhlesi B, Tulaimat A, Faibussowitsch I, et al. Obesity hypoventilation syndrome: prevalence and predictors in patients with obstructive sleep apnea. Sleep Breath 2007;11:117–24.

16. Javaheri S, Colangelo G, Lacey W, et al. Chronic hypercapnia in obstructive sleep apnea-hypopnea syndrome. Sleep 1994;17:416–23.

17. Considine R, Sinha MK, Heiman ML, et al. Serum immunoreactive-leptin concentrations in normal-weight and obese humans. N Engl J Med 1996; 334:292–5.

18. Kalra S. Central leptin insufficiency syndrome: an interactive etiology for obesity, metabolic and neural diseases and for designing new therapeutic interventions. Peptides 2008;29:127–38.

19. Tankersley C, O'Donnell C, Daood MJ, et al. Leptin attenuates respiratory complications associated with the obese phenotype. J Appl Physiol 1998; 85:2261–9.

20. Gilbert R, Sipple JH, Auchincloss JH Jr. Respiratory control and work of breathing in obese subjects. J Appl Physiol 1961;16:21–6.

21. Kress J, Pohlman AS, Alverdy J, et al. The impact of morbid obesity on oxygen cost of breathing (VO2(RESP)) at rest. Am J Respir Crit Care Med 1999;160:883–6.

22. Phipps P, Starritt E, Caterson I, et al. Association of serum leptin with hypoventilation in human obesity. Thorax 2002;57:75–6.

23. Shimura R, Tatsumi K, Nakamura A, et al. Fat accumulation, leptin, and hypercapnia in obstructive sleep apnea-hypopnea syndrome. Chest 2005; 127:543–9.

24. Berger KI, Goldring RM, Rapoport DM. Obesity hypoventilation syndrome. Semin Respir Crit Care Med 2009;30:253–61.

25. Ayappa I, Berger KI, Norman RG, et al. Hypercapnia and ventilatory periodicity in obstructive sleep apnea syndrome. Am J Respir Crit Care Med 2002;166:1112–5.

26. Norman R, Goldring RM, Clain JM, et al. Transition from acute to chronic hypercapnia in patients with periodic breathing: predictions from a computer model. J Appl Physiol 2006;100: 1733–41.

27. Lin C, Wu KM, Chou CS, et al. Oral airway resistance during wakefulness in eucapnic and hypercapnic sleep apnea syndrome. Respir Physiol Neurobiol 2004;139:215–24.

28. Adesanya A, Lee W, Greilich NB, et al. Perioperative management of obstructive sleep apnea. Chest 2010;138:1489–98.

29. Seet E, Chung F. Management of sleep apnea in adults - functional algorithms for the perioperative period. Can J Anaesth 2010;57:849–64.

30. Lee M, Lin CC, Shen SY, et al. Work of breathing in eucapnic and hypercapnic sleep apnea syndrome. Respiration 2009;77:146–53.

31. Sharp J, Henry JP, Sweany SK, et al. The total work of breathing in normal and obese men. J Clin Invest 1964;43:728–39.

32. Steier J, Jolley CJ, Seymour J, et al. Neural respiratory drive in obesity. Thorax 2009;64:719–25.

33. Lopata M, Onal E. Mass loading, sleep apnea, and the pathogenesis of obesity hypoventilation. Am Rev Respir Dis 1982;126:640–5.

34. Sampson M, Grassino K. Neuromechanical properties in obese patients during carbon dioxide rebreathing. Am J Med 1983;75:81–90.

35. Zwillich CW, Sutton FD, Pierson DJ, et al. Decreased hypoxic ventilatory drive in the obesity-hypoventilation syndrome. Am J Med 1975;59:343–8.

36. Kessler R, Chaouat A, Schinkewitch P, et al. The obesity-hypoventilation syndrome revisited: a prospective study of 34 consecutive cases. Chest 2001;120:369–76.

37. Marik P, Desai H. Characteristics of patients with the "malignant obesity hypoventilation syndrome" admitted to an ICU. J Intensive Care Med 2012. http://dx.doi.org/10.1177/0885066612444261.

38. Sugerman HJ, Baron PL, Fairman RP, et al. Hemodynamic dysfunction in obesity hypoventilation syndrome and the effects of treatment with surgically induced weight loss. Ann Surg 1988;207: 604–13.

39. de Divitiis O, Fazio S, Petitto M, et al. Obesity and cardiac function. Circulation 1981;64:477–82.

40. Arzt M, Young T, Finn L, et al. Association of sleep-disordered breathing and the occurrence of stroke. Am J Respir Crit Care Med 2005;172: 1447–51.

41. Coughlin S, Mawdsley L, Mugarza JA, et al. Obstructive sleep apnoea is independently associated with an increased prevalence of metabolic syndrome. Eur Heart J 2004;25:735–41.

42. Peker Y, Kraiczi H, Hedner J, et al. An independent association between obstructive sleep apnoea and coronary artery disease. Eur Respir J 1999;14: 179–84.

43. Sin D, Fitzgerald F, Parker JD, et al. Relationship of systolic BP to obstructive sleep apnea in patients with heart failure. Chest 2003;123:1536–43.

44. Tung A. Anaesthetic considerations with the metabolic syndrome. Br J Anaesth 2010;105:24–33.

45. Chung S, Yuan H, Chung F. A systemic review of obstructive sleep apnea and its implications for anesthesiologists. Anesth Analg 2008;107: 1543–63.

46. Kaw R, Pasupuleti V, Walker E, et al. Postoperative complications in patients with obstructive sleep apnea. Chest 2011;141:436–41.

47. Liao P, Yegneswaran B, Vairavanathan S, et al. Postoperative complications in patients with obstructive sleep apnea: a retrospective matched cohort study. Can J Anaesth 2009;56:819–28.

48. Nowbar S, Burkart KM, Gonzales R, et al. Obesity-associated hypoventilation in hospitalized patients: prevalence, effects, and outcome. Am J Med 2004; 116:1–7.

49. Perez de Llano LA, Golpe R, Ortiz Piquer M, et al. Short-term and long-term effects of nasal intermittent positive pressure ventilation in patients with obesity-hypoventilation syndrome. Chest 2005; 128:587–94.

50. Sugerman HJ, Fairman RP, Sood RK, et al. Long-term effects of gastric surgery for treating respiratory insufficiency of obesity. Am J Clin Nutr 1992; 55:597S–601S.

51. Efthimiou E, Sampalis J, Christou N. Validation of obesity surgery mortality risk score in patients undergoing gastric bypass in a Canadian center. Surg Obes Relat Dis 2009;5:643–7.

52. Lin C. Effect of nasal CPAP on ventilatory drive in normocapnic and hypercapnic patients with obstructive sleep apnoea syndrome. Eur Respir J 1994;7:2005–10.

53. Perez de Llano LA, Golpe R, Piquer MO, et al. Clinical heterogeneity among patients with obesity hypoventilation syndrome: therapeutic implications. Respiration 2008;75:34–9.

54. Piper AJ, Sullivan CE. Effects of short-term NIPPV in the treatment of patients with severe obstructive sleep apnea and hypercapnia. Chest 1994;105:434–40.

55. Banerjee D, Yee BJ, Piper AJ, et al. Obesity hypoventilation syndrome: hypoxemia during continuous positive airway pressure. Chest 2007;131: 1678–84.

56. Chouri-Pontarollo N, Borel JC, Tamisier R, et al. Impaired objective daytime vigilance in obesity-hypoventilation syndrome: impact of noninvasive ventilation. Chest 2007;131:148–55.

57. Budweiser S, Riedl SG, Jörres RA, et al. Mortality and prognostic factors in patients with obesity-hypoventilation syndrome undergoing noninvasive ventilation. J Intern Med 2007;261:375–83.

58. de Lucas-Ramos P, de Miguel-Díez J, Santacruz-Siminiani A, et al. Benefits at 1 year of nocturnal intermittent positive pressure ventilation in patients with obesity-hypoventilation syndrome. Respir Med 2004;98:961–7.

59. Heinemann F, Budweiser S, Dobroschke J, et al. Non-invasive positive pressure ventilation improves lung volumes in the obesity hypoventilation syndrome. Respir Med 2007;101:1229–35.

60. Han F, Chen E, Wei H, et al. Treatment effects on carbon dioxide retention in patients with obstructive sleep apnea-hypopnea syndrome. Chest 2001;119:1814–9.

61. Priou P, Hamel JF, Person C, et al. Long-term outcome of noninvasive positive pressure ventilation for obesity hypoventilation syndrome. Chest 2010;138:84–90.

62. Schafer H, Ewig S, Hasper E, et al. Failure of CPAP therapy in obstructive sleep apnoea syndrome: predictive factors and treatment with bilevel-positive airway pressure. Respir Med 1998;92: 208–15.

63. Piper A, Wang D, Yee BJ, et al. Randomised trial of CPAP versus bilevel support in the treatment of obesity hypoventilation syndrome without severe nocturnal desaturation. Thorax 2008;63: 395–401.

64. American Academy of Sleep Medicine. Clinical guidelines for the manual titration of positive airway pressure in patients with obstructive sleep apnea. J Clin Sleep Med 2008;4:157–71.

65. Contal O, Adler D, Borel JC, et al. Impact of different back-up respiratory rates on the efficacy of non-invasive positive pressure ventilation in obesity hypoventilation syndrome: a randomized trial. Chest 2012. http://dx.doi.org/10.1378/chest.11-2848.

66. Storre JH, Seuthe B, Fiechter R, et al. Average volume-assured pressure support in obesity hypoventilation: a randomized crossover trial. Chest 2006;130:815–21.

67. Murphy P, Davidson C, Hind MD, et al. Volume targeted versus pressure support non-invasive ventilation in patients with super obesity and chronic respiratory failure: a randomised controlled trial. Thorax 2012;67:727–34.

68. Berry RB, Chediak A, Brown LK, et al. Best clinical practices for the sleep center adjustment of noninvasive positive pressure ventilation (NPPV) in stable chronic alveolar hypoventilation syndromes. J Clin Sleep Med 2010;6:491–509.

69. Aubier M, Murciano D, Milic-Emili J, et al. Effects of the administration of O2 on ventilation and blood gases in patients with chronic obstructive pulmonary disease during acute respiratory failure. Am Rev Respir Dis 1980;122:747–54.

70. Robinson T, Freiberg DB, Regnis JA, et al. The role of hypoventilation and ventilation-perfusion redistribution in oxygen-induced hypercapnia during acute exacerbations of chronic obstructive pulmonary disease. Am J Respir Crit Care Med 2000;161: 1524–9.

71. Wijesinghe M, Williams M, Perrin K, et al. The effect of supplemental oxygen on hypercapnia in subjects with obesity-associated hypoventilation: a randomized, crossover, clinical study. Chest 2011;139:1018–24.

72. Mokhlesi B, Tulaimat A, Parthasarathy S. Oxygen for obesity hypoventilation syndrome: a double-edged sword? Chest 2011;139:975–7.

73. Marti-Valeri C, Sabate A, Masdevall C, et al. Improvement of associated respiratory problems in morbidly obese patients after open Roux-en-Y gastric bypass. Obes Surg 2007;17:1102–10.

74. Greenburg D, Lettieri CJ, Eliasson AH. Effects of surgical weight loss on measures of obstructive sleep apnea: a meta-analysis. Am J Med 2009; 122:535–42.

75. Buchwald H, Avidor Y, Braunwald E, et al. Bariatric surgery: a systematic review and meta-analysis. JAMA 2004;292:1724–37.

76. Fernandez AJ, Demaria EJ, Tichansky DS, et al. Multivariate analysis of risk factors for death following gastric bypass for treatment of morbid obesity. Ann Surg 2004;239:698–702.

77. Flum D, Belle SH, King WC, et al. Perioperative safety in the longitudinal assessment of bariatric surgery. N Engl J Med 2009;361:445–54.

78. Bayliss D, Millhorn DE. Central neural mechanisms of progesterone action: application to the respiratory system. J Appl Physiol 1992;73:393–404.

79. Sutton FJ, Zwillich CW, Creagh CE, et al. Progesterone for outpatient treatment of Pickwickian syndrome. Ann Intern Med 1975;83:476–9.

80. Poulter N, Chang CL, Farley TM, et al. Risk of cardiovascular diseases associated with oral progestagen preparations with therapeutic indications [letter]. Lancet 1999;354:1610.

81. Tojima H, Kunitomo F, Kimura H, et al. Effects of acetazolamide in patients with the sleep apnoea syndrome. Thorax 1988;43:113–9.

82. Whyte K, Gould GA, Airlie MA, et al. Role of protriptyline and acetazolamide in the sleep apnea/hypopnea syndrome. Sleep 1988;11:463–72.

83. Raurich J, Rialp G, Ibáñez J, et al. Hypercapnic respiratory failure in obesity-hypoventilation syndrome: CO2 response and acetazolamide treatment effects. Respir Care 2010;55:1442–8.

84. Pedersen T, Møller AM, Pedersen BD. Pulse oximetry for perioperative monitoring: systematic review of randomized, controlled trials. Anesth Analg 2003;96:426–31.

85. Kaw R, Hernandez AV, Walker E, et al. Determinants of hypercapnia in obese patients with obstructive sleep apnea: a systematic review and meta-analysis of cohort studies. Chest 2009;136:787–96.

86. Chung F, Yegneswaran B, Liao P, et al. STOP questionnaire: a tool to screen patients for obstructive sleep apnea. Anesthesiology 2008;108:812–21.

87. Chung F, Yegneswaran B, Liao P, et al. Validation of the Berlin questionnaire and American Society of Anesthesiologists checklist as screening tools for obstructive sleep apnea in surgical patients. Anesthesiology 2008;108:822–30.

88. Abrishami A, Khajehdehi A, Chung F. A systematic review of screening questionnaires for obstructive sleep apnea. Can J Anaesth 2010;57:423–38.

89. Chung F, Subramanyam R, Liao P, et al. High STOP-Bang score indicates a high probability of obstructive sleep apnoea. Br J Anaesth 2012;108: 768–75.

90. Lee T, Marcantonio ER, Mangione CM, et al. Derivation and prospective validation of a simple index for prediction of cardiac risk of major noncardiac surgery. Circulation 1999;100:1043–9.

91. Fleisher LA, Beckman JA, Brown KA, et al. ACC/AHA 2007 guidelines on perioperative cardiovascular evaluation and care for noncardiac surgery: a report of the American College of Cardiology/American Heart Association Task Force on Practice Guidelines (Writing Committee to Revise the 2002 Guidelines on Perioperative Cardiovascular Evaluation for Noncardiac Surgery): developed in collaboration with the American Society of Echocardiography, American Society of Nuclear Cardiology, Heart Rhythm Society, Society of Cardiovascular Anesthesiologists, Society for Cardiovascular Angiography and Interventions, Society for Vascular Medicine and Biology, and Society for Vascular Surgery. Circulation 2007;116: 418–99.

92. Gallagher M, Franklin BA, Ehrman JK, et al. Comparative impact of morbid obesity vs heart failure on cardiorespiratory fitness. Chest 2005; 127:2197–203.

93. McCullough P, Gallagher MJ, Dejong AT, et al. Cardiorespiratory fitness and short-term complications after bariatric surgery. Chest 2006;130:517–25.

94. Smetana G. Preoperative pulmonary evaluation. N Engl J Med 1999;340:937–44.

95. Memtsoudis S, Liu SS, Ma Y, et al. Perioperative pulmonary outcomes in patients with sleep apnea after noncardiac surgery. Anesth Analg 2011;112: 113–21.

96. Qaseem A, Snow V, Fitterman N, et al. Risk assessment for and strategies to reduce perioperative pulmonary complications for patients undergoing noncardiothoracic surgery: a guideline from the American College of Physicians. Ann Intern Med 2006;144:575–80.

97. Siyam M, Benhamou D. Difficult endotracheal intubation in patients with sleep apnea syndrome. Anesth Analg 2002;95:1098–102.

98. Kim J, Lee JJ. Preoperative predictors of difficult intubation in patients with obstructive sleep apnea syndrome. Can J Anaesth 2006;53:393–7.

99. Langeron O, Masso E, Huraux C, et al. Prediction of difficult mask ventilation. Anesthesiology 2000; 92:1229–36.

100. Rose D, Cohen MM. The airway: problems and predictions in 18,500 patients. Can J Anaesth 1994;41:372–83.

101. Brodsky J, Lemmens HJ, Brock-Utne JG, et al. Morbid obesity and tracheal intubation. Anesth Analg 2002;94:732–6.

102. Mashour G, Kheterpal S, Vanaharam V, et al. The extended Mallampati score and a diagnosis of diabetes mellitus are predictors of difficult laryngoscopy in the morbidly obese. Anesth Analg 2008; 107:1919–23.

103. Kheterpal S, Han R, Tremper KK, et al. Incidence and predictors of difficult and impossible mask ventilation. Anesthesiology 2006;105:885–91.

104. Cattano D, Melnikov V, Khalil Y, et al. An evaluation of the rapid airway management positioner in obese patients undergoing gastric bypass or laparoscopic gastric banding surgery. Obes Surg 2010;20:1436–41.

105. Murgu S, Pecson J, Colt HG. Bronchoscopy during noninvasive ventilation: indications and technique. Respir Care 2010;55:595–600.

106. Wong D, Wang J, Venkatraghavan L. Awake bronchoscopic intubation through an air-Q® with the application of BIPAP. Can J Anaesth 2012;59: 915–6.

107. Rothfleisch R, Davis LL, Kuebel DA, et al. Facilitation of fiberoptic nasotracheal intubation in a morbidly obese patient by simultaneous use of nasal CPAP. Chest 1994;106:287–8.

108. Gander S, Frascarolo P, Suter M, et al. Positive end-expiratory pressure during induction of general anesthesia increases duration of nonhypoxic apnea in morbidly obese patients. Anesth Analg 2005;100:580–4.

109. Gupta A, Stierer T, Zuckerman R, et al. Comparison of recovery profile after ambulatory anesthesia with propofol, isoflurane, sevoflurane and desflurane: a systematic review. Anesth Analg 2004;98:632–41.

110. Cashman J, Dolin SJ. Respiratory and haemodynamic effects of acute postoperative pain management: evidence from published data. Br J Anaesth 2004;93:212–23.

111. Gali B, Whalen FX, Schroeder DR, et al. Identification of patients at risk for postoperative respiratory complications using a preoperative obstructive sleep apnea screening tool and post-anesthesia care assessment. Anesthesiology 2009;110:869–77.

112. Macintyre P, Loadsman JA, Scott DA. Opioids, ventilation and acute pain management. Anaesth Intensive Care 2011;39:545–58.

113. Ready L, Oden R, Chadwick HS, et al. Development of an anesthesiology-based postoperative pain management service. Anesthesiology 1988; 68:100–6.

114. Vila HJ, Smith RA, Augustyniak MJ, et al. The efficacy and safety of pain management before and after implementation of hospital-wide pain management standards: is patient safety compromised by treatment based solely on numerical pain ratings? Anesth Analg 2005;101:474–80.

115. American Society of Anesthesiologists Task Force on Neuraxial Opioids, Horlocker TT, Burton AW, Connis RT, et al. Practice guidelines for the prevention, detection, and management of respiratory depression associated with neuraxial opioid administration. Anesthesiology 2009;110:218–30.

116. Rennotte M, Baele P, Aubert G, et al. Nasal continuous positive airway pressure in the perioperative management of patients with obstructive sleep apnea submitted to surgery. Chest 1995;107: 367–74.

117. El-Solh A, Aquilina A, Pineda L, et al. Noninvasive ventilation for prevention of post-extubation respiratory failure in obese patients. Eur Respir J 2006;28:588–95.

118. Carr G, Mokhlesi B, Gehlbach BK. Acute cardiopulmonary failure from sleep-disordered breathing. Chest 2012;141:798–808.

Evaluation of the Child with Sleep-Disordered Breathing Scheduled for Adenotonsillectomy

Karen A. Brown, MD

KEYWORDS

- Pediatrics • Obstructive sleep apnea syndrome • Oximetry
- Perioperative adverse respiratory events

KEY POINTS

- The primary treatment of pediatric obstructive sleep apnea syndrome (OSAS) is adenotonsillectomy, and the safety of ambulatory adenotonsillectomy programs is predicated on the admission of the child with severe OSAS.
- The challenge is to identify the child with severe OSAS in the preoperative period.
- Preoperative evaluation with a combination of sleep-disordered breathing questionnaires plus an assessment with nocturnal oximetry has several advantages.
- It aligns with the diagnostic approach recommended by sleep physicians.
- It provides a useful prediction of perioperative respiratory adverse events and the medical interventions required to manage them.

INTRODUCTION: THE NATURE OF THE PROBLEM

Sleep-disordered breathing (SDB) is a nonspecific term encompassing a continuum from habitual benign snoring to the obstructive sleep apnea syndrome (OSAS). The prevalence of parent-reported snoring in children is 7.5%,[1] The gold standard to diagnose the severity of SDB is polysomnography (PSG). Recorded during a sleep study, PSG measures indices of apnea (defined as >90% reduction in tidal volume), hypopnea (defined as >50% reduction in tidal volume), hypoxia (defined as a saturation <92%), and hypoventilation.[2] The apnea-hypopnea index (AHI) and respiratory disturbance index (RDI) are measures of both central and obstructive apnea and hypopnea. Both are expressed as the number of events per hour of sleep. The nadir saturation ($nSaO_2$) and cumulative times below saturation thresholds provide an assessment of hypoxia. Hypoventilation is assessed by the cumulative times above a threshold carbon dioxide (CO_2) level.[2,3] An elevated bicarbonate level on a blood gas drawn on awakening is also consistent with a diagnosis of OSAS.[4] The prevalence of test-positive OSAS is 1% to 4%.[2,5] Pediatric OSAS is therefore as prevalent as childhood asthma.

PATIENT HISTORY
Diagnostic Features of Sleep-Disordered Breathing in Children

A consensus statement for diagnostic criteria in pediatric OSAS has yet to be achieved. However, PSG findings in OSAS are often an AHI greater than 2 and $nSaO_2$ less than 92%. Dayyat and colleagues[2] proposed a classification of OSAS severity based on PSG measures of obstructive airway events, sleep disruption, hypoxia, and

Department of Pediatric Anesthesia, Montreal Children's Hospital, McGill University Health Centre, 2300 Tupper Street, Room C-1118, Montreal, Quebec H3H 1P3, Canada
E-mail address: karen.brown@mcgill.ca

Sleep Med Clin 8 (2013) 149–155
http://dx.doi.org/10.1016/j.jsmc.2012.11.010

hypoventilation (**Table 1**). SDB also includes habitual snoring, the upper airway resistance syndrome, and obstructive alveolar hypoventilation. The PSG findings in these entities are an AHI less than 2 and nadir SaO_2 greater than 92%. Obstructive alveolar hypoventilation is also accompanied by hypercarbia. As SDB has been linked to neurocognitive dysfunction, poor school performance, and metabolic derangements including childhood obesity and cardiovascular sequelae, and as therapeutic options vary, all nuances of SDB are of interest to sleep physicians.[1,2] The primary treatment of SDB is adenotonsillectomy (T&A), and it has long been recognized that a diagnosis of OSAS increases the risk for perioperative respiratory adverse events (PRAEs). Herein the agendas of sleep physicians and anesthesiologists diverge. Whereas sleep physicians consider an AHI score greater than 10 diagnostic of severe pediatric OSAS,[2] the American Academy of Pediatrics recommends a higher threshold (AHI >24) to exclude children with OSAS from ambulatory T&A programs.[6] The goal of anesthesiologists is to identify the child at risk for PRAEs and to implement risk-reduction strategies.

In the 1980s, ambulatory programs for T&A were developed in North America. From the onset the OSAS was an exclusion criterion for day surgery.[7] However, 3 decades ago SDB was the indication for T&A in only 20% of the caseload.[8] The diagnosis of OSAS was based on parent questioning, and admission of children with obstructive breathing symptoms was not a burden. In 2005, obstructive breathing represented 75% to 80% of the annual caseload of T&As.[8] Admission of all children with positive symptoms for SDB threatens to overburden North American health care systems.

Evaluation of the Child with SDB

In 1976 Guilleminault and colleagues[9] reported 8 snoring children with PSG evidence of severe OSAS and symptoms of daytime somnolence, morning headaches, poor school performance, behavioral disturbances, and new-onset enuresis. Over the subsequent 3 decades dozens of SDB questionnaires (SBD-Q) have been developed with the aim of diagnosing pediatric OSAS from clinical criteria alone. Loud snoring, parental reports of cyanosis and apnea during sleep, an impression that their child is struggling to breathe, and fearfulness while watching their child sleep are key questions.

The pitfalls of a diagnosis based on clinical criteria alone are well published. Many SBD-Qs are able to distinguish normal children from snoring children. Chervin and colleagues[10] compared results from PSG with responses from a 22-item SDB-Q, the Sleep-Related Breathing Disorder (SRBD), and reported correct classification of 85%. However, when applied to a population of snoring children, SDB-Qs are of limited value. Carroll and colleagues[11] compared the historical features in children with primary snoring (AHI <1) and OSAS (AHI ≥1). In the primary snoring group 83% of parents reported extremely loud snoring, 96% reported snoring most nights, and 50% were fearful of their child's breathing pattern during sleep. In the OSAS children, parents reported positive responses respectively 91%, 97%, and 90% of the time. Brietzke and colleagues[12] calculated the combined positive predictive value for OSAS from 10 different SDB-Qs. Overall, SDB-Qs agreed with PSG only 55% of the time, and clinical criteria tended to overdiagnose OSAS. Constantin and colleagues[13] reported that OSAS-18, an 18-item SDB-Q, missed 60% of children with OSAS severe enough to cause repetitive oxygen desaturation during sleep. Despite these limitations, the use of clinical criteria was endorsed by the American Society of Anesthesiologists.[3] In a preoperative assessment of more than 2000 children, parents reported snoring in 940 (46%).[14] The ratios between habitual snoring and

Table 1
Classification of OSAS severity proposed by Dayyat and colleagues

OSAS Severity	Obstructive Breathing OAHI (#/h)	Sleep Disruption RAI (#/h)	Hypoxia nSaO2 (%)	Hypoventilation T_{EtCO2} >50 mm Hg (%TST)
Mild	2–5	2–5	88–92	10–15
Moderate	5–10	5–8	80–88	15–20
Severe	>10	>8	<80	>20

Abbreviations: EtCO2, end-tidal CO_2; nSaO2, nadir saturation; OAHI, obstructive apnea-hypopnea index; RAI, respiratory arousal index; TST, total sleep time.

From Dayyat E, Kheirandish-Gozal L, Gozal D. Childhood obstructive sleep apnea: one or two distinct disease entities? Sleep Med Clin 2007;2:433–44; with permission.

OSAS in children range from 4:1 to 6:1.[15] It is likely, therefore, that the American Society of Anesthesiologists score results in an overdiagnosis of OSAS in children.

Medical complexity

Children with neurologic disorders, especially those associated with brainstem involvement, and children with inborn errors of metabolism may develop OSAS.[6,16] Numerous studies report a higher risk for PRAEs in the medically complex child.[17–21] The authors reported the adjusted odds ratio for any medical complexity was 2.4.[20] Biavati and colleagues[19] reported high odds ratios for specific medical conditions: seizure disorder = 5.2, cerebral palsy = 6.8, cardiac = 3.3, and prematurity = 1.9. McGowan and colleagues[21] also reported a higher risk in the former premature child.

Young age

Don and colleagues[22] evaluated 363 otherwise healthy children who had been referred for evaluation of SDB. There was a predilection for children younger than 3 years to have more severe OSAS (AHI >5, $nSaO_2$ <85%, and end-tidal CO_2 tension >54 mm Hg). In a surgical referral population of 334 children, 37% of young children (<5 years) demonstrated recurrent hypoxia during sleep, and for each 1-year decrease in age, the odds of having desaturation during sleep increased by 17%.[13]

Young age is also a risk factor for PRAEs following T&A. The adjusted odds ratio for PRAE for age younger than 3 years ranges from 2.5 to 3.5.[17–20,23] Two decades ago McColley and colleagues[18] estimated the probability of PRAEs for the combination of age younger than 3 years plus an AHI greater than 10 to be 60% to 82%.

Ethnicity is another risk factor for OSAS. In young African Americans, SDB is almost twice as prevalent as in young Caucasians.[24,25] Stepanski and colleagues[26] reported that African American children exhibit more profound desaturation with obstructive events than do Caucasian children. Boss and colleagues[27] also reported that African American ethnicity was associated with more profound desaturation indices and persistent SDB following T&A.

Perioperative adverse respiratory events

In a prospective study of more than 2000 pediatric anesthetics, Parnis and colleagues[14] reported that 22% of children experienced an adverse event, although their definition of adverse events included nonrespiratory complications such as vomiting. A history of snoring increased the probability of an adverse event from 22% to approximately 30%. Adverse respiratory events, which they defined as coughing, desaturation below 95%, and airway obstruction, each represented 4% of events during recovery. A diagnosis of OSAS increases the perioperative risk, such that 25% to 60% of children with OSAS will experience a PRAE following T&A.[4,17,18,20,28] The PRAEs may be delayed in onset, and major life-threatening events may occur during sleep.[28,29]

Consultants for the American Academy of Pediatrics recommend that children who exhibit an AHI greater than 24, and/or hypercapnia on the preoperative PSG, and/or saturation below 80% in the preoperative assessment or postoperative period be admitted and observed following T&A.[6] This recommendation is of limited value, as few children are assessed with PSG in the preoperative period. As a consequence, many advocate a 2-step assessment process combining an SDB-Q with an additional non-PSG test.

Tests in Addition to the SDB-Q

Physical examination

A positive SDB-Q plus a large neck circumference, hypertension, and/or obesity are strongly suggestive of OSAS in adult patients.[30] Children with OSAS may exhibit adenotonsillar hypertrophy, a long oval-shaped face with a small triangular chin, a high palate, a long soft palate, and retro position of the mandible.[31,32] Tonsillar size, however, correlates poorly with the severity of OSAS.[3] The presence of systemic hypertension in children should alert the clinician to the possibility of severe OSAS.[9] Yilmaz and colleagues[33] measured pulmonary artery pressures in 52 otherwise healthy children aged 7 years, randomly selected from a T&A list. A positive history for OSAS was reported in 59%. Elevated pulmonary artery pressures (>20 mm Hg) were recorded in 27 children, and mean pulmonary artery pressures decreased following T&A. However, pulmonary hypertension and ventricular hypertrophy are usually asymptomatic.

Response to general anesthesia

The additional test may be the child's response to anesthesia. A propensity for airway collapse in children with OSAS is unmasked during general anesthesia. During halothane anesthesia, Waters and colleagues,[34] comparing children with severe OSAS (AHI 30) with controls, reported a higher closing pressure of the pharynx, supporting the notion of a more collapsible upper airway in children with OSAS. Strauss and colleagues[35] reported a blunted response to hypercarbia in children with obstructive SDB. Waters and colleagues[34] compared ventilation during steady-state 1%

halothane anesthesia and reported a greater decrease in minute ventilation in children with severe OSAS. In addition, they reported a heightened respiratory sensitivity to a small dose of fentanyl (50 µg/kg), which resulted in apnea in 46% of children with severe OSAS. This heightened respiratory sensitivity to fentanyl is consistent with a heightened analgesic sensitivity to opioids in children with severe OSAS.[36,37]

The additional test may be the occurrence of respiratory complications in the immediate postoperative period. In an adult population, the combination of a positive SDB-Q plus the occurrence of recurrent respiratory events in the postanesthesia care unit was strongly predictive of subsequent respiratory complications.[30] Although the use of preoperative SBD-Qs plus the occurrence of postoperative respiratory events may be useful in inpatient populations, the approach is of limited value to ambulatory programs whereby the period of observation in the postoperative period may be brief. The challenge for ambulatory programs is to distinguish SDB from severe OSAS in the preoperative period. Indeed, a decade ago the American Academy of Pediatrics identified the development of a low-cost, high-sensitivity, and high-specificity screening method for OSAS as a research area of interest.[16]

SDB-Qs Plus Preoperative Oximetry

The authors have found the combination of SDB-Qs and preoperative evaluation with overnight oximetry helpful.[38–40] Children referred for evaluation of SDB are assessed initially with oximetry. Those with abnormal oximetry require no additional testing to establish the diagnosis of OSAS.[39] Brouillette and colleagues[38] determined the probability that an abnormal oximetry study would be associated with PSG evidence of OSAS (AHI >1). In a surgical referral population of otherwise healthy children with only adenotonsillar hypertrophy as the explanation for SDB, an abnormal oximetry trend graph had a likelihood ratio of 43 and the posttest probability of having OSAS was 99%. Nixon and colleagues[39] developed an OSAS severity score, the McGill Oximetry Score (MOS). The investigators defined an abnormal oximetry trend graph as one with 3 or more clusters of desaturation and an intercluster saturation returning to baseline. The clusters coincide with rapid eye movement sleep when skeletal hypotonia promotes collapse of the pharyngeal airway. Three levels of severity (MOS2, MOS3, and MOS4) were identified from the $nSaO_2$ in at least 3 clusters (<90%, <85%, and <80%, respectively). The $nSaO_2$ during sleep inversely correlated with the AHI such that MOS2 and MOS3 had an AHI greater than 10 and MOS4 had an AHI greater than 40.[39] Preoperative evaluation of children referred for SDB with the combination of SDB-Q plus a MOS aligns with recent recommendations by sleep physicians.[41] In addition, the MOS correlates with the OSAS severity scale proposed in **Table 1**.[2] A MOS4 with $nSaO_2$ less than 80% is consistent with the proposed hypoxia criteria of severe OSAS. It is noteworthy that in an unselected surgical population of children (n = 44) awaiting T&A, 34% showed baseline saturations below 90% and/or episodic hypoxemia during sleep.[42]

Oximetry as a predicator of PRAEs following T&A

Removal of the tonsils and adenoids does not immediately cure the OSAS, and desaturation on the initial night following T&A is extremely common in these children.[4,20,28,29] Therefore, the clinical relevance of PRAEs following T&A is often stratified by the medical interventions required to treat them.[4,17,18,20] As the risk for PRAEs and medical intervention correlates inversely with the severity of nocturnal hypoxemia in the preoperative sleep study,[4,17,18,20,39,43] the authors have found the MOS useful to stratify the risk for PRAEs. The odds ratio for a medical intervention ranges from 3.7 to 5.5 if the preoperative $nSaO_2$ is less than 80%.[4,20] The likelihood ratio (LR) for a medical intervention for a preoperative $nSaO_2$ less than 80% is approximately 3, increasing the posttest probability of a PRAE from 20% to 50%. The LR for a medical intervention for a preoperative $nSaO_2$ greater than 80% is 0.5, decreasing the posttest probability of a PRAE from 20% to 10%. Inclusion of a measure of OSAS risk to age and medical risk model for PRAE doubled the Nagelkerke pseudo R^2 value to 0.3. Comparing an Age, Medical, and AHI Risk model with an Age, Medical, and Saturation Risk model showed similar statistics.[20] A MOS of 2 or more detected 6 of the 7 (sensitivity: 86%) children who required a major respiratory intervention following T&A.[39]

An advantage of a 2-stage preoperative assessment (ie, SBD-Q plus MOS) is that it allows identification of the high-risk child before surgery and prioritization of children with severe OSAS (ie, MOS4).[39] Furthermore, the combination of SBD-Qs plus the MOS stratifies the risk for PRAEs. Targeted risk-reduction strategies become possible. Ragavendran and colleagues[44] reported that an anesthetic regimen for children with MOS4, which included a reduced opioid dosing and airway doses of dexamethasone, decreased the incidence of PRAEs without compromising patient analgesia. Children with profound hypoxemia demonstrate a heightened respiratory[34] and analgesic[36,37] sensitivity to opioids, and the mechanism underlying this heightened sensitivity may involve oxygen-sensitive gene regulation.[45–47]

Of note, Urschitz and colleagues[5] also used the combination of SDB-Qs plus oximetry to screen a population of primary school children for SDB, and reported that an abnormal oximetry of less than 90% had a sensitivity of 0.7, a specificity of 0.8, and a positive likelihood ratio of 4.

A positive SDB-Q is not pathognomonic for OSAS. The late-onset central hypoventilation syndrome (LO-CHS) and Prader-Willi Syndrome (PWS) may masquerade as OSAS. The LO-CHS is a rare syndrome, but 2 published pediatric cases report delayed emergence following anesthesia as the presenting sign. Profound hypoventilation and an inability to wean from mechanical ventilation were problematic.[48,49] Typically LO-CHS present in children older than 2 years with sleep-related breathing difficulties and hypothalamic abnormalities. However, Weese-Mayer and colleagues[50] reported the case of a 35-year-old man with a life-long history of snoring, nocturnal gasping, and "stopping breathing and turning blue" while asleep. The PSG study revealed an AHI of 77 and a nadir saturation of 65%. A central apnea index of 16, profound hypercarbia during wakefulness, and the Congenital Central Hypoventilation Syndrome mutation in PHOX2b distinguished LO-CHS from OSAS.

The PWS is characterized by hypothalamic obesity, mental retardation, hypotonia and hypogonadism, and abnormalities of chromosome 15. The physical findings of obesity, hypotonia, and hypogonadism with a positive SDB-Q should alert the clinician to the possibility of the PWS. Formal testing often reveals a blunted chemoresponsiveness to both hypercarbia and hypoxia and autonomic dysfunction, features that distinguish PWS from the OSAS.[51]

Incomplete resolution of OSAS

In a prospective study of more than 500 children studied before and 40 to 720 days after T&A, only 27% had normalized their respiratory pattern. In children with severe OSAS, only 40% had complete resolution of their OSAS.[52] Mitchell and Kelly[53,54] reported that 34% of children with severe OSAS continued to have OSAS following T&A. Suen and colleagues[55] reported that an RDI greater than 19 was associated with residual OSAS following T&A. Children older than 7 years and obese children were more likely to have persistent OSAS. A positive SDB-Q plus a validated test for OSAS severity identifies children with SDB who need to be monitored more closely following T&A.

SUMMARY

Pediatric OSAS is as prevalent as childhood asthma. The primary treatment is T&A. The safety of ambulatory T&A programs is predicated on the exclusion of high-risk children from these programs. As PRAEs may be delayed in onset and life-threatening, a diagnosis of severe OSAS (AHI >24 and nSaO$_2$ <80%) excludes the child with severe OSAS from ambulatory programs. Whereas young age, medical complexity, and African American ethnicity are easily recognized in the preoperative evaluation, the severity of SDB is not. Preoperative evaluation with a combination of SDB-Qs plus the MOS has several advantages. It aligns with the diagnostic approach recommended by sleep physicians, and provides a useful prediction of PRAEs and the medical interventions required to manage the PRAEs. Oximetry is potentially more widely available and cost effective than PSG. Furthermore, preoperative evaluation with a combination of SDB-Qs plus the MOS allows (1) triage of patients, (2) inclusion of the low-risk child in ambulatory T&A programs, (3) admission of the child with severe OSAS to hospital, and (4) implementation of risk-reduction strategies.

REFERENCES

1. Lumeng JC, Chervin RD. Epidemiology of pediatric obstructive sleep apnea. Proc Am Thorac Soc 2008;5:242–52.
2. Dayyat E, Kheirandish-Gozal L, Gozal D. Childhood obstructive sleep apnea: one or two distinct disease entities? Sleep Med Clin 2007;2:433–44.
3. Practice guidelines for the perioperative management of patients with obstructive sleep apnea: a report by the American Society of Anesthesiologists Task Force on Perioperative Management of patients with obstructive sleep apnea [article]. Anesthesiology 2006;104:1081–93.
4. Brown K, Morin I, Hickey C, et al. Urgent adenotonsillectomy: an analysis of risk factors associated with postoperative respiratory morbidity. Anesthesiology 2003;99:586–95.
5. Urschitz MS, Brockmann PE, Schlaud M, et al. Population prevalence of obstructive sleep apnoea in a community of German third graders. Eur Respir J 2010;36:556–68.
6. Marcus CL, Brooks LJ, Davidson Ward S, et al. Diagnosis and management of childhood obstructive sleep apnea syndrome. Pediatrics 2012;130: e714–55.

7. Shott SR, Myer CM III, Cotton RT. Efficacy of tonsillectomy and adenoidectomy as an outpatient procedure: a preliminary report. Int J Pediatr Otorhinolaryngol 1987;13:157–63.

8. Erickson BK, Larson DR, St. Sauveur JL, et al. Changes in incidence and indications of tonsillectomy and adenotonsillectomy, 1970-2005. Otolaryngol Head Neck Surg 2009;140:894–901.

9. Guilleminault C, Eldridge FL, Simmons FB, et al. Sleep apnea in eight children. Pediatrics 1976;58: 23–31.

10. Chervin RD, Hedger K, Dillon JE, et al. Pediatric sleep questionnaire (PSQ): validity and reliability of scales for sleep-disordered breathing, snoring, sleepiness, and behavioral problems. Sleep Med 2000;1:21–32.

11. Carroll JL, McColley SA, Marcus CL, et al. Inability of clinical history to distinguish primary snoring from obstructive sleep apnea syndrome in children. Chest 1995;108:610–8.

12. Brietzke SE, Katz ES, Roberson DW. Can history and physical examination reliably diagnose pediatric obstructive sleep apnea/hypopnea syndrome? A systematic review of the literature. Otolaryngol Head Neck Surg 2004;131:827–32.

13. Constantin E, Tewfik TL, Brouillette RT. Can the OSA-18 quality-of-life questionnaire detect obstructive sleep apnea in children? Pediatrics 2010;125:e162–8.

14. Parnis SJ, Barker DS, Van Der Walt JH. Clinical predictors of anaesthetic complications in children with respiratory tract infections. Paediatr Anaesth 2001;11:29–40.

15. Dayyat E, Kheirandish-Gozal L, Capdevila OS, et al. Obstructive sleep apnea in children. Chest 2009; 136:137–44.

16. Marcus CL, Brooks LJ, Jones J, et al. Clinical practice guideline: diagnosis and management of childhood obstructive sleep apnea syndrome. Pediatrics 2002;109:704–12.

17. Rosen GM, Muckle RP, Mahowald MW, et al. Postoperative respiratory compromise in children with obstructive sleep apnea syndrome: can it be anticipated? Pediatrics 1994;93:784–8.

18. McColley SA, April MM, Carroll JL, et al. Respiratory compromise after adenotonsillectomy in children with obstructive sleep apnea. Arch Otolaryngol Head Neck Surg 1992;118:940–3.

19. Biavati MJ, Manning SC, Phillips DL. Predictive factors for respiratory complications after tonsillectomy and adenoidectomy in children. Arch Otolaryngol Head Neck Surg 1997;123:517–21.

20. Wilson K, Lakheeram I, Morielli A, et al. Can assessment for obstructive sleep apnea help predict postadenotonsillectomy respiratory complications? Anesthesiology 2002;96:313–22.

21. McGowan FX, Kenna MA, Fleming JA, et al. Adenotonsillectomy for upper airway obstruction carries increased risk in children with a history of prematurity. Pediatr Pulmonol 1992;13:222–6.

22. Don DM, Geller KA, Koempel JA, et al. Age specific differences in pediatric obstructive sleep apnea. Int J Pediatr Otorhinolaryngol 2009;73:1025–8.

23. Wiatrak BJ, Myer CM III, Andrews TM. Complications of adenotonsillectomy in children under 3 years of age. Am J Otolaryngol 1991;12:170–2.

24. Redline S, Tishler PV, Schluchter M, et al. Risk factors for sleep-disordered breathing in children: associations with obesity, race, and respiratory problems. Am J Respir Crit Care Med 1999;159: 1527–32.

25. Redline S, Tishler PV, Hans MG. Racial differences in sleep-disordered breathing in African-Americans and Caucasians. Am J Respir Crit Care Med 1997; 155:186–92.

26. Stepanski E, Zayyad A, Nigro C, et al. Sleep-disordered breathing in a predominantly African-American pediatric population. J Sleep Res 1999; 8:65–70.

27. Boss EF, Smith DF, Ishman SL. Racial/ethnic and socioeconomic disparities in the diagnosis and treatment of sleep-disordered breathing in children. Int J Pediatr Otorhinolaryngol 2011;75:299–307.

28. Koomson A, Morin I, Brouillette RT, et al. Children with severe OSAS who have adenotonsillectomy in the morning are less likely to have postoperative desaturation than those operated in the afternoon. Can J Anaesth 2004;51:62–7.

29. Nixon GM, Kermack AS, McGregor CD, et al. Sleep and breathing on the first night after adenotonsillectomy for obstructive sleep apnea. Pediatr Pulmonol 2005;39:332–8.

30. Gali B, Whalen FX, Schroeder DR, et al. Identification of patients at risk for postoperative respiratory complications using a preoperative obstructive sleep apnea screening tool and postanesthesia care assessment. Anesthesiology 2009;110:869–77.

31. Guilleminault C, Pelayo R, Leger D, et al. Recognition of sleep-disordered breathing in children. Pediatrics 1996;98:871–82.

32. Schwengel DA, Sterni LM, Tunkel DE, et al. Perioperative management of children with obstructive sleep apnea. Anesth Analg 2009;109:60–75.

33. Yilmaz MD, Onrat E, Altuntas A, et al. The effects of tonsillectomy and adenoidectomy on pulmonary arterial pressure in children. Am J Otolaryngol 2005;26:18–21.

34. Waters KA, McBrien F, Stewart P, et al. Effects of OSA, inhalational anesthesia, and fentanyl on the airway and ventilation of children. J Appl Physiol 2002;92:1987–94.

35. Strauss SG, Lynn AM, Bratton SL, et al. Ventilatory response to CO_2 in children with obstructive sleep apnea from adenotonsillar hypertrophy. Anesth Analg 1999;89:328–32.

36. Brown KA, Laferrière A, Moss IR. Recurrent hypoxemia in young children with obstructive sleep apnea is associated with reduced opioid requirements for analgesia. Anesthesiology 2004;100:806–10.

37. Brown KA, Laferrière A, Lakheeram I, et al. Recurrent hypoxemia in children is associated with increased analgesic sensitivity to opiates. Anesthesiology 2006;105:665–9.

38. Brouillette RT, Morielli A, Leimanis A, et al. Nocturnal pulse oximetry as an abbreviated testing modality for pediatric obstructive sleep apnea. Pediatrics 2000;105:405–12.

39. Nixon GM, Kermack AS, Davis GM, et al. Planning adenotonsillectomy in children with obstructive sleep apnea: the role of overnight oximetry. Pediatrics 2004;113:e19–25.

40. Brown KA. Outcome, risk, and error and the child with obstructive sleep apnea. Paediatr Anaesth 2011;21:771–80.

41. Muzumdar H, Arens R. Diagnostic issues in pediatric obstructive sleep apnea. Proc Am Thorac Soc 2008;5:263–73.

42. van Someren V, Hibbert J, Stothers JK, et al. Identification of hypoxaemia in children having tonsillectomy and adenoidectomy. Clin Otolaryngol 1990; 15:263–71.

43. Schroeder JW, Anstead AS, Wong H. Complications in children who electively remain intubated after adenotonsillectomy for severe obstructive sleep apnea. Int J Pediatr Otorhinolaryngol 2009;73:1095–9.

44. Raghavendran S, Bagry H, Detheux G, et al. An anesthetic management protocol to decrease respiratory complications after adenotonsillectomy in children with severe sleep apnea. Anesth Analg 2010;110:1093–101.

45. Laferrière A, Liu JK, Moss IR. Neurokinin-1 versus mu-opioid receptor binding in rat nucleus tractus solitarius after single and recurrent intermittent hypoxia. Brain Res Bull 2003;59:307–13.

46. Peng PH, Huang HS, Lee YJ, et al. Novel role for the delta-opioid receptor in hypoxic preconditoning in rat retinas. J Neurochem 2009;108:741–54.

47. Hambrecht VS, Vlisides PE, Row BW, et al. G proteins in rat prefrontal cortex (PFC) are differentially activated as a function of oxygen status and PFC region. J Chem Neuroanat 2009;37:112–7.

48. Mahmoud M, Bryan Y, Gunter J, et al. Anesthetic implications of undiagnosed late onset central hypoventilation syndrome in a child: from elective tonsillectomy to tracheostomy. Paediatr Anaesth 2007; 17:1001–5.

49. Mahfouz AK, Rashid M, Khan MS, et al. Late onset congenital central hypoventilation syndrome after exposure to general anesthesia. Can J Anaesth 2011;58:1105–9.

50. Weese-Mayer DE, Berry-Kravis EM, Zhou L. Adult identified with congenital central hypoventilation syndrome-mutation in PHOX2b gene and late-onset CHS. Am J Respir Crit Care Med 2005;171:88.

51. Grob GN. The rise and decline of tonsillectomy in twentieth-century America. J Hist Med Allied Sci 2007;62:383–421.

52. Bhattacharjee R, Kheirandish-Gozal L, Spruyt K, et al. Adenotonsillectomy outcomes in treatment of obstructive sleep apnea in children. Am J Respir Crit Care Med 2010;182:676–83.

53. Mitchell RB, Kelly J. Outcome of adenotonsillectomy for obstructive sleep apnea in obese and normal-weight children. Otolaryngol Head Neck Surg 2007;137:43–8.

54. Mitchell RB. Adenotonsillectomy for obstructive sleep apnea in children: outcome evaluated by pre- and postoperative polysomnography. Laryngoscope 2007;117:1844–54.

55. Suen JS, Arnold JE, Brooks LJ. Adenotonsillectomy for treatment of obstructive sleep apnea in children. Arch Otolaryngol Head Neck Surg 1995;121:525–30.

Curricular Elements for Circadian Rhythm and Sleep Disorders in Anesthesiology Training Programs

Norman Bolden, MD[a], Kingman P. Strohl, MD[b],*

KEYWORDS

- Sleep • Sleep disorders • Upper airway physiology • Sleep apnea • Chronopharmacology
- Sleepiness

KEY POINTS

- The concepts of sleep neurophysiology and knowledge of sleep disorders are used in an anesthetic practice.
- Training programs for general anesthesiology should incorporate this knowledge system into didactic and practical curriculum in a deliberate fashion.
- Competencies should be linked to formative assessments.
- There are opportunities for research into the principles of sleep and chronobiology in the clinical practice of anesthesiology and its subspecialties of obstetrics and pain management.

INTRODUCTION

Sleep disorders and circadian rhythm are fundamental to the biology of many human illnesses. Particularly relevant to the experience and practice of anesthesiology are the topics of consciousness, anesthetic pharmacology, management of the upper airway, and clinical management and recognition of sleep disorders, in particular obstructive sleep apnea/hypopnea, in the perioperative arena.[1–3]

Implementation of some or the whole of this curriculum will present challenges for program directors who already have to comply with several directives and an increasing number of subspecialty areas, for example, pain, obstetrics, and cardiac anesthesiology. The greatest likelihood of success will be achieved if the competencies are seamlessly integrated into existing training methods and experience, and assessed by in-service examinations.

Sleep apnea is probably the most common disorder encountered in anesthetic practice because it is the most common chronic sleep disorder in primary care[4,5] and in tertiary sleep centers.[6] Other knowledge and skills concerning adequate sleep, recovery sleep, and circadian rhythm are also important not only for clinical performance in residency training,[7] but also for practice professionalism and learning.[1–3,7–12]

A learning system for sleep and chronobiology in medical education is beginning to emerge, but exposure is inconsistent not only across undergraduate programs in the United States but also across international programs. There is increasing need for knowledge about sleep and chronobiology in undergraduate medical education,[13] as

[a] Department of Anesthesiology, MetroHealth Medical Center, Case Western Reserve University, 2500, Metro Health Drive, Cleveland, OH 44109, USA; [b] Center for Sleep Disorders Research, Louis Stokes Cleveland DVA Medical Center, Case Western Reserve University, 111j(w) VAMC, 10701 East Boulevard, Cleveland, OH 44106, USA
* Corresponding author.
E-mail address: KPSTROHL@aol.com

Sleep Med Clin 8 (2013) 157–164
http://dx.doi.org/10.1016/j.jsmc.2012.11.008
1556-407X/13/$ – see front matter Published by Elsevier Inc.

the topics are listed in various content areas of American Board of Internal Medicine examinations,[14,15] and also identified as goals for undergraduate medical education.[16] Questions on knowledge of sleep and chronobiology appear in standardized testing. The United States Medical Licensing Examination (USMLE) Step 1 assesses knowledge and application of the sciences basic to the practice of medicine, and its content now includes the ontogeny of sleep, circadian rhythm, and the impact of sleepiness on human behavior. USMLE Step 2 assesses the application of medical knowledge, skills, and clinical science essential for the provision of patient care (under supervision), and now explicitly considers recognition of sleep apnea, narcolepsy and idiopathic hypersomnolence, insomnia, and other sleep disturbances under the content area of "paroxysmal disorders." USMLE Step 3 assesses application of medical knowledge and understanding of clinical science essential for the unsupervised practice of medicine. It now explicitly identifies sleep disorders in the context of the nervous system disease/disorders, as well as the traditional topics on patient presentations and clinical assessments.[17] Thus in the course of postgraduate training, the anesthesiology resident will have studied or is likely to encounter some of this content area in formalized testing.

Competencies in topics in sleep and chronobiology are articulated for residency training in internal medicine practice[15] and for pulmonary and critical care medicine (American Thoracic Society). For these programs, the range of expected instructional topics is updated regularly by the Accreditation Council of Graduate Medical Education (ACGME). Over the past 10 years all ACGME programs have needed to document instruction in fatigue, the effects of extended hours, and effective and ineffective countermeasures to sleep loss, and the ACGME assesses programs for the presence of this instruction.[18,19] Regardless of attitudes about the duty hours,[20] this instruction is generally perceived as useful.[21]

METHODOLOGY

To refocus concepts and expected behaviors into the context of training in anesthesia, the authors derived educational competencies for sleep and circadian rhythm using existing methodology.[22,23] Sleep curricula and commentary[13,16,24] for other postgraduate programs were examined. The publicly available information on the content of the American Board of Anesthesiology (ABA) in-service examinations was reviewed. Subsequent discussions included review of existing ACGME

guidelines for Anesthesiology residency programs, the literature on perioperative management and sleep disorders, and interactions with board members of the Society for Anesthesia and Sleep Medicine.

CONTENT IN CURRENT PRACTICE

An estimate of current knowledge and skills used in the management of sleep and sleep disorders in anesthetic practice was compiled. One focal point for the start of this search was articles on the emerging importance of the anesthesiologist in preoperative and perioperative management.[25,26] Of interest, these articles from 2002 do not explicitly or implicitly mention sleep or sleep apnea. At this point in time, however, one might assume that the magnitude of sleep apnea was not generally appreciated, and indeed the seminal article on complications related to known and unknown obstructive sleep apnea (OSA) appeared the next year.[27,28] Contrast this to the subsequent articles[29] and commentary, as well as societal statements of the importance of recognition and optimal management.[30–32]

On review of this literature and discussions among colleagues, a table was compiled using 3 headings correlating with the areas of basic science, procedures, and management (**Box 1**). The outline presented in **Box 1** identifies a broad range of subjects. Not all are used in daily practice, nor do all anesthesiologists have or should expect training in all subjects. There are at present no studies detailing which are the most used or useful in clinical practice, except as suggested by expert opinion.[30,32] However, there is a range of knowledge and skills identified as being relevant.

PROPOSED COMPETENCIES

Considering the aforementioned themes, there may be 6 "core proficiencies" (**Table 1**). The first 3 are based on knowledge about sleep physiology, pharmacology, and risk factors related to respiratory depression. This content is often delivered through lectures or reading assignments, and assessed by having the trainee take a short, written examination. The next 3 "core proficiencies" involve management, and could be delivered in problem-based learning discussions or practice settings. Assessments are more dynamic and applicable to clinical activities. One skill would be the ability to derive an appropriate differential diagnosis after eliciting a sleep complaint as a comorbid condition during a preoperative encounter. A second skill is the interpretation of the polysomnography report as it might come from a sleep center or laboratory. As is done for chest radiographs, the anesthesiologist should understand how and what data is collected, and the strengths and limitations of the summary measures, rather than rely solely on the diagnosis and recommendation contained as a summary interpretation. There may be risk factors such as the level of oxygenation, for example, percent time less than an oxygen saturation of 90%, that is not captured by the apnea-hypopnea index (AHI) or respiratory disturbance index (RDI). The third skill articulated is the identification and management of central and upper airway apneas in the perioperative setting. Assessments of these skills will require attention to the broad range of clinical decision making and patient-based experiences, including economic and legal ramifications of care pathways. Skills should be assessed during the conduct of patient care using both formal and informal assessment of trainee proficiency.

Articulation of competency in the area of sleep in the anesthesia training program creates an understanding of program expectations, as well as a plan consistent with the ACGME goals as to the expected knowledge and skills of a trainee. However, competency should be revisited periodically to ensure relevance to patient needs.

CURRICULAR RESOURCES

Knowledge and acquisition of skills can be accomplished by several models and modes of instruction.[23] As anesthesia residency programs vary in size and scope and also the expertise available in the management of sleep disorder, the manner of instruction will vary according to local resources. Furthermore, varying formats are useful in accommodating all types of learners.[33] A lecture can be reinforced by case-based instruction modules, interactive instructional programs or models, and one-on-one instruction. **Box 2** is a list of objectives identified during the course of discussions or in review of this document by other individuals. The authors would encourage programs to share case materials, and share experiences in delivery of content.

Current sources for content include the sleep textbooks in the field; however, there are recent reviews that identify material more relevant to anesthesia. There are Internet resources that could be modified or adapted by training programs to enhance learning.

ASSESSMENT TOOLS

Knowledge is generally tested by written examination, but there is increasing interest in complementary assessments such as observed patient interactions, simulated patients, structured clinical encounters, or chart review as outcomes for assessment during training.[17] An array of assessment tools is available[34–36] or can be constructed from the competency objectives.

Regarding national programs for assessment, information is reported for content areas labeled as "key words" in the ABA in-service examinations. In searching these terms there were questions noted on distinguishing central sleep apnea from OSA (57% answered correctly in 2012), OSA (94% answered correctly in 2008 and 85% answered correctly in 2009), and rapid desaturation in morbid obesity (51% answered correctly in 2009, 55% in 2012). Under the key word "Airway" there were questions about airway anesthesia anatomy and obesity airway evaluation.

If the content and competencies areas suggested here are to be recognized as part of anesthetic training, additional categories of questions, for example, sleep physiology or the neurophysiologic interactions between sleep and anesthesia or the impact of sleepiness on professional development, might be appropriate.

ADVANCED ACTIVITIES AND RESEARCH OPPORTUNITIES

Research in sleep disorders and the related topic of chronobiology is expected by the ACGME to be conducted within most residency programs. **Box 3** lists some of the ideas that arose out of discussions. Local practitioners in sleep medicine, as well as physician-scientists who conduct research in sleep and chronobiology, could be identified as mentors and advisors.

Finally, there is the opportunity to proceed to advanced training in an accredited ACGME fellowship for Sleep Medicine.[37] It must be emphasized that this entails a commitment to learning and patient care not just for sleep apnea but for some 93 other sleep problems and disorders, and the provision of care for patients with chronic sleep disorders, including narcolepsy, insomnia, restless legs syndrome, and circadian misalignment. This body of knowledge and skills includes assessments and management of children, neonates, and adults. The specialty is outpatient oriented, and as currently implemented is often based in one of several departments: internal medicine, neurology, psychiatry, pediatrics, and so forth. There is no academic or nonacademic practice plan for Sleep Medicine that is based in a department of anesthesia. The choice of pursuing certification in Sleep Medicine requires a 1-year commitment to fellowship training during

Box 1
Content relevant to the practice of anesthesiology

1. PHYSIOLOGY OF SLEEP AND CIRCADIAN RHYTHM

   a. Basic elements

      i. Neural pathways for initiating and maintaining sleep with implications for how anesthetic agents work

      ii. Effects of common drugs on respiratory control

      iii. Functional anatomy of the upper airway and chest wall

   b. Pathophysiologic mechanisms and consequences

      i. Obstructive sleep apnea

      ii. Central sleep apnea and Cheyne-Stokes respiration

      iii. Nocturnal hypoventilation in other diseases (chronic obstructive pulmonary disease [COPD], restrictive diseases, asthma)

   c. Clinical epidemiology of anesthetic complications in sleep apnea

2. DIAGNOSTIC METHODS AND PROCEDURES

   a. Sleep-related history and physical examination

      i. History, including the use of patient-based tools such as STOP-Bang and the Berlin Questionnaire

      ii. Prescribed medications

      iii. Directed examination of the patient (airway/chest wall/body mass index)

      iv. Comorbidity: hypoventilation, obesity, congestive heart failure, gastroesophageal reflux disease, panic attacks

   b. Testing, its indications, and clinical utility

      i. Cardiorespiratory monitoring over time

         1. Airflow and respiratory effort measurements

         2. Continuous oximetry and end-tidal CO_2 measurements

      ii. Polysomnography

         1. Indications for testing

         2. How to read an interpretation

3. BROAD-SENSE CLINICAL MANAGEMENT

   a. Obstructive sleep apnea

      i. Medical/surgical treatment

         1. Ventilatory support: continuous positive airway pressure, bilevel treatment, oxygen

         2. Surgical management including uvulopalatopharyngoplasty and bariatric surgery

         3. Behavioral and pharmacologic options

      ii. Intraoperative anesthetic management considerations

         1. Airway management

         2. Impact of local and regional anesthesia

         3. Choice of anesthetic agents

         4. Postoperative pain control considerations

      iii. Definitions of quality outcomes with regard to perioperative care

   b. Central sleep apnea (Cheyne-Stokes respiration)

      i. Correlations with heart disease and stroke

      ii. Similarities and differences with opioid-induced central apnea

c. Sleep-related breathing in medical disorders

  i. Pulmonary diseases: respiratory failure, COPD, restrictive lung disease, asthma

  ii. Cardiac disease: congestive heart failure, angina, hypertension

  iii. Neuromuscular diseases

d. Assessments of the hospitalized patient

  i. Recognition of sleep-disordered breathing

  ii. Postoperative management and treatment

4. ADMINISTRATIVE AND PROFESSIONAL ISSUES

a. Instruction in sleep and circadian rhythm in residency training

b. Comanagement with sleep specialists and across departments

which time there would be little room for a continuity of practice of anesthesiology. Thus, one would need to balance outpatient visits for sleep disorders, interpretations of diagnostic studies, and a practice of anesthesia, and experience some degree of competition from other practitioners. Furthermore, the career pathway for the anesthesiologist with sleep certification will need negotiations among departments or specialists and hospital appointments that recognize the need for a novel mix of practice skills of both sleep and anesthesiology.

IMPLEMENTATION IN THE SHORT TERM

In the role of perioperative physician, anesthesiologists must evaluate patients preoperatively by ensuring that they are in their optimal state before surgery, use the knowledge of the patients' underlying medical condition and comorbidities in

Table 1
Objectives for competency with instructional methods and assessments

Following Completion of an Accredited Training Program in Anesthesiology, the Physician Will:	Suggested Instructional Methods	Recommended Assessment Methods
Contrast the effects of sleep, sleep loss, and anesthesia on cognitive functioning	Reading assignments or lecture-based presentation	Standardized written and/or oral examination
Describe the pharmacology of medications used to treat sleep disorders or that have impact on sleep disorders	Reading assignments or lecture-based presentation	Standardized written and/or oral examination
Describe the risk factors for respiratory depression	Problem-based cases, lecture series, or reading assignments	Standardized written and/or oral examination
Describe the pathophysiology and consequences of obstructive sleep apnea/hypopnea syndrome and the obesity hypoventilation syndrome	Problem-based cases, lecture series, or reading assignments	Oral examination or observations in teaching medical students
Formulate an appropriate perioperative plan for management of recognized and previously unrecognized sleep apnea	Clinic-based experiences, preceptor Teaching	Behavioral checklists, global rating scales using standardized patients and real patients
Assess a polysomnography report	Examples and case management	Checklist evaluation and/or standardized encounters

---

Box 2
Examples of presentations to achieve competency objectives

- Sleep and Anesthetic Practice
  - Describe the Two-Process Model of Vigilance and how it relates to shift work, on-call clinical work, and clinical presentations of sleepiness and inattention
  - Describe the impact of one night of total sleep loss, chronic partial sleep loss, and sleep inertia on cognitive function
  - Contrast the tools used for pretest probability for clinical decision making with those used for management of sleep-disordered breathing in the perioperative period
  - Contrast treatment options for patients with recognized sleep apnea in regard of planning for anesthetic agents during the operative procedure
- Impact of Sleep and Sleep Apnea on Perioperative Practice
  - List the management issues raised by sleep apnea in the preoperative and postoperative care of the surgical patient
  - Describe the features of the surgical intensive care unit environment that enhance or inhibit the restorative effects of sleep and circadian rhythm
  - List the role of oxygen therapy in masking recognition of sleep-disordered breathing
  - Identify the role of intrathoracic pressure swings occurring in sleep apnea on cardiovascular functions
- General Knowledge and Clinical Management
  - Demonstrate the use of a sleep history
  - Explain the importance of and expectations for follow-up to a patient whose sleep apnea is recognized in the perioperative period

---

establishing an anesthetic plan, and ensure safe management of the patient following the surgical procedure.[38,39] Therefore, the practical implications for inclusion of a curriculum incorporating circadian rhythm and sleep within anesthesiology training programs are easily discernible.

Many patients will have some degree of OSA that will be first recognized on presentation in the preoperative period.[40] Thus, patients scheduled for elective surgery as well as those requiring urgent/emergency surgery will be at risk for upper-airway management problems and

---

Box 3
Examples of topics for in-depth study or research

- Fundamentals of Clinical Management
  - Expression of sleep versus circadian rhythm in pain management
  - Clinical management of central sleep apnea
  - Sleep and sleep behavior following local anesthesia
  - Role of sleep-disordered breathing in all-cause cardiopulmonary adverse postoperative events
- Art and Science
  - Discrimination of sleepiness, fatigue, and inattention in neurocognitive features of pain management
  - Strategy for follow-up of newly diagnosed sleep apnea in the postoperative period
- Other Areas
  - Systems management of sleepiness in anesthesia training
  - Sleep apnea and policy
  - Medical economics of sleep apnea management in anesthetic practice

instability, and adverse cardiopulmonary events following surgery. The quantitative impact of mild, moderate, and severe sleep apnea may be different, as it has been the high-profile dramatic cases whereby known severe sleep apnea is underappreciated and intervention has been delayed that currently dominate the informal conversations and the quality-assurance committees in many hospitals.

In any event, a resident in general anesthesiology should be aware of the symptoms of OSA and be familiar with screening tools to identify patients at high risk for OSA, and appropriately act to mitigate risk. The preoperative encounter also allows the anesthesiologist to initiate a plan tailored to pathophysiologic processes associated with various sleep disorders. This approach includes use of regional anesthesia (when appropriate) and use of anesthetic agents that would cause the least amount of respiratory depression for the least amount of time. A multimodal approach to postoperative analgesia would also allow for the limited use of parenteral narcotics, which can exacerbate respiratory depression in patients with sleep disorders in the postoperative period.

Finally, immediate instruction is needed in regard of familiarity with interpretation of sleep studies (polysomnography), medical management therapies for sleep-disordered breathing including positive pressure therapies, and the limitations of surgical treatment for OSA (core competencies, see **Table 1**).

OSA has long-term health implications and, if left untreated, leads to increased morbidity and mortality. The identification of patients with OSA during the preoperative consultation leads to decreased morbidity and mortality long after recovery from the surgical encounter. The implementation of this knowledge in sleep disorders therefore has immediate short-term and potential long-term benefit to the patient.

ACKNOWLEDGMENTS

The authors would like to thank the board of the Society for Anesthesia and Sleep Medicine for support and commentary on this article.

REFERENCES

1. Brown EN, Lydic R, Schiff ND. General anesthesia, sleep, and coma. N Engl J Med 2010;363(27): 2638–50.
2. Chung F, Hillman D, Lydic R. Sleep medicine and anesthesia: a new horizon for anesthesiologists. Anesthesiology 2011;114(6):1261–2.
3. Lydic R, Baghdoyan HA. Sleep, anesthesiology, and the neurobiology of arousal state control. Anesthesiology 2005;103(6):1268–95.
4. Ohayon MM, Guilleminault C, Priest RG, et al. Snoring and breathing pauses during sleep: telephone interview survey of a United Kingdom population sample. BMJ 1997;314(7084):860–3.
5. Netzer NC, Hoegel JJ, Loube D, et al. Prevalence of symptoms and risk of sleep apnea in primary care. Chest 2003;124(4):1406–14.
6. Punjabi NM, Welch D, Strohl K. Sleep disorders in regional sleep centers: a national cooperative study. Coleman II Study Investigators. Sleep 2000;23(4): 471–80.
7. Cao CG, Weinger MB, Slagle J, et al. Differences in day and night shift clinical performance in anesthesiology. Hum Factors 2008;50(2):276–90.
8. Laurenson J. Sleep disruption and performance. Anaesthesia 2003;58(10):1026.
9. Merry AF, Warman GR. Fatigue and the anaesthetist. Anaesth Intensive Care 2006;34(5):577–8.
10. Murray D, Dodds C. The effect of sleep disruption on performance of anaesthetists—a pilot study. Anaesthesia 2003;58(6):520–5.
11. Nelson CS, Dell'Angela K, Jellish WS, et al. Residents' performance before and after night call as evaluated by an indicator of creative thought. J Am Osteopath Assoc 1995;95(10):600–3.
12. Parker JB. The effects of fatigue on physician performance—an underestimated cause of physician impairment and increased patient risk. Can J Anaesth 1987;34(5):489–95.
13. Strohl KP. Concerning the sleep curriculum in a pulmonary training program. Sleep Breath 2001; 5(2):53–6.
14. Sateia MJ, Owens J, Dube C, et al. Advancement in sleep medicine education. Sleep 2000;23(8):1021–3.
15. Rosen RC, Zozula R, Jahn EG, et al. Low rates of recognition of sleep disorders in primary care: comparison of a community-based versus clinical academic setting. Sleep Med 2001;2(1):47–55.
16. Strohl KP, Veasey S, Harding S, et al. Competency-based goals of a medical curriculum for sleep and chronobiology. Sleep 2003;26(3):333–6.
17. Accreditation Council for Graduate Medical Education. Available at: http://www.acgme.org/acgmeweb. Accessed December 18, 2012.
18. Proposed general ACGME requirements for resident duty hours and supervision. Neurocirugia (Astur) 2002;13(2):154.
19. Nasca TJ, Day SH, Amis ES Jr. The new recommendations on duty hours from the ACGME Task Force. N Engl J Med 2010;363(2):e3.
20. Antiel RM, Thompson SM, Hafferty FW, et al. Duty hour recommendations and implications for meeting the ACGME core competencies: views of residency directors. Mayo Clin Proc 2011;86(3):185–91.

21. Myers JS, Bellini LM, Morris JB, et al. Internal medicine and general surgery residents' attitudes about the ACGME duty hours regulations: a multicenter study. Acad Med 2006;81(12):1052–8.

22. Stone DH. A method of deriving definitions of specific medical competencies: a framework for curriculum planning and evaluation. Med Teach 1987;9(2):155–9.

23. Carraccio C, Wolfsthal SD, Englander R, et al. Shifting paradigms: from Flexner to competencies. Acad Med 2002;77(5):361–7.

24. Harding SM, Hawkins JW. What is a necessary knowledge base for sleep professionals? Sleep Breath 2001;5(3):101–8.

25. Dedrick DF. The perioperative physician. ASA Newsletter 2002;66(11):4.

26. Hepner DL. The anesthesiologist as perioperative physician. ASA Newsletter 2002;66(11):5–15.

27. Gupta RM, Parvizi J, Hanssen AD, et al. Postoperative complications in patients with obstructive sleep apnea syndrome undergoing hip or knee replacement: a case-control study. Mayo Clin Proc 2001; 76(9):897–905.

28. Liao P, Yegneswaran B, Vairavanathan S, et al. Postoperative complications in patients with obstructive sleep apnea: a retrospective matched cohort study. Can J Anaesth 2009;56(11):819–28. http://dx.doi.org/10.1007/s12630-009-9190-y. PubMed PMID: 19774431.

29. Adesanya AO, Lee W, Greilich NB, et al. Perioperative management of obstructive sleep apnea. Chest 2010; 138(6):1489–98.

30. Fleetham J, Ayas N, Bradley D, et al. Canadian Thoracic Society 2011 guideline update: diagnosis and treatment of sleep disordered breathing. Can Respir J 2011;18(1):25–47.

31. Blackman A, McGregor C, Dales R, et al. Canadian Sleep Society/Canadian Thoracic Society position paper on the use of portable monitoring for the diagnosis of obstructive sleep apnea/hypopnea in adults. Can Respir J 2010;17(5):229–32.

32. Joshi GP, Ankichetty SP, Gan TJ, et al. Society for ambulatory anesthesia consensus statement on preoperative selection of adult patients with obstructive sleep apnea scheduled for ambulatory surgery. Anesth Analg 2012;115(5):1060–8.

33. Taylor RM. Defining, constructing and assessing learning outcomes. Rev Sci Tech 2009;28(2):779–88.

34. American Academy of Sleep Medicine. Available at: www.aasmnet.org. Accessed December 18, 2012.

35. Zozula R, Bodow M, Yatcilla D, et al. Development of a brief, self-administered instrument for assessing sleep knowledge in medical education: "the ASKME Survey". Sleep 2001;24(2):227–33.

36. Papp KK, Erokwu BO, Decker MJ, et al. Medical student competence in eliciting a history for "chronic fatigue". Sleep and Breathing 2001;5:123–9.

37. Strohl KP. Sleep medicine training across the spectrum. Chest 2011;139(5):1221–31.

38. Hepner DL, Bader AM. The perioperative physician and professionalism: the two must go together! Anesth Analg 2001;93(5):1088–90.

39. Adesanya AO, Joshi GP. Hospitalists and anesthesiologists as perioperative physicians: are their roles complementary? Proc (Bayl Univ Med Cent) 2007; 20(2):140–2.

40. Fleetham JA. Waking up to sleep-disordered breathing. Thorax 2010;65(9):762–3.

Unanswered Questions in Sleep and Anesthesia

Eswar Sundar, MD[a],*, Atul Malhotra, MD[b]

KEYWORDS

- Obstructive sleep apnea • Perioperative screening and triaging for OSA
- Anesthesia, sleep, and sedation • Extubation failure • Sedation in the ICU

KEY POINTS

- Several major questions remain regarding the potential links between anesthesia and sleep medicine.
- Basic science needs to focus on the neurobiological mechanisms underlying sleep and anesthesia, such that pharmacology could ultimately recapitulate the benefits of natural sleep.
- Physiologists should continue efforts to define mechanisms underlying upper airway motor control and ventilatory control that are important in obstructive sleep apnea (OSA) and can potentially be targeted in the perioperative and intensive care setting, for example, to prevent extubation failure.
- Clinical trials should focus on the potential benefits of screening, diagnosing, and treating OSA in the perioperative setting.

INTRODUCTION

Before we embark on a discussion of unanswered questions about sleep and anesthesia, here are some questions that have been answered. OSA is a widespread disorder that affects the cardiovascular, respiratory, and neurologic systems. Hypertension, coronary artery disease, stroke, diabetes, and congestive heart failure are highly prevalent in patients with OSA.[1–5] OSA is also associated with increased incidence of motor vehicle and occupational accidents.[6,7] Consistent continuous positive airway pressure (CPAP) use improves neurocognitive function, quality of life, and hypertension.[8–13] A meta-analysis of observational studies also shows that CPAP treatment reduces the rate of motor vehicle crashes.[14] Although studies showing a reduction in cardiovascular events such as myocardial infarction and stroke risk after CPAP treatment are sparse, evolving data, including that from recent trials, show a beneficial effect of CPAP in retarding atherosclerosis in the carotid intima.[15] Despite this knowledge, OSA is underdiagnosed and CPAP adherence is quite variable.[16]

DOES OSA INCREASE PERIOPERATIVE COMPLICATIONS?

Although an increased risk of perioperative and postoperative complications associated with OSA has not been conclusively proven, there are numerous reports and observational studies to support increased perioperative morbidity in OSA.[17] Nader and colleagues[18] compared autoadjusting positive airway pressure treatment to oxygen therapy or no therapy in hospitalized patients with symptoms suggesting OSA and found no difference in short-term morbidity. However, this study did not focus on surgical patients. Kaw and colleagues[19] studied 471 patients who had undergone PSG in a 3-month

Conflict of interest and Financial disclosures: None.
[a] Department of Anesthesia, Critical Care and Pain Medicine, Beth Israel Deaconess Medical Center, Harvard Medical School, 1 Deaconess Road, CC539, Boston, MA 02215, USA; [b] Department of Medicine, Brigham and Women's Hospital, Harvard Medical School, 75 Francis Street, Boston, MA 02115, USA
* Corresponding author.
E-mail address: esundar@bidmc.harvard.edu

Sleep Med Clin 8 (2013) 165–175
http://dx.doi.org/10.1016/j.jsmc.2012.11.001

period before a surgical procedure. About 60% of the patients had an apnea–hypopnea index (AHI) greater than 5 per hour, diagnostic of OSA. Patients with OSA had a higher incidence of postoperative hypoxemia, intensive care unit (ICU) transfers, and longer length of stay. However, given that desaturation is used to define AHI, one could question the importance of hypoxemia per se as a postoperative outcome measure.

Joint surgery in patients with OSA has been investigated in at least 2 studies.[20,21] Both studies have found an increased incidence of delirium in patients with OSA. The study by Gupta and colleagues[20] from the Mayo Clinic suggests that patients with OSA undergoing major joint surgery had a higher incidence of unplanned admissions and reintubations, compared with non-OSA subjects, even when postoperative narcotic use was similar between subjects with and without OSA. However, one major limitation of this study was that the investigators did not control for body mass index (BMI), calculated as the weight in kilograms divided by the height in meters squared, differences between the groups; therefore, the effects of obesity versus OSA are unclear. In a more recent case-control retrospective study of 234 ambulatory surgery patients with known OSA, Sabers and colleagues[22] from Mayo Clinic found that the diagnosis of OSA did not increase the rate of unplanned admissions. The investigators, however, noted that the rate of readmission (23.9% in the OSA group and 18.8% in the non-OSA group) was high in their study for both groups compared with their institution's general readmission rate after surgery. The reason for this increase is not clear and may relate to the lack of PSGs in the control group. In theory, undetected OSA in the control group could bias toward the null hypothesis because outcomes may then be similar between OSA and (misclassified) controls. Thus, careful, well-controlled studies will be required to draw definitive conclusions.

In a nonblinded study of patients undergoing elective surgery under general anesthesia, patients were screened for possible OSA. In this study from Australia, the investigators attempted to overcome statistical noninclusion bias by screening patients using a combination of the Epworth Sleepiness Scale, BMI, hypertension, and an airway examination. In the immediate postoperative period, patients who were considered to be at risk of OSA had significantly more obstructive respiratory events and spent longer time with lower oxygen saturations compared with low-risk patients. BMI and a longer time in the supine position were factors associated with respiratory obstruction, whereas daytime sleepiness was not

predictive of postoperative respiratory compromise. Opioid use was significantly associated with central respiratory depression in both groups.[23] Although this study showed a significant risk of airway obstruction and desaturation in the screen-positive group, this finding should be expected because OSA diagnosis requires these elements. As such, focus on hard outcomes such as duration of hospitalization, myocardial infarction, and mortality would be preferable.

One of the largest studies to address the possible risk of perioperative complications was the study by Memtsoudis and colleagues[24] in 2011. The investigators used National Inpatient Sample data to identify patients with a coded diagnosis of sleep apnea for each year between 1998 and 2007 and chose demographically matched subjects without the disease. Only patients who underwent orthopedic and general surgery were included in the study. Over 6 million patients' data were included in the study. The average yearly incidence of coding for "sleep apnea" was 2.5% for patients who underwent orthopedic surgery and 1.4% for those who underwent general surgery increasing over time to reach 5.5% and 2.7%, respectively, by the end of the study period. There was an increased incidence of aspiration, postoperative intubation, and mechanical ventilation in subjects coded with sleep apnea compared with those without the coding diagnosis. The incidence of pulmonary embolism was higher in patients with sleep apnea undergoing orthopedic procedures compared with subjects without sleep apnea. Although the group without the diagnosis of sleep apnea were not necessarily screened and excluded for OSA, the sheer number of patients likely minimized the influence of small numbers of patients with undetected OSA. The only significant difference between the groups was the prevalence of obesity, the group with sleep apnea having a fivefold higher prevalence of obesity compared with controls. Like most studies using large administrative databases, there is lack of detailed information such as severity of illness and specificity of diagnosis. Moreover, one could argue that a known diagnosis of OSA may lower the threshold for reintubation (eg, to facilitate sedation/analgesia) such that OSA per se may not cause respiratory failure in this context. However, this study provides the strongest evidence to date that OSA probably increases postoperative pulmonary complications and increases the resource use in hospitals.

In aggregate, data suggest that postoperative patients with OSA probably have a higher incidence of obstructive apneas, oxygen desaturation, aspiration, and pulmonary embolism, perhaps leading to increased incidence of delirium, postoperative intubation, and mechanical ventilation. Postoperative opioid use probably exacerbates these complications, and these events seem to increase resource use in health care institutions.

IF OSA DOES INCREASE PERIOPERATIVE COMPLICATIONS, THEN DOES POSTOPERATIVE CPAP REDUCE THEM?

The American Society of Anesthesiologists (ASA) practice guidelines on the perioperative management of patients suspected or known to have OSA is equivocal on the postoperative use of CPAP.[25] However, there is one study showing that the incidence of total in-hospital postoperative complications including desaturations is the highest among a group of non-CPAP-compliant patients with known OSA. In fact, this group of patients required CPAP institution as well as other interventions more frequently in the face of complications.[26] Drummond and colleagues,[27] however, demonstrated that in unselected patients undergoing major abdominal surgery, oxygen supplementation rather than CPAP administration reduced the frequency of oxygen desaturation during the first 24 hours postoperatively. However, this study was not directed at patients with OSA or even patients who screened high risk for OSA.

Clearly, oxygen desaturation is the most common postoperative "event" observed in patients with OSA in the postoperative period. Desaturations alone may not constitute a complication or adverse effect because patients with OSA or those who are at risk for it by definition should have desaturations. Even if oxygen desaturations were deemed to be a complication, there is still not enough evidence to suggest that CPAP will prevent them. However, it is quite possible that patients with known OSA who are noncompliant with CPAP treatment probably represent a group that may most benefit from CPAP in the postoperative period. Thus, further work is clearly required in this area, including randomized trials to draw rigorous conclusions about lack of CPAP use.

WHAT ARE WE SCREENING FOR IN THE PERIOPERATIVE PERIOD: RISK OF OSA OR RISK OF ADVERSE EVENTS ASSOCIATED WITH OSA?

The gold standard for the diagnosis of OSA is currently an overnight sleep study. However, sending patients to an overnight sleep study preoperatively like one would send patients for a chest radiograph or even a stress test is not practical in the current model of health care

delivery. It is clear that OSA is associated with complications such as hypertension, desaturations, arrhythmias, and upper airway obstruction and that these could potentially affect perioperative outcomes. So an alternative method of screening is required. Unlike most other screening tests that rely on a single test, preoperative screening for OSA relies largely on questionnaires.[28] The following screening tools for OSA are referenced in the literature for use in the perioperative setting: the Berlin questionnaire[29–32] (**Table 1**), STOP and STOP-BANG[33] (**Table 2**), the ASA checklist[25,31] (**Table 3**), the Perioperative Sleep Apnea Prediction (P-SAP) study[34] (**Table 4**), and Sleep Apnea Clinical Score (SACS)[35,36] (**Table 5**). All these screening tools have used a PSG to validate their respective questionnaires except the SACS study. However, the prospective studies validating the Berlin questionnaire, STOP, and ASA checklist report only 8.5% of their screened subjects completing an overnight PSG[28,31,33] with a high degree of self-selection bias. The P-SAP study, however, validated a derived sleep apnea score in patients who happened to have a PSG in the 6-month period before the derivation. The P-SAP retrospective observational study showed better sensitivity for the diagnosis of OSA than the STOP questionnaire, which was prospective. The SACS study from the Mayo Clinic did not validate using overnight PSG but instead assessed the ability of a sleep apnea clinical score combined with recurrent Post Anesthesia Care Unit (PACU) respiratory events to predict higher oxygen desaturation index and respiratory complications on the surgical floor. Thus, clearly, these various questionnaires are screening for different outcomes.

Given the fact that patients with OSA have an increased postoperative incidence of obstructive apneas, oxygen desaturation, and pulmonary complications that increase resource use,[20,24] would it be more appropriate to screen and triage for the potential trigger, oxygen desaturation on the floor, rather than preoperatively screening for the presence or absence of an actual condition, that is, OSA? Perioperative screening for OSA is primarily about risk stratification and appropriate management to prevent adverse events associated with OSA. The other comorbidities associated with OSA such as daytime sleepiness, hypertension, and arrhythmias have not been studied adequately in the perioperative period and probably have less of an impact on complications and hospital resource use.

Screening by its very nature will tend to include mild and moderate forms of the disease. None of the studies that show an increased incidence of

Table 1
The Berlin questionnaire

Height_____ m; Weight_____ Kg; Age_____ male/female	Please choose only one correct response to each question	
Category 1	*Points assignments*	*Points tally*
1. Do you snore? a. Yes b. No	1 point for a	
If you do snore		
2. Your snoring is? a. Slightly louder than breathing b. As loud as talking c. Louder than talking d. Very loud-can be heard in adjacent rooms	1 point for c 1 point for d	
3. How often do you snore? a. Nearly every day b. 3-4 times a week c. 1-2 times a week d. 1-2 times a month e. Never or nearly never	1 point for a 1 point for b	
4. Has your snoring ever bothered other people? a. Yes b. No c. Don't know	1 point for a	
5. Has anyone noticed that you quit breathing during your sleep a. Nearly every day b. 3-4 times a week c. 1-2 times a week d. 1-2 times a month e. Never or nearly never	2 points for a 2 points for b	
Category 1 is positive if total score is 2 or more points	Total for category 1 ⇨	
Category 2		
6. How often do you feel tired or fatigued after your sleep? a. Nearly every day b. 3-4 times a week c. 1-2 times a week d. 1-2 times a month e. Never or nearly never	1 point for a 1 point for b	
7. During your waking time, do you feel tired, fatigued or not up to par? a. Nearly every day b. 3-4 times a week c. 1-2 times a week d. 1-2 times a month e. Never or nearly never	1 point for a 1 point for b	
8. Have you ever nodded off or fallen asleep while driving a vehicle? a. Yes b. No	1 point for a	
9. If you ever nodded off or fallen asleep while driving a vehicle, how often does this occur? a. Nearly every day b. 3-4 times a week c. 1-2 times a week d. 1-2 times a month e. Never or nearly never	Do not score for Question 9	

(continued on next page)

Table 1		
(continued)		
Category 2 is positive if total score is 2 or more points	Total for category 2 ⇨	
Category 3		
10. Do you have high blood pressure		
a. Yes	1 point for a	
b. No		
c. Don't know		

High risk of OSA: two or more categories scored as positive.
Low risk of OSA: only one or two categories scored as positive.
    Adapted from Chung F, Yegneswaran B, Liao P, et al. Validation of the Berlin questionnaire and American Society of Anesthesiologists checklist as screening tools for obstructive sleep apnea in surgical patients. Anesthesiology 2008;108:822–30; with permission.

pulmonary complication in the postoperative period in patients with a diagnosis of OSA show if the severity of OSA has any influence in this association. It is still not known if mild and moderate OSA is associated with an increase in adverse perioperative outcomes. Most of the screening questionnaires for OSA in the perioperative setting define about 25% of the population as high risk for OSA (**Table 6**). This high positive screening rate could substantially increase the resource use in the recovery room and on the floors. In addition, workup biases in the studies by Chung and colleagues[31,33] artificially depress the false-positive rate possibly leading to further increases in resource use.[28] At this point, application of CPAP or intensive monitoring on the floors is the most viable option in caring for those patients who screen high risk for OSA. Hence it is of utmost importance that additional triage be undertaken to identify a further subpopulation

among the high-risk patients who may really benefit from these interventions.[28,36]

SLEEP, SEDATION, AND ANESTHESIA: DIFFERENT STATES ON A SPECTRUM OR JUST DIFFERENT STATES?

Brown and colleagues[37] published a superb review of sleep and anesthesia, the neural pathways associated with these states, and the different drugs used to produce sedation and general anesthesia. However, considerable uncertainty still exists if sleep, sedation, and anesthesia are the same or vastly different states. Sleep and anesthesia differ in that one is spontaneous, whereas the other is drug induced. Anesthesia can always be induced and maintained, whereas onset and maintenance of sleep is not always guaranteed.[38] Despite differences, anesthesia and sleep also seem to have a degree of interplay. Sleep deprivation seems to

Table 2			
The STOP-BANG questionnaire			
	Circle Yes or No to the Following Questions		
Snoring	Do you snore loudly (louder than talking or loud enough to be heard through closed doors)?	Yes	No
Tired	Do you often feel tired, fatigued, or sleepy during daytime?	Yes	No
Observed apneas	Has anyone observed you stop breathing during your sleep?	Yes	No
Blood pressure	Do you have or are you being treated for high blood pressure?	Yes	No
BMI	BMI more than 35 kg/m^2?	Yes	No
Age	Age over 50 y old?	Yes	No
Neck circumference	Neck circumference greater than 40 cm?	Yes	No
Gender	Male?	Yes	No

High risk of OSA: if answering YES to 3 or more items.
Low risk of OSA: if answering YES to 2 or less items.
    Adapted from Chung F, Yegneswaran B, Liao P, et al. STOP questionnaire: a tool to screen patients for obstructive sleep apnea. Anesthesiology 2008;108:812–21; with permission.

Table 3
The ASA obstructive sleep apnea checklist

	Category Result
Category 1: Predisposing physical characteristics	
a. BMI ≥35 b. Neck circumference >45 cm/17 in. (men) or 40 cm/16 in. (women) c. Craniofacial abnormalities affecting the airway d. Anatomic nasal obstruction e. Tonsils nearly touching or touching the midline	If 2 or more items in this category are present, then this category is positive.
Category 2: History of apparent airway obstruction during sleep	
a. Snoring loud enough to be heard through closed doors b. Frequent snoring c. Observed pauses in breathing during sleep d. Awakens from sleep with a choking sensation e. Frequent arousals from sleep	If 2 or more items are present (or 1 item if patients live alone), then this category is positive.
Category 3: Somnolence	
a. Frequent somnolence or fatigue despite adequate "sleep" b. Falls asleep easily in a nonstimulating environment (eg, watching TV, reading, riding in or driving a car) despite adequate sleep c. Parent or teacher comments that child appears sleepy during the day, is easily distracted, is overly aggressive or has difficulty concentrating d. Child often difficult to arouse at usual awakening time	If one or more items in this category are present, then this category is positive.

High risk of OSA if 2 or more categories are scored positive.
Low risk of OSA if only 1 or no category is positive.
Adapted from Gross JB, Bachenberg KL, Benumof JL, et al. Practice guidelines for the perioperative management of patients with obstructive sleep apnea: a report by the American Society of Anesthesiologists Task Force on Perioperative Management of patients with obstructive sleep apnea. Anesthesiology 2006;104:1081–93; with permission.

Table 4
The P-SAP score

Score 1 Point for Every Item Answered Yes	Points
Male gender	Yes/No
History of snoring	Yes/No
"Thick" neck	Yes/No
Mallampatti 3 or 4	Yes/No
Hypertension (treated or untreated)	Yes/No
Type II diabetes (treated or untreated)	Yes/No
BMI >30	Yes/No
Age >43	Yes/No
Thyromental distance <4 cm	Yes/No
Total points	

P-SAP score >4 has a sensitivity of 0.667 and a specificity of 0.773, PPV 0.19, and NPV 0.97 for the diagnosis of OSA.
Abbreviations: NPV, negative predictive value; PPV, positive predictive value.
Adapted from Ramachandran SK, Kheterpal S, Consens F, et al. Derivation and validation of a simple perioperative sleep apnea prediction score. Anesth Analg 2010;110:1007–15; with permission.

Table 5
Flemons Sleep Apnea Clinical Score (SACS)

Hypertension	Do you have high blood pressure or have you been told to take medication for high blood pressure? ☐ Yes ☐ No
Historical question 1	If you snore people who have shared or are sharing my bedroom tell me that (pick 1 answer) ☐ Usually (3-5 times a week) ☐ Always (every night)
Historical question 2	If you gasp or choke in your sleep, the frequency of these symptoms are ☐ Usually (3-5) times a week ☐ Always (every night)
Neck circumference	Neck circumference is _____ cm (we will measure you)

Sleep Apnea Clinical Score (SACS) Prediction Chart

Not Hypertensive				Hypertensive		
No Historical Features	1 Historical Feature Present	Both Historical Features Present	Neck Circumference (cm)	No Historical Features	1 Historical Feature Present	Both Historical Features Present
0	0	1	<30	0	1	2
0	0	1	30-31	1	2	4
0	1	2	32-33	1	3	5
1	2	3	34-35	2	4	8
1	3	5	36-37	4	6	11
2	4	7	38-39	5	9	16
3	6	10	40-41	8	13	22
5	8	14	42-43	11	18	30
7	12	20	44-45	15	25	42
10	16	28	46-47	21	35	58
14	23	38	48-49	29	48	80
19	32	53	>49	40	66	110

Probability of sleep apnea is low if SACS is <15.
Probability of sleep apnea is high if SACS is ≥15.
Adapted from Gali B, Whalen FX, Schroeder DR, et al. Identification of patients at risk for postoperative respiratory complications using a preoperative obstructive sleep apnea screening tool and ostanesthesia care assessment. Anesthesiology 2009;110:869–77; with permission.

increase the potency of anesthetic agents and may explain why patients with OSA display increased sensitivity to anesthetics.[38,39] The ventrolateral preoptic nucleus (VLPO) in the hypothalamus is intimately associated with the initiation and maintenance of sleep. However, VLPO-lesioned rats that become sleep deprived still seem to be susceptible to many anesthetics.[39] Although there may be some overlap of the neuronal pathways for sleep and anesthesia, it has not been conclusively proven that anesthetics act solely through endogenous sleep state control systems.[40] Different anesthetic drugs produce their effects in slightly different manners. For example, sedation produced by ketamine differs from that produced by propofol.

Ketamine induces N-methyl-D-aspartate receptors in the inhibitory interneurons on the cortex and limbic system resulting in increased neural activity and unconsciousness. Propofol predominantly induces chloride currents through γ-aminobutyric acid receptor activation of inhibitory interneurons in the pyramidal cortex and subcortical area, which can be reversed with centrally acting cholinomimetic agents.[37] One key function of sleep is the dissipation of homeostatic sleep drive (ie, less tired after sleeping) such that a sleep-deprived individual normalizes after recovery sleep. One study did show that sleep-deprived animals did show improvement after anesthesia,[41] although only minimal data suggest that anesthesia serves the

Table 6
Characteristics of studies used to screen for OSA in the surgical population

	ASA Checklist	STOP-BANG	Berlin Questionnaire	P-SAP Study	
Validating author	Chung et al,[31] 2008	Chung et al,[33] 2008	Chung et al,[31] 2008	Ramachandran et al,[34] 2010	
Number of items	14 questions in 3 categories including calculated and measured items	8 items including calculated and measured items	10 questions in 3 categories. No calculated or measured items	9 items including calculated and measured items and a specialized airway examination	

				PSG and AHI	
Validating Test	PSG and AHI	PSG and AHI	PSG and AHI	P-SAP>2	P-SAP>6
AHI 5–15					
Sensitivity	0.72	0.84	0.69	0.95	0.22
Specificity	0.38	0.56	0.56	0.26	0.91
PPV	0.72	0.81	0.78	0.80	0.84
NPV	0.38	0.60	0.45	0.60	0.27
Likelihood ratio	1.16	1.90	1.56	1.28	2.4
AHI >15					
Sensitivity	0.79	0.93	0.79	0.97	0.26
Specificity	0.37	0.43	0.50	0.17	0.87
PPV	0.45	0.52	0.51	0.48	0.62
NPV	0.73	0.90	0.78	0.89	0.60
Likelihood ratio	1.25	1.63	1.58	1.16	2.00
AHI >30					
Sensitivity	0.87	1.00	0.87	0.98	0.32
Specificity	0.36	0.37	0.46	0.13	0.85
PPV	0.27	0.31	0.35	0.24	0.38
NPV	0.91	1.00	0.93	0.96	0.82
Likelihood ratio	1.35	1.58	1.61	1.12	2.13
Notes	Subjects for the ASA checklist, STOP questionnaire, and Berlin questionnaire studies were mostly the same patients, 18 y or older and who were recruited at surgical preoperative clinics in Toronto. The authors, however, publish the results in two separate publications.[31,33] Only 211 (8.5%) of 2467 patients who were screened with the ASA checklist, STOP questionnaire, and Berlin questionnaire underwent PSG.			The screening test was administered to a general surgical group and a group of surgical patients who happened to have a PSG in the 6 mo leading up to surgery	

Abbreviations: AHI, apnea-hypopnea index; NPV, negative predictive value; PPV, positive predictive value; PSG, polysomnography.

From Sundar E, Chang J, Smetana G. Perioperative screening for and management of patients with obstructive sleep apnea. J Clin Outcome Manag 2011;18:1–13; with permission.

same restorative functions as natural sleep. Thus, the current state of knowledge favors the notion that sleep is separate, whereas sedation and anesthesia may be a continuum. So the next time an anesthesiologist says to a patient "you will be asleep while we take your gall bladder out" it may not be entirely accurate, albeit reassuring to patients.

IS EXTUBATION FAILURE AN UPPER AIRWAY DISEASE?

Weakness or dysfunction of the genioglossus and other dilator muscles of the airway after prolonged intubation could lead to airway collapse and extubation failure. So if this statement is true, its stand to reason that obese patients who have reduced airway caliber and OSA would benefit the most from CPAP application postextubation. Esteban and colleagues[42] in his study from Spain originally showed that in patients who had been extubated after respiratory failure, noninvasive ventilation (NIV) did not reduce the incidence of subsequent reintubations compared with patients who received standard therapy after an extubation failure. Although the time period to reintubation was longer in the NIV group compared with controls, the incidence of death was higher in the intervention group. However, the patients in this study were all randomized after postextubation respiratory distress had occurred and NIV was not used prophylactically as a bridge but rather as a rescue intervention. A more recent study of extubation failures after cardiac surgery also found that NIV did not prevent reintubations in about 50% of patients after extubation. However, in this study a BMI greater than 30 kg/m^2 was associated with NIVs preventing reintubations.[43] All patients with sleep apnea had successfully staved off reintubation with NIV.

Nava and colleagues[44] elegantly showed that use of NIV immediately after extubation reduces the incidence of extubation failures and reintubations compared with administration of standard therapy after extubation. A few other studies have shown the usefulness of NIV and CPAP in preventing pulmonary complications as well.[43,45] The reason for this benefit is not clear but may be due to the ability of CPAP to preserve upper airway patency.[46–49] Another study assessed the utility of NIV in liberating patients with chronic obstructive pulmonary disease (COPD) from the ventilator. In these patients, there was a significant reduction in ICU mortality and time to discharge compared with NIV in patients without COPD and hypercapnic respiratory failure.[50] A comprehensive analysis of the role of NIV recommends that NIV be used in weaning only patients with COPD with hypercapnic respiratory failure.[51] Thus it seems promising that an NIV bridge might reduce the rate of reintubations in patients in the ICU, especially the obese, patients with COPD, and those with OSA. One purported mechanism for this benefit is via relief of upper airway obstruction postextubation, although further data are clearly required. However, NIV as a rescue strategy after extubation failure has been associated with complications,[41,42] emphasizing the role of NIV as a preemptive rather than rescue strategy.[42,43]

SLEEPING IN THE ICU

Sleep is a reversible physiologic state of unconsciousness. Rapid eye movement (REM) sleep is characterized by rapid eye movements, a desynchronized electroencephalogram (EEG), and reduction in muscle tone. Non-REM sleep on the contrary is symbolized by a synchronized brain EEG pattern and increase in muscle tone. Sleep deprivation is associated with considerable neurocognitive defects including delirium.[52] A recent study from Italy[53] showed that there was significant sleep disruption in patients in the ICU. Delirium and benzodiazepine use was associated with severe REM sleep reduction. REM sleep is believed to have restorative function, and thus the observed reduction in REM sleep could in theory account for ICU-related delirium. In addition, 2 studies have suggested a link between OSA and postoperative delirium in elderly patients undergoing knee replacements.[20,21] Conceivably, the frequent episodes of airway collapse in OSA lead to hypoxemia, disrupted sleep, sleep inertia, and daytime sleepiness, all of which may be precipitating and/or augmenting factors of delirium.[54] Sedation with dexmedetomidine rather than with lorazepam was, however, associated with more days free of delirium or coma in the ICU. Patients sedated with dexmedetomidine tended to stay closer to the target sedation level compared with patients sedated with benzodiazepines.[55] In theory, dexmedetomidine has a somewhat unique pharmacology that promotes sleep via the VLPO rather than nonspecific sedation. However, the Midazolam/Dexmedetomidine/Propofol/Dexmedetomidine (MIDEX/PRODEX) multicenter trial did not show dexmedetomidine to be superior to propofol or midazolam in reducing the total duration of mechanical ventilation. Hypotension was also quite common with dexmedetomidine.[56] Definitive data still remain sparse that improving sleep in the ICU prevents delirium or clinical outcomes.

SUMMARY

Several major questions remain regarding the potential links between anesthesia and sleep medicine. We have chosen a few topics to emphasize but recognize that there are countless other examples of unanswered questions that should be addressed. Basic science needs to focus on the neurobiological mechanisms underlying sleep and anesthesia, ideally such that pharmacology could ultimately recapitulate the benefits of natural sleep. Physiologists can continue efforts to define mechanisms underlying upper airway motor control and ventilatory control that are important in OSA and can potentially be targeted in the anesthesia setting, for example, to prevent extubation failure. Clinical trials can focus on the potential benefits of screening, diagnosing, and treating OSA in the perioperative setting. Medical education needs to target awareness of OSA and its consequences such that patients and practitioners are aware of the potential risk associated with undiagnosed OSA. Thus, we all have work to do.

REFERENCES

1. Shahar E, Whitney CW, Redline S, et al. Sleep-disordered breathing and cardiovascular disease: cross-sectional results of the Sleep Heart Health Study. Am J Respir Crit Care Med 2001;163:19–25.
2. Peppard PE, Young T, Palta M, et al. Prospective study of the association between sleep-disordered breathing and hypertension. N Engl J Med 2000; 342:1378–84.
3. Plantinga L, Rao MN, Schillinger D. Prevalence of self-reported sleep problems among people with diabetes in the United States, 2005-2008. Prev Chronic Dis 2012;9:E76.
4. Iyer SR, Iyer RR. Sleep, ageing and stroke–newer directions in management of stroke. J Assoc Physicians India 2010;58:442–6.
5. Arzt M, Young T, Finn L, et al. Association of sleep-disordered breathing and the occurrence of stroke. Am J Respir Crit Care Med 2005;172:1447–51.
6. Teran-Santos J, Jimenez-Gomez A, Cordero-Guevara J. The association between sleep apnea and the risk of traffic accidents. Cooperative Group Burgos-Santander. N Engl J Med 1999;340:847–51.
7. Lindberg E, Carter N, Gislason T, et al. Role of snoring and daytime sleepiness in occupational accidents. Am J Respir Crit Care Med 2001;164: 2031–5.
8. Butt M, Dwivedi G, Shantsila A, et al. Left ventricular systolic and diastolic function in obstructive sleep apnea: impact of continuous positive airway pressure therapy. Circ Heart Fail 2012;5:226–33.
9. Vanderveken OM, Boudewyns A, Ni Q, et al. Cardiovascular implications in the treatment of obstructive sleep apnea. J Cardiovasc Transl Res 2011;4:53–60.
10. Pendharkar SR, Tsai WH, Eves ND, et al. CPAP increases exercise tolerance in obese subjects with obstructive sleep apnea. Respir Med 2011; 105:1565–71.
11. Monahan K, Redline S. Role of obstructive sleep apnea in cardiovascular disease. Curr Opin Cardiol 2011;26:541–7.
12. Magalang UJ, Richards K, McCarthy B, et al. Continuous positive airway pressure therapy reduces right ventricular volume in patients with obstructive sleep apnea: a cardiovascular magnetic resonance study. J Clin Sleep Med 2009;5:110–4.
13. Coughlin SR, Mawdsley L, Mugarza JA, et al. Cardiovascular and metabolic effects of CPAP in obese males with OSA. Eur Respir J 2007;29:720–7.
14. Tregear S, Reston J, Schoelles K, et al. Continuous positive airway pressure reduces risk of motor vehicle crash among drivers with obstructive sleep apnea: systematic review and meta-analysis. Sleep 2010;33:1373–80.
15. Drager LF, Bortolotto LA, Figueiredo AC, et al. Effects of continuous positive airway pressure on early signs of atherosclerosis in obstructive sleep apnea. Am J Respir Crit Care Med 2007;176:706–12.
16. Malhotra A, White DP. Obstructive sleep apnoea. Lancet 2002;360:237–45.
17. Chung SA, Yuan H, Chung F. A systemic review of obstructive sleep apnea and its implications for anesthesiologists. Anesth Analg 2008;107:1543–63.
18. Nader NZ, Steinel JA, Auckley DH. Newly identified obstructive sleep apnea in hospitalized patients: analysis of an evaluation and treatment strategy. J Clin Sleep Med 2006;2:431–7.
19. Kaw R, Pasupuleti V, Walker E, et al. Postoperative complications in patients with obstructive sleep apnea. Chest 2012;141:436–41.
20. Gupta RM, Parvizi J, Hanssen AD, et al. Postoperative complications in patients with obstructive sleep apnea syndrome undergoing hip or knee replacement: a case-control study. Mayo Clin Proc 2001; 76:897–905.
21. Flink BJ, Rivelli SK, Cox EA, et al. Obstructive sleep apnea and incidence of postoperative delirium after elective knee replacement in the nondemented elderly. Anesthesiology 2012;116:788–96.
22. Sabers C, Plevak DJ, Schroeder DR, et al. The diagnosis of obstructive sleep apnea as a risk factor for unanticipated admissions in outpatient surgery. Anesth Analg 2003;96:1328–35 [table of contents].
23. Blake DW, Chia PH, Donnan G, et al. Preoperative assessment for obstructive sleep apnoea and the prediction of postoperative respiratory obstruction and hypoxaemia. Anaesth Intensive Care 2008;36: 379–84.
24. Memtsoudis S, Liu SS, Ma Y, et al. Perioperative pulmonary outcomes in patients with sleep apnea after noncardiac surgery. Anesth Analg 2011;112:113–21.
25. Gross JB, Bachenberg KL, Benumof JL, et al. Practice guidelines for the perioperative management of patients with obstructive sleep apnea: a report by the American Society of Anesthesiologists Task Force on Perioperative Management of patients with obstructive sleep apnea. Anesthesiology 2006;104:1081–93 [quiz: 117–8].

26. Liao P, Yegneswaran B, Vairavanathan S, et al. Post-operative complications in patients with obstructive sleep apnea: a retrospective matched cohort study. Can J Anaesth 2009;56:819–28.

27. Drummond GB, Stedul K, Kingshott R, et al. Automatic CPAP compared with conventional treatment for episodic hypoxemia and sleep disturbance after major abdominal surgery. Anesthesiology 2002;96:817–26.

28. Sundar E, Chang J, Smetana G. Perioperative screening for and management of patients with obstructive sleep apnea. J Clin Outcome Manag 2011;18:399–411.

29. Netzer NC, Stoohs RA, Netzer CM, et al. Using the Berlin Questionnaire to identify patients at risk for the sleep apnea syndrome. Ann Intern Med 1999; 131:485–91.

30. Ahmadi N, Chung SA, Gibbs A, et al. The Berlin questionnaire for sleep apnea in a sleep clinic population: relationship to polysomnographic measurement of respiratory disturbance. Sleep Breath 2008;12:39–45.

31. Chung F, Yegneswaran B, Liao P, et al. Validation of the Berlin questionnaire and American Society of Anesthesiologists checklist as screening tools for obstructive sleep apnea in surgical patients. Anesthesiology 2008;108:822–30.

32. Sharma SK, Vasudev C, Sinha S, et al. Validation of the modified Berlin questionnaire to identify patients at risk for the obstructive sleep apnoea syndrome. Indian J Med Res 2006;124:281–90.

33. Chung F, Yegneswaran B, Liao P, et al. STOP questionnaire: a tool to screen patients for obstructive sleep apnea. Anesthesiology 2008;108:812–21.

34. Ramachandran SK, Kheterpal S, Consens F, et al. Derivation and validation of a simple perioperative sleep apnea prediction score. Anesth Analg 2010; 110:1007–15.

35. Gali B, Whalen FX Jr, Gay PC, et al. Management plan to reduce risks in perioperative care of patients with presumed obstructive sleep apnea syndrome. J Clin Sleep Med 2007;3:582–8.

36. Gali B, Whalen FX, Schroeder DR, et al. Identification of patients at risk for postoperative respiratory complications using a preoperative obstructive sleep apnea screening tool and postanesthesia care assessment. Anesthesiology 2009;110:869–77.

37. Brown EN, Lydic R, Schiff ND. General anesthesia, sleep, and coma. N Engl J Med 2010;363:2638–50.

38. Tung A, Mendelson WB. Anesthesia and sleep. Sleep Med Rev 2004;8:213–25.

39. Eikermann M, Vetrivelan R, Grosse-Sundrup M, et al. The ventrolateral preoptic nucleus is not required for isoflurane general anesthesia. Brain Res 2011;1426: 30–7.

40. Chamberlin NL, Eikermann M. This is no humbug: anesthetic agent-induced unconsciousness and sleep are visibly different. Anesthesiology 2010; 113:1007–9.

41. Tung A, Bergmann BM, Herrera S, et al. Recovery from sleep deprivation occurs during propofol anesthesia. Anesthesiology 2004;100:1419–26.

42. Esteban A, Frutos-Vivar F, Ferguson ND, et al. Noninvasive positive-pressure ventilation for respiratory failure after extubation. N Engl J Med 2004;350: 2452–60.

43. Garcia-Delgado M, Navarrete I, Garcia-Palma MJ, et al. Postoperative respiratory failure after cardiac surgery: use of noninvasive ventilation. J Cardiothorac Vasc Anesth 2012;26:443–7.

44. Nava S, Gregoretti C, Fanfulla F, et al. Noninvasive ventilation to prevent respiratory failure after extubation in high-risk patients. Crit Care Med 2005;33:2465–70.

45. Boeken U, Schurr P, Kurt M, et al. Early reintubation after cardiac operations: impact of nasal continuous positive airway pressure (nCPAP) and noninvasive positive pressure ventilation (NPPV). Thorac Cardiovasc Surg 2010;58:398–402.

46. Basner RC. Continuous positive airway pressure for obstructive sleep apnea. N Engl J Med 2007;356:1751–8.

47. Eckert DJ, Malhotra A. Pathophysiology of adult obstructive sleep apnea. Proc Am Thorac Soc 2008;5:144–53.

48. Fleetham JA. Upper airway imaging in relation to obstructive sleep apnea. Clin Chest Med 1992;13: 399–416.

49. Corda L, Redolfi S, Montemurro LT, et al. Short- and long-term effects of CPAP on upper airway anatomy and collapsibility in OSAH. Sleep Breath 2009;13:187–93.

50. Prasad SB, Chaudhry D, Khanna R. Role of noninvasive ventilation in weaning from mechanical ventilation in patients of chronic obstructive pulmonary disease: an Indian experience. Indian J Crit Care Med 2009;13:207–12.

51. Ferreyra G, Fanelli V, Del Sorbo L, et al. Are guidelines for non-invasive ventilation during weaning still valid? Minerva Anestesiol 2011;77:921–6.

52. Goel N, Rao H, Durmer JS, et al. Neurocognitive consequences of sleep deprivation. Semin Neurol 2009;29:320–39.

53. Trompeo AC, Vidi Y, Locane MD, et al. Sleep disturbances in the critically ill patients: role of delirium and sedative agents. Minerva Anestesiol 2011;77:604–12.

54. Bateman BT, Eikermann M. Obstructive sleep apnea predicts adverse perioperative outcome: evidence for an association between obstructive sleep apnea and delirium. Anesthesiology 2012;116:753–5.

55. Pandharipande PP, Pun BT, Herr DL, et al. Effect of sedation with dexmedetomidine vs lorazepam on acute brain dysfunction in mechanically ventilated patients: the MENDS randomized controlled trial. JAMA 2007;298:2644–53.

56. Jakob SM, Ruokonen E, Grounds RM, et al. Dexmedetomidine vs midazolam or propofol for sedation during prolonged mechanical ventilation: two randomized controlled trials. JAMA 2012;307:1151–60.

Index

Note: Page numbers of article titles are in **boldface** type.

A

Abdominal surgery, postoperative positive airway pressure protocols for, 124

Adenotonsillectomy, evaluation of child with sleep-disordered breathing scheduled for, **149–155**

Airway management. *See also* Respiratory management *and* Upper airway.
  in obesity hyperventilation syndrome, 141

Ambulatory surgery, for patients with obstructive sleep apnea patients, 116–117
    perioperative complications *vs.* inpatient surgery, 132–133

Anesthesia, postoperative disposition of known and suspected obstructive sleep apnea patients after general, 114–116

  sleep medicine and, 1–175
    circadian rhythm and sleep disorders in anesthesiology training programs, **157–164**
    common mechanisms of action, **1–9**
      anesthetics in sleep pathways, 2–3
      arousal pathways, 1
      circadian control of immune function, 5
      circadian rhythm, 3–5
      sleep disruption and cognitive dysfunction in sedated ICU patients, 5–6
      sleep pathways, 1–2
    differences and similarities in, **23–28**
      collapsibility, 24–25
      common narcotic switch, 24
      crossing the consciousness divide, 25–26
      difficult airways, 25
      in patients with obstructive sleep apnea, 26–28
    in children with sleep-disordered breathing in for adenotonsillectomy, **149–155**
    obesity hyperventilation syndrome and, **135–147**
    obstructive sleep apnea and, medical sedation and, **43–58**
      perioperative clinical pathways to manage sleep-disordered breathing, **105–120**
      perioperative complications in patients with, **93–103, 129–134**
      perioperative positive airway pressure therapy, **121–128**
      perioperative respiratory management of obese patients with, **59–64**
      preoperative evaluation of, **73–91**
      role of inflammation in chronic sleep restriction and, **11–21**
      screening tool for, **65–72**
      similarities and differences in, **23–28**
    unanswered questions in, **165–175**
      CPAP and postoperative complications, 167
      extubation failure and upper airway disease, 173
      obstructive sleep apnea and postoperative complications, 165–167
      sleeping in the ICU, 173
      spectrum of sleep, sedation, and anesthesia, 169–172
      what are we screening for, 167–169
    upper airway physiology in sleep and, **29–41**
      clinical risk factors and pharyngeal collapsibility, 33–35
      control of patency, 29–32
      neuromuscular control, 32–33
      pharmacological modulation of pharyngeal collapsibility, 35–38
      structural/mechanical loads, 32

Anesthesiology training programs, curricular elements for circadian rhythm and sleep disorders in, **157–164**
    advanced and research opportunities, 159–161
    assessment tools, 159
    content in current practice, 158
    curricular resources, 159
    implementation in the short term, 161–163
    methodology, 158
    proposed competencies, 158–159

Arousal pathways, 1

B

Bariatric surgery, for obesity hyperventilation syndrome, 138–139
    perioperative complications in, 132
    postoperative positive airway pressure protocols for, 125–126
    use of STOP-Bang questionnaire in, 69

Benzodiazepine GABA$_A$ receptor antagonists, for sedation in patients with obstructive sleep apnea, 45–50

Bicarbonate, serum, and specificity of STOP-Bang questionnaire, 70

C

Cardiac surgery, postoperative positive airway
pressure protocols for, 124–125
Cardiothoracic surgery, postoperative noninvasive
ventilation protocols for, 126
Cardiovascular disorders, obstructive sleep apnea
and chronic sleep restriction and, 13–14
Children. *See* Pediatrics.
Chronic sleep restriction. *See* Sleep restriction,
chronic.
Circadian rhythms, 3–4
anesthesia and, 4–5
control of immune function, 5
curricular elements for, in anesthesiology training
programs, **157–164**
Clinical pathways, perioperative, to manage
obstructive sleep apnea, **105–120**
ambulatory surgery for patients with, 116–117
comorbidities associated with, 106
diagnostic criteria, 106
intraoperative risk mitigation strategies for,
113–114
methods for perioperative screening for, 110
portable polysomnography and overnight
oximetry, 112
postoperative complications in patients with,
106–107
postoperative disposition after general
anesthesia, 114–116
preoperative evaluation, 107–112
of patient with diagnosed, 107–110
of patient with suspected, 110–112
principles of management, 107
Coexisting diseases, associated with obstructive
sleep apnea, 106
obstructive sleep apnea and, perioperative
complications due to, 95
Cognitive dysfunction, due to sleep disruption in
sedated patients in ICU, 5–6
Complications, perioperative, in patients with
obstructive sleep apnea, **93–103, 129–134,** 167
for ambulatory *vs.* inpatient surgery, 132–133
for bariatric surgery, 132
mechanisms for, 95–96
coexisting diseases, 95
heart rate variability and conduction
abnormalities, 93–94
inflammation, 95
metabolic dysfunction, 95
oxidative stress, 95
respiratory depression, 95–96
risk modification, 96–99
sympathetic activation, 94–95
postoperative, positive airway pressure for,
123–126
risk modification, 96–99

opioid reduction strategies, 97–98
patient selection, 96–97
perioperative CPAP therapy, 97
postoperative CPAP therapy, 97
postoperative monitoring and surveillance,
98
postoperative pulmonary management,
98–99
Conduction abnormalities, obstructive sleep apnea
and, 93–94
Continuous positive airway pressure (CPAP) therapy,
perioperative risk modification in patients with
obstructive sleep apnea, 97
postoperative, 97
preoperative, 97
postoperative, effect on perioperative
complications in patients with obstructive
sleep apnea, 167
Curriculum. *See* Anesthesiology training programs.

D

Dexmedetomidine, common mechanism as with
sleep, 3

E

Education. *See* Anesthesiology training programs.
Endoscopy, use of STOP-Bang questionnaire in
patients undergoing, 69
Endothelial dysfunction, in obstructive sleep apnea
and chronic sleep restriction, 13–14
Eszopiclone, in obstructive sleep apnea, 50–51
Evaluation, preoperative. *See* Preoperative
evaluation.
Extubation failure, as an upper airway disease in
obstructive sleep apnea patients, 173

F

Flurazepam, in obstructive sleep apnea, 47

G

GABA$_A$ receptor antagonists, for sedation in patients
with obstructive sleep apnea, 45–51
benzodiazepines, 45–50
non-benzodiazepine, 50–51
Gastric bypass surgery, postoperative positive
airway pressure protocols for, 125–126
General anesthesia, postoperative disposition of
known and suspected obstructive sleep apnea
patients after, 114–116

H

Heart rate variability, obstructive sleep apnea and,
93–94

Home sleep testing, for preoperative evaluation of obstructive sleep apnea, **73–91**

Hypercapnia, acute, in obesity hyperventilation syndrome, 136

Hypnotics, in patients with obstructive sleep apnea, **43–58**
    benzodiazepine GABA$_A$ receptor antagonists, 45–50
    non-benzodiazepine GABA$_A$ receptor antagonist hypnotics, 50–51
    novel, 51

Hypoxemia, perioperative constant, in obese patients, 60–61
    postoperative intermittent, in obese patients with sleep apnea, 61–62

I

Inflammation, obstructive sleep apnea and, 95
    role in sleep apnea and chronic sleep restriction, **11–21**
        cardiovascular disorders and, 13–14
        mechanisms for endothelial dysfunction in, 14–17
        metabolic syndrome and, 11–13

L

Laboratory polysomnography, *vs.* home sleep testing for preoperative evaluation of obstructive sleep apnea, **73–91**

Leptin resistance, in obesity hyperventilation syndrome, 136

Lung function, in obese patients, 60

M

Medical sedation. See Sedation.

Metabolic dysfunction, obstructive sleep apnea and, 95

Metabolic syndrome, obstructive sleep apnea and chronic sleep restriction and, 11–13

Methadone, for sedation in patients with obstructive sleep apnea, 54

Midazolam, in obstructive sleep apnea, 47

Monitoring, for obstructive sleep apnea. See Portable monitoring.

Morphine, for sedation in patients with obstructive sleep apnea, 54

N

Nitrazepam, in obstructive sleep apnea, 47

Noninvasive ventilation, postoperative protocols for, 126

O

Obesity, perioperative respiratory management of obstructive sleep apnea with, **59–64**
    airway management strategies, 63
    burden of obesity on respiratory functions, 60
    fat deposition around pharyngeal airway, 61
    lung function in, 60
    perioperative constant hypoxemia in, 60–61
    possible changes of loop gain in, 62–63
    postoperative lung volume reduction and intermittent episodic hypoxemia, 61–62

Obesity hyperventilation syndrome, anesthesia and, **135–147**
    distinguishing clinical features, 136–137
    intraoperative management, 141–142
        airway management, 141
        emergence from anesthesia, 141–142
    morbidity and mortality, 137
    pathophysiology, 136
        impaired compensation of acute hypercapnia, 136
        impairment in respiratory mechanics, 136
        leptin resistance, 136
    postoperative management, 142–143
        opioid-induced ventilatory impairment, 142
        positive airway pressure therapy, 142–143
    preoperative assessment of patients with, 139–141
        risk stratification and cardiopulmonary testing, 141
        screening for, 139–140
        screening for obstructive sleep apnea, 140–141
    treatment, 137–139
        bariatric surgery, 138–139
        pharmacotherapy, 139
        positive airway pressure therapy, 137–138
        supplemental oxygen, 138

Obstructive sleep apnea, chronic sleep restriction and, role of inflammation in, **11–21**
    cardiovascular disorders and, 13–14
    mechanisms for endothelial dysfunction in, 14–17
    metabolic syndrome and, 11–13
    medical sedation and, **43–58**
        benzodiazepine GABA$_A$ receptor antagonists, 45–50
        non-benzodiazepine GABA$_A$ receptor antagonist hypnotics, 50–51
        opioids, 51–55
        pathophysiologic mechanisms, 44–45
    perioperative clinical pathways to manage, **105–120**
        ambulatory surgery for patients with, 116–117
        comorbidities associated with, 106
        diagnostic criteria, 106

Obstructive (*continued*)
  intraoperative risk mitigation strategies for,
    113–114
  methods for perioperative screening for, 110
  portable polysomnography and overnight
    oximetry, 112
  postoperative complications in patients with,
    106–107
  postoperative disposition after general
    anesthesia, 114–116
  preoperative evaluation, 107–112
    of patient with diagnosed, 107–110
    of patient with suspected, 110–112
  principles of management, 107
perioperative complications in patients with,
  93–103, 129–134
  in ambulatory *vs.* inpatient surgery, 132–133
  in bariatric surgery, 132
  mechanisms for, 95–96
    coexisting diseases, 95
    heart rate variability and conduction
      abnormalities, 93–94
    inflammation, 95
    metabolic dysfunction, 95
    oxidative stress, 95
    respiratory depression, 95–96
    sympathetic activation, 94–95
  risk modification, 96–99
    opioid reduction strategies, 97–98
    patient selection, 96–97
    perioperative CPAP therapy, 97
    postoperative CPAP therapy, 97
    postoperative monitoring and surveillance,
      98
    postoperative pulmonary management,
      98–99
perioperative respiratory management of obese
  patients with, **59–64**
  airway management strategies, 63
  burden of obesity on respiratory functions, 60
  fat deposition around pharyngeal airway, 61
  lung function in, 60
  perioperative constant hypoxemia in, 60–61
  possible changes of loop gain in, 62–63
  postoperative lung volume reduction and
    intermittent episodic hypoxemia, 61–62
positive airway pressure therapy for perioperative
  patients, **121–128**
  historical perspective, 121–122
  noninvasive ventilation, 126
  postoperative protocols, 123–126
  preoperative protocols, 122–123
preoperative evaluation with home testing *vs.*
  laboratory testing, **73–91**
  differences between, 74–76
    scoring and interpretation, 75–76
    signal collection, 74–75

  integration of assessment in the preoperative
    clinic, 85–90
  portable monitoring devices, 76–85
    advantages and limitations of, 83–84
    outcomes based on, *vs.* in-laboratory
      testing algorithms, 85
    patient selection for *vs.* polysomnography,
      84–85
    selection of, 78–81
    types of, 76–78
    validation of with polysomnography, 81–83
similarities and differences in sleep and
  anesthesia, **23–28**
  crossing the consciousness divide, 25–26
  difficult airways, 25
  perioperative management, 26–28
  perioperative problems in, 26
  shared neurobiology, 24
  upper airway collapsibility, during anesthesia,
    25
    during sleep, 24
STOP-Bang questionnaire as screening tool for,
  65–72
  development of, 66–68
  in bariatric surgical patients, 69
  in patients undergoing endoscopy, 69
  referring patients for further workup, 70
  score on, and postoperative complications, 70
  serum bicarbonate and specificity of, 70
  to identify undiagnosed apnea in medical
    patients, 69–70
  validation of, 68–69
upper airway physiology in, **29–41**
Obstructive sleep apnea syndrome, evaluation of
  child with sleep-disordered breathing scheduled
  for adenotonsillectomy, **149–155**
Opioids, for sedation in patients with obstructive
  sleep apnea, 51–55
  opioid-induced ventilatory impairment in obesity
    hyperventilation syndrome, 142
  reduction of, for perioperative risk modification in
    patients with obstructive sleep apnea, 97–98
Orthopedic patients, postoperative positive airway
  pressure protocols for, 124
Oxidative stress, obstructive sleep apnea and, 95
Oximetry, preoperative, in children scheduled for
  adenotonsillectomy, 152–153
Oxygen, supplemental, for obesity hyperventilation
  syndrome, 138

P

Pediatrics, evaluation of child with sleep-disordered
  breathing scheduled for adenotonsillectomy,
  149–155
Pharmacotherapy, for obesity hyperventilation
  syndrome, 139

Pharyngeal collapse. *See also* Upper Airway.
  impact of clinical risk factors on, 33–35
  pharmacologic modulation of, 35–38
    in patients with obstructive sleep apnea,
      33–38
Physiology, upper airway, in sleep and anesthesia,
  23–28, 29–41
Polysomnography, portable, and overnight oximetry,
  112
  vs. home sleep testing for preoperative evaluation
    of obstructive sleep apnea, **73–91**
Portable monitoring, for preoperative evaluation of
  obstructive sleep apnea, **73–91**
    differences between laboratory testing and,
      74–76
      scoring and interpretation, 75–76
      signal collection, 74–75
    home sleep testing devices, 76–85
      advantages and limitations of, 83–84
      outcomes based on, *vs.* in-laboratory
        testing algorithms, 85
      patient selection for *vs.* polysomnography,
        84–85
      selection of, 78–81
      types of, 76–78
      validation of with polysomnography, 81–83
    integration of assessment in the preoperative
      clinic, 85–90
Positive airway pressure therapy. *See also*
  Continuous positive airway pressure.
  for obesity hyperventilation syndrome, 137–138
    postoperative, for prevention and treatment of
      respiratory failure in, 142–143
  for perioperative patients, **121–128**
    historical perspective, 121–122
    noninvasive ventilation, 126
    postoperative protocols, 123–126
    preoperative protocols, 122–123
Postoperative disposition, of known and suspected
  obstructive sleep apnea patients after general
  anesthesia, 114–116
Preoperative evaluation, of patients with obesity
  hyperventilation syndrome, 139–141
  of patients with obstructive sleep apnea, home *vs.*
    laboratory testing, **73–91**
    in diagnosed cases, 107–110
    in suspected cases, 110–112
    methods for, 110
Pulmonary management, postoperative, as risk
  modification in patients with obstructive sleep
  apnea, 98–99

Q

Questionnaires, for sleep-disordered breathing in
  children scheduled for adenotonsillectomy,
  150–151

STOP-Bang, screening for obstructive sleep
  apnea with, **65–72**

R

Ramelteon, in obstructive sleep apnea, 51
Remifentanil, for sedation in patients with obstructive
  sleep apnea, 54
Respiratory depression, obstructive sleep apnea and,
  perioperative complications due to, 95–96
Respiratory failure, in obesity hyperventilation
  syndrome, prevention of, 143
    treatment of, 143–144
Respiratory management, perioperative, of obese
  patients with obstructive sleep apnea, **59–64**
    airway management strategies, 63
    burden of obesity on respiratory functions, 60
    fat deposition around pharyngeal airway, 61
    lung function in, 60
    perioperative constant hypoxemia in, 60–61
    possible changes of loop gain in, 62–63
    postoperative lung volume reduction and
      intermittent episodic hypoxemia, 61–62
Risk modification, for perioperative complications in
  patients with obstructive sleep apnea, 96–99,
  113–114
    intraoperative strategies, 113–114
    opioid reduction strategies, 97–98
    patient selection, 96–97
    perioperative CPAP therapy, 97
    postoperative CPAP therapy, 97
    postoperative monitoring and surveillance, 98
    postoperative pulmonary management, 98–99

S

Screening tools. *See also* Preoperative evaluation.
  for obstructive sleep apnea, **65–72,** 110, 167–169
Sedation, in patients with obstructive sleep apnea,
  43–58
    benzodiazepine GABA$_A$ receptor antagonists,
      45–50
    non-benzodiazepine GABA$_A$ receptor
      antagonist hypnotics, 50–51
    opioids, 51–55
    pathophysiologic mechanisms, 44–45
Sleep, and anesthesia, 1–175
    circadian rhythm and sleep disorders in
      anesthesiology training programs, **157–164**
    common mechanisms of action, **1–9**
      anesthetics in sleep pathways, 2–3
      arousal pathways, 1
      circadian control of immune function, 5
      circadian rhythm, 3–5
      sleep disruption and cognitive dysfunction
        in sedated ICU patients, 5–6
      sleep pathways, 1–2

Sleep (*continued*)
    differences and similarities, **23–28**
        common narcotic switch, 24
        crossing the consciousness divide, 25–26
        difficult airways, 25
        in patients with obstructive sleep apnea,
           26–28
        upper airway collapsibility, 24–25
    in children with sleep-disordered breathing in
        for adenotonsillectomy, **149–155**
    in the ICU, 173
    obesity hyperventilation syndrome and,
        135–147
    obstructive sleep apnea and, medical sedation
        and, **43–58**
        perioperative clinical pathways to manage
           sleep-disordered breathing, **105–120**
        perioperative complications in patients
           with, **93–103, 129–134**
        perioperative positive airway pressure
           therapy, **121–128**
        perioperative respiratory management of
           obese patients with, **59–64**
        preoperative evaluation of, **73–91**
        role of inflammation in chronic sleep
           restriction and, **11–21**
        screening tool for, **65–72**
        similarities and differences in, **23–28**
    unanswered questions in, **165–175**
    upper airway physiology in, **29–41**
        clinical risk factors and pharyngeal
           collapsibility, 33–35
        control of patency, 29–32
        neuromuscular control, 32–33
        pharmacological modulation of pharyngeal
           collapsibility, 35–38
        structural/mechanical loads, 32
Sleep apnea. *See* Obstructive sleep apnea.
Sleep restriction, chronic, role of inflammation in
    sleep apnea and, **11–21**
    cardiovascular disorders and, 13–14
    mechanisms for endothelial dysfunction in,
        14–17
    metabolic syndrome and, 11–13
Sleep-disordered breathing. *See also* Obstructive
    sleep apnea.
    evaluation of child scheduled for
        adenotonsillectomy with, **149–155**
STOP-Bang questionnaire, for obstructive sleep
    apnea screening, **65–72,** 110, 167, 169
    development of, 66–68
    in bariatric surgical patients, 69
    in patients undergoing endoscopy, 69

    or screening for risk of adverse events
        associated with apnea, 167, 169
    referring patients for further workup, 70
    score on, and postoperative complications, 70
    serum bicarbonate and specificity of, 70
    to identify undiagnosed apnea in medical
        patients, 69–70
    validation of, 68–69
Sympathetic activation, obstructive sleep apnea and,
    94–95

T

Temazepam, in obstructive sleep apnea, 47
Training programs, curricular elements for circadian
    rhythm and sleep disorders in anesthesiology,
    157–164
        advanced and research opportunities,
           159–161
        assessment tools, 159
        content in current practice, 158
        curricular resources, 159
        implementation in the short term, 161–163
        methodology, 158
        proposed competencies, 158–159
Tramadol, for sedation in patients with obstructive
    sleep apnea, 54
Triazolam, in obstructive sleep apnea, 47, 50

U

Upper airway, differences and similarities in sleep and
    anesthesia, **23–28**
        collapsibility, 24–25
        common narcotic switch, 24
        crossing the consciousness divide, 25–26
        difficult airways, 25
        in patients with obstructive sleep apnea, 26–28
    fat deposition around, in obesity and sleep apnea,
        61
    is extubation failure a disease of, 173
    physiology in sleep and anesthesia, **29–41**
        clinical risk factors and pharyngeal
           collapsibility, 33–35
        control of patency, 29–32
        neuromuscular control, 32–33
        pharmacological modulation of pharyngeal
           collapsibility, 35–38
        structural/mechanical loads, 32

Z

Zaleplon, in obstructive sleep apnea, 50
Zolpidem, in obstructive sleep apnea, 50

Moving?

Make sure your subscription moves with you!

To notify us of your new address, find your **Clinics Account Number** (located on your mailing label above your name), and contact customer service at:

Email: **journalscustomerservice-usa@elsevier.com**

800-654-2452 (subscribers in the U.S. & Canada)
314-447-8871 (subscribers outside of the U.S. & Canada)

Fax number: **314-447-8029**

Elsevier Health Sciences Division
Subscription Customer Service
3251 Riverport Lane
Maryland Heights, MO 63043

*To ensure uninterrupted delivery of your subscription, please notify us at least 4 weeks in advance of move.

Printed and bound by CPI Group (UK) Ltd, Croydon, CR0 4YY

03/10/2024

01040332-0014